EYE MOVEMENT DISORDERS

Monographs in Ophthalmology

P.C. Maudgal and L. Missotten (eds.), Superficial Keratitis. 1981.
ISBN 90-6193-801-5.

P.F.J. Hoyng, Pharmacological Denervation and Glaucoma. A Clinical Trial Report with Guanethidine and Adrenaline in One Eye Drop. 1981.
ISBN 90-6193-802-3.

N.W.H.M. Dekkers, The Cornea in Measles. 1981. ISBN 90-6193-803-1.

P. Leonard and J. Rommel, Lens Implantation – 30 years of progress. 1982.
ISBN 90-6193-804-X.

C.E. van Nouhuys, Dominant Exudative Vitreoretinopathy and Other Vascular Developmental Disorders of the Peripheral Retina. 1982. ISBN 90-6193-805-8.

L. Evens (ed.), Convergent Strabismus. 1982. ISBN 90-6193-806-6.

A. Neetens, A. Löwenthal and J.J. Martin (eds.), The Visual System in Myelin Disorders. 1984. ISBN 90-6193-807-4.

H.J.M. Völker-Dieben, The Effect of Immunological and Non-Immunological Factors on Corneal Graft Survival. 1984. ISBN 90-6193-808-2.

J.A. Oosterhuis, Ophthalmic Tumours. 1985. ISBN 90-6193-528-8.

O. van Nieuwenhuizen, Cerebral Visual Disturbance in Infantile Encephalopathy. 1987.
ISBN 0-89838-860-0.

E.A.C.M. Sanders, R.J.W. de Keizer and D.S. Zee (eds.), Eye Movement Disorders.
1987. ISBN 0-89838-874-0.

Eye Movement Disorders

Edited by

E.A.C.M. SANDERS

Department of Neurology, Guy's Hospital,
London, United Kingdom

R.J.W. DE KEIZER

Department of Ophthalmology, Leiden University Hospital,
Leiden, The Netherlands

D.S. ZEE

Department of Neurology, The Johns Hopkins University,
School of Medicine, Baltimore, U.S.A.

1987

MARTINUS NIJHOFF/DR W. JUNK PUBLISHERS
A MEMBER OF THE KLUWER ACADEMIC PUBLISHERS GROUP
DORDRECHT / BOSTON / LANCASTER

Distributors

for the United States and Canada: Kluwer Academic Publishers, P.O. Box 358,
Accord Station, Hingham, MA 02018-0358, USA
for the UK and Ireland: Kluwer Academic Publishers, MTP Press Limited,
Falcon House, Queen Square, Lancaster LA1 1RN, UK
for all other countries: Kluwer Academic Publishers Group, Distribution Center,
P.O. Box 322, 3300 AH Dordrecht, The Netherlands

Library of Congress Cataloging in Publication Data

```
Eye movement disorders.

    (Monographs in opthalmology)
    Includes index.
    1. Eye--Movement disorders.  I. Sanders, E. A. C. M.
II. Keizer, Robert Jan Willem de.  III. Zee, David S.
IV. Series.  [DNLM: 1. Eye Manifestations.  2. Eye
Movements.  3. Oculomotor Muscles--physiopathology.
4. Vision Disorders.  W1 MO568D / WW 410 E972]
RE731.E914 1987        617.7'62          87-5540
```

ISBN-13: 978-94-010-7989-1   e-ISBN-13: 978-94-009-3317-0
DOI: 10/1007/978-94-009-3317-0

Copyright

Preface

There is perhaps no area of neuro-ophthalmology that is advancing more rapidly with respect to an understanding of its anatomy and physiology than the ocular motor system. For this reason, it is difficult not only to keep up with the latest information concerning the basic mechanisms involved in the control of eye movements but also to remain up to date regarding the pathophysiology of specific disorders of eye movement. The material in this book is derived from a two-day course on eye movements held in The Netherlands in 1986. The course was designed as an introduction to the normal ocular motor system and to disorders of eye movements and was aimed toward orthoptists, ophthalmologists, optometrists, neurologists, and neurosurgeons. The chapters in this book were compiled by a trio of experts in the field of eye movements and contain discussions of anatomy and physiology of the ocular motor system, techniques of examination of patients with diplopia, and pathophysiology of specific disorders of ocular motility. Many of the authors of these chapters are among the most active investigators of eye movements in the world today, and their comments thus reflect the latest information in the field. This text is both basic and comprehensive and thus has something for everyone, from the student just beginning a study of the ocular motor system to the seasoned 'veteran' who wishes to know the latest information regarding central ocular motor control mechanisms.

Neil R. Miller MD
Baltimore, Maryland

Table of contents

VIII

List of abbreviations

AION   anterior ischemic optic neuropathy
CCF   carotid cavernous fistula
CK   creatine-kinase
CNS   central nervous system
CPEO   chronic progressive external ophthalmoplegia
CR   corneal reflexion
CT-scan   computed tomography scan
DLPN   dorsolateral pontine nuclei
DMI   double magnetic induction
EEG   electro-encephalography
EMG   electromyography
ENG   electronystagmography
ENT   ear, nose and throat
EOG   electro-oculography
ESR   erythrocyte sedimentation rate
FEF   frontal eye fields
GPD   glycerophosphatase dehydrogenase
iC   nucleus interstitials of Cajal
INC   interstitial nucleus of Cajal
INO   internuclear ophthalmoplegia
IR   infrared
IRIS   iris-scleral reflexion (method)
iv-DSA   intravenous digital subtraction angiography
MI   magnetic induction
MLF   medial longitudinal fascicle
MRI   magnetic resonance imaging
nD   nucleus Darkschewitsch
NMR   nuclear magnetic resonance
NOT   prefectal nucleus of the optic tract
OKN   optokinetic nystagmus (reflex)
OPG   oculoplethysmography
PPRF   paramedian pontine reticular formation
PS   pupil scanning (method)
PSP   progressive supranuclear palsy
riMLF   rostral interstitial nucleus of the MLF
SC   superior colliculus
SEM   saccadic eye movements
TIA   transient ischemic attack
TV   television
VOR   vestibulo-ocular reflex

List of contributors

A.Th.M. van Balen
Department of Ophthalmology, Free University Hospital, De Boelelaan 1117, 1007 MB Amsterdam, The Netherlands

L.A.K. Bastiaensen
Department of Ophthalmology, St. Elizabeth Hospital, Hilvarenbeekseweg 60, 5022 GC Tilburg, The Netherlands

J.J.M. Bierlaagh
Orthoptic Department, Leiden University Hospital, Rijnsburgerweg 10, 2333 AA Leiden, The Netherlands

W. Bles
ENT Department, Free University Hospital, De Boelelaan 1117, 1007 MB Amsterdam, The Netherlands

E.L.E.M. Bollen
Department of Neurology, Leiden University Hospital, Rijnsburgerweg 10, 2333 AA Leiden, The Netherlands

O.J.S. Buruma
Department of Neurology, Leiden University Hospital, Rijnsburgerweg 10, 2333 AA Leiden, The Netherlands

U. Büttner
Department of Neurology, Grosshadern Clinic, Ludwig Maximilian University, Marchionistrasse 15, 8000 Munich 70, F.R.G.

J.A. Büttner-Ennever
Department of Neuropathology, Grosshadern Clinic, Ludwig Maximilian University, Marchionistrasse 15, 8000 Munich 70, F.R.G.

H. Collewijn

Department of Physiology I, Erasmus University, Dr. Molewaterplein 50, 3015 GE Rotterdam, The Netherlands

J.G. van Dijk

Department of Neurology, Leiden University Hospital, Rijnsburgerweg 10, 2333 AA Leiden, The Netherlands

M.H. Gobin

Department of Ophthalmology, Leiden University Hospital, Rijnsburgerweg 10, 2333 AA Leiden, The Netherlands

J. van Gijn

Department of Neurology, Utrecht University Hospital, P.O. Box 16250, 3500 CG Utrecht, The Netherlands

J.C. den Heyer

Department of Neurology, Leiden University Hospital, Rijnsburgerweg 10, 2333 AA Leiden, The Netherlands

T.U. Hoogenraad

Department of Neurology, Utrecht University Hospital, P.O. Box 16250, 3500 CG Utrecht, The Netherlands

W. van der Kamp

Department of Neurology, Leiden University Hospital, Rijnsburgerweg 10, 2333 AA Leiden, The Netherlands

R.J.W. de Keizer

Department of Ophthalmology, Leiden University Hospital, Rijnsburgerweg 10, 2333 AA Leiden, The Netherlands

L. Koornneef

Orbital Center, Department of Ophthalmology, Academic Medical Center, University of Amsterdam, Meibergdreef 9, 1105 AZ Amsterdam, The Netherlands

N.R. Miller

Wilmer Insitute, Johns Hopkins University School of Medicine, Baltimore, MD, U.S.A.

J.A. Oosterhuis

Department of Ophthalmology, Leiden University Hospital, Rijnsburgerweg 10, 2333 AA Leiden, The Netherlands

G. Padberg
Department of Neurology, Leiden University Hospital, Rijnsburgerweg 10,
2333 AA Leiden, The Netherlands

J.P.H. Reulen
Department of Medical Physics, Free University of Amsterdam, De Boelelaan 1117, 1007 MB Amsterdam, The Netherlands

R.A.C. Roos
Department of Neurology, Leiden University Hospital, Rijnsburgerweg 10,
2333 AA Leiden, The Netherlands

E.A.C.M. Sanders
Department of Neurology, Guy's Hospital, St. Thomas Street, SE1 9RT,
London, United Kingdom (presently at: Department of Neurology, Utrecht
University Hospital, P.O. Box 16250, 3500 CG Utrecht, The Netherlands)

C.C. Sterk
Department of Ophthalmology, Leiden University Hospital, Rijnsburgerweg
10, 2333 AA Leiden, The Netherlands

M. Swart-van den Berg
Department of Ophthalmology, Leiden University Hospital, Rijnsburgerweg
10, 2333 AA Leiden, The Netherlands

R.T.W.M. Thomeer
Department of Neurosurgery, Leiden University Hospital, Rijnsburgerweg
10, 2333 AA Leiden, The Netherlands

A.G.M. van Vliet
Department of Neurology, Dijkzigt Hospital, Erasmus University, Dr. Molewaterplein 40, 3015 GD Rotterdam, The Netherlands

J. Voogd
Department of Anatomy, Erasmus University, Dr. Molewaterplein 50, 3015
GE Rotterdam, The Netherlands

A.R. Wintzen
Department of Neurology, Leiden University Hospital, Rijnsburgerweg 10,
2333 AA Leiden, The Netherlands

D.S. Zee
Department of Neurology, Johns Hopkins University School of Medicine, 600
North Wolfe Street, Baltimore MD 21205, U.S.A.

Section I

Anatomy and physiology

Anatomy of the oculomotor system

J. VOOGD

The anatomy of the oculomotor system includes the eye muscles, their innervation by the 3rd, 4th and 6th cranial nerves and the pre-oculomotor centers in the brainstem with their tectal, neocortical and cerebellar afferent paths. The primate oculomotor system was reviewed by Wolff [1], Nieuwenhuys et al. [2], Henn et al. [3, 4] and Leigh and Zee [5].

1. Eye muscles

The four recti muscles with the superior oblique and the levator palpebrae muscle arise from a common tendinous ring in the apex of the orbit and from the inferior surface of the lesser wing of the sphenoid bone. The recti are inserted into the bulb in front of the equator. The tendon of the superior oblique passes through the cartilaginous trochlea and bends backwards to insert behind the equator (Fig. 1). The inferior oblique muscle arises near the inferior border of the orbit. It passes backwards under the same angle as the reflected tendon of the superior oblique and also inserts behind the equator.

Three axis, passing through the center of the eyeball, can be used to describe the movements of the eye. Wheel rotation takes place around the anterior-posterior (visual) axis (medial rotation of the upper part of the eye or intorsion; lateral rotation or extorsion). Movements around the transverse axis are elevation and depression of the center of the cornea. Abduction and adduction of the center of the cornea take place around the vertical axis.

The lines of traction of the medial and lateral recti are located in the same plane as the visual axis. Contraction of these muscles therefore leads to pure abduction or adduction of the eye. The lines of traction of the superior and inferior recti, however, make an angle of approximately 23° with the visual axis [6]. Because this angle is less than 45°, the main actions of these muscles for the eye in primary position are elevation and depression. The angle of the lines of traction of the superior and inferior oblique with the visual line is 51°, i.e. more than 45°. The

4

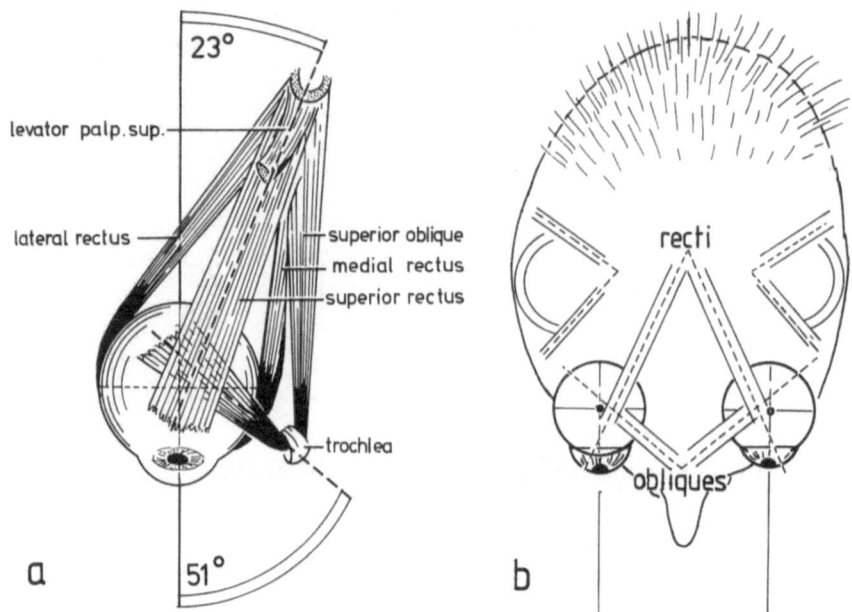

Figure 1. a. Extrinsic eyemuscles of the left eye. b. Diagram showing the lines of traction of the superior and inferior recti and the oblique muscles and the planes of the anterior and posterior semicircular canals. Angles according to Simpson and Graf (1981).

main action of these muscles increases when the eye is abducted. When the eye is adducted the action of the oblique muscles becomes almost pure elevation and depression and the superior and inferior recti become pure rotators of the eye. Moreover the superior and inferior recti adduct, and the oblique muscles abduct the eye, because the lines of traction of these four muscles pass medial to the vertical axis of the eye.

The superior and inferior recti and the oblique muscles exert their actions in two, approximately perpendicular planes. In conjugated gaze movements the synergists of the superior and inferior recti of one eye therefore are the oblique muscles of the other eye (Figs. 1 and 2).

2. Nerve supply

The external eye muscles are innervated by the 3rd, 4th and 6th cranial nerves. Proprioceptive innervation is supplied by the ophthalmic branch of the trigeminal nerve.

The nucleus of the abducens nerve is located in the tegmentum of the pons under the floor of the fourth ventricle (Fig. 5). The fibers of the genu of the facial nerve pass around it on its medial side, separating it from the medial longitudinal

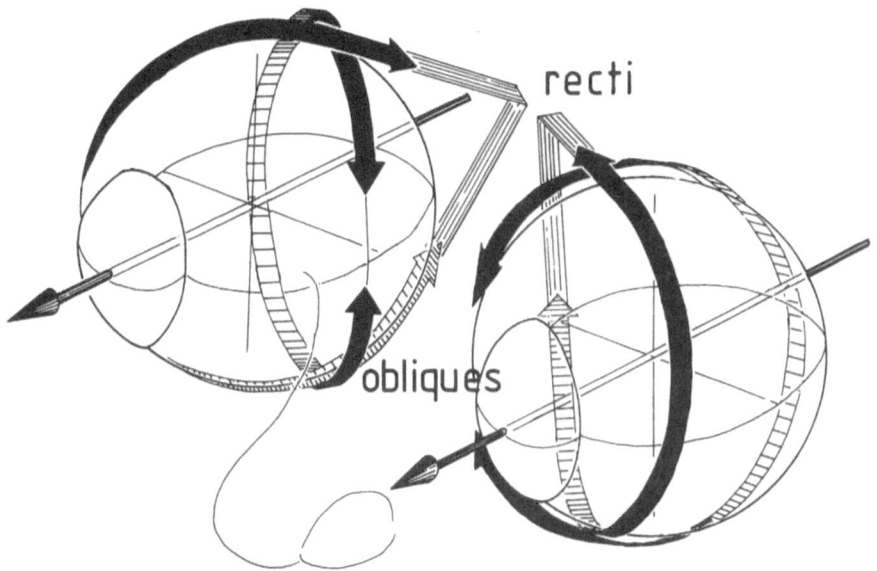

Figure 2. Diagram showing the planes of action of the inferior and superior recti and the oblique muscles of both eyes. In conjugated movements the recti of one eye are the synergists of the oblique muscles of the other eye.

fascicle. Bundles of nerve fibers leave the nucleus on its ventromedial aspect, pass ventrally through the medial lemniscus and the trapezoid body to exit along the caudal margin of the pons at the lateral border of the pyramidal tract. Here the nerve turns forward, through the pontine cistern, where it is crossed by the anterior inferior cerebellar artery (Fig. 3). It pierces the dura over the basi occipital bone and then bends forwards over the apex of the petrosal bone to enter the sinus cavernosus together with the inferior petrosal sinus. Within the sinus it is located lateral to the internal carotid artery. The abducens nerve enters the orbit through the tendinous ring, which is located over the medial, wide portion of the superior orbital fissure. Within the muscular cone it terminates on the lateral rectus muscle (Fig. 4).

The abducens nucleus contains the motor neurons innervating the lateral rectus muscle and interneurons whose axons constitute the internuclear pathway which connects the abducent nucleus with the motor neurons innervating the contralateral medial rectus located within the oculomotor nucleus. The internuclear fibers ascend within the contralateral medial longitudinal fascicle (Figs. 5e and 10a).

The nucleus of the trochlear nerve is located in the caudal mesencephalon (Fig. 5) ventral to the central grey, embedded in the medial longitudinal fascicle. The nerve passes caudally within the central grey to cross and exit in the anterior medullary velum. The nerve follows the superior cerebellar artery to emerge at

6

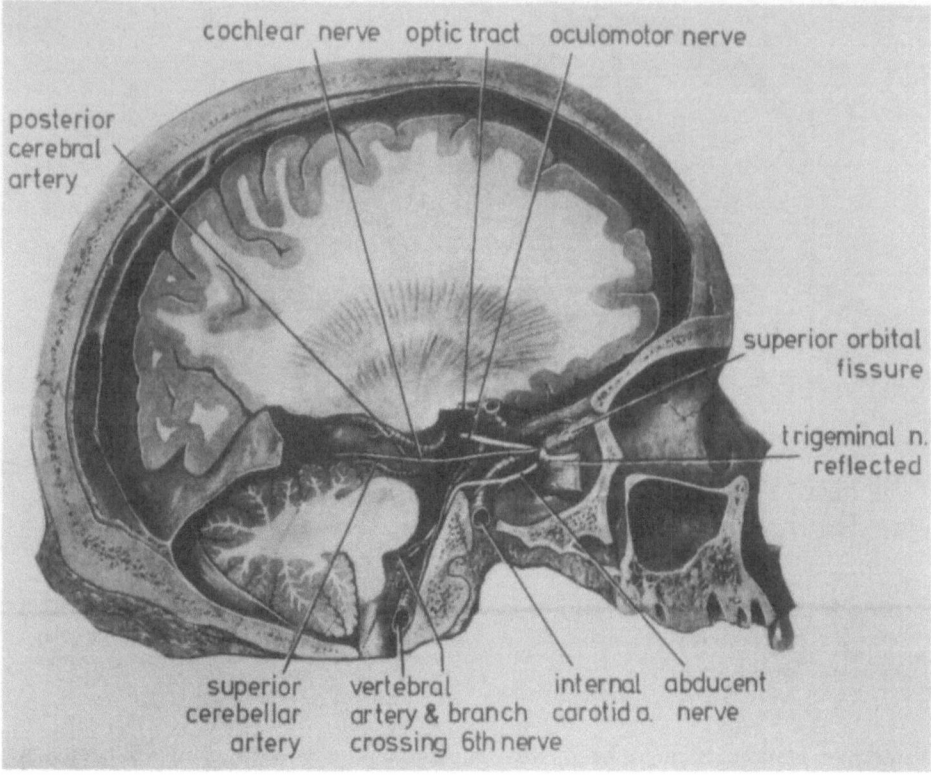

Figure 3. Intracranial course of the 3rd, 4th and 6th cranial nerves. Reproduced from E. Wolff, Anatomy of the Eye and Orbit, London, Lewis & Co, 1986.

the ventral surface of the brain (Fig. 3). It pierces the dura over the sinus cavernosus and crosses the oculomotor nerve in the lateral wall of the sinus. It enters the orbit, through the lateral part of the superior orbital fissure, passing outside the muscular cone to terminate on the superior oblique muscle (Fig. 4).

The oculomotor nuclei are located more rostrally at the level of the superior colliculus (Fig. 5). They occupy the V-shaped space between the two medial longitudinal fasciculi, ventral to the central grey matter. The fibers of the oculomotor nerve pass ventrally, medial and through the red nucleus to exit medial to the cerebral peduncle in the interpeduncular fossa.

The oculomotor nerve passes rostrally through the interpeduncular cistern, in between the superior cerebellar and posterior cerebral arteries and alongside the posterior communicating artery (Fig. 3). It pierces the dura in between posterior and anterior clinoidal processes, passes in the lateral wall of the sinus cavernosus to enter the orbit through the medial wide portion of the superior orbital fissure and the tendinous ring. Here it divides into superior and inferior branches. The superior branch innervates the superior rectus and the levator palpeprae muscles.

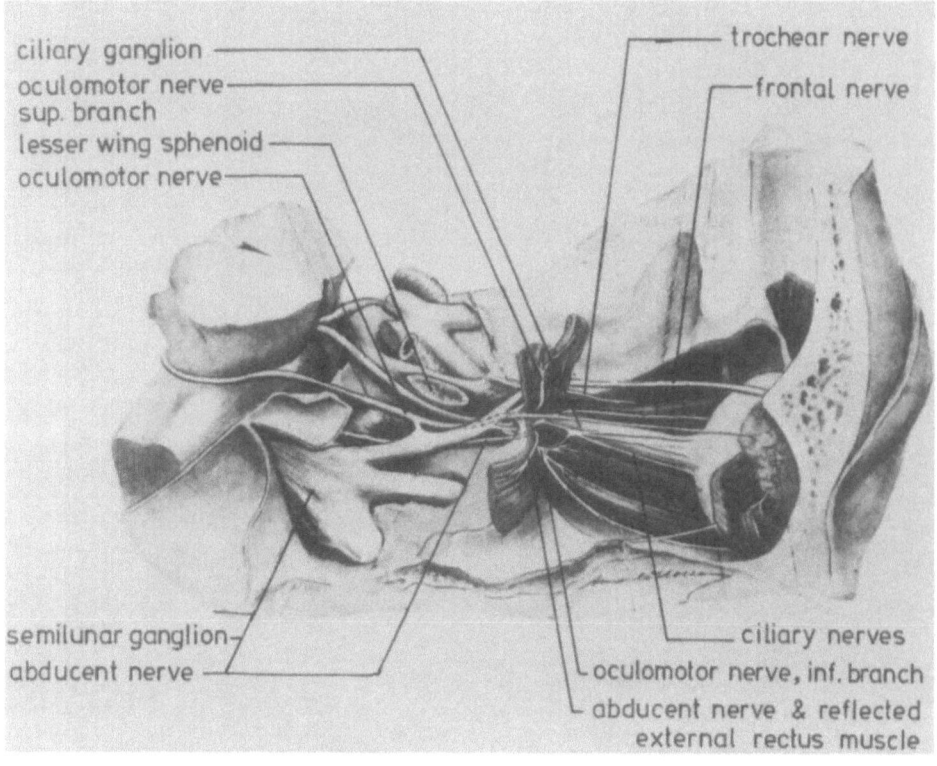

Figure 4. Entrance of the 3rd, 4th and 6th cranial nerves into the orbit. Reproduced from H. Rouvière, Anatomie Humaine, T.I. Masson & cie, Paris, 1924.

The inferior branch supplies the medial and inferior recti and the inferior obliques and terminates in the ciliary ganglion (Fig. 4).

The intranuclear topography of the motor neurons of the oculomotor nucleus innervating the different eye muscles was originally described by Warwick [7] (Fig. 6) and updated by Büttner-Ennever et al. [8], both in the monkey. One of the main features of Warwick's diagram is the crossing of the fibers innervating the superior rectus muscle. The oculomotor nucleus also contains internuclear neurons, projecting to the contralateral abducens nucleus. In the monkey these are mainly located among the motor neurons of the oculomotor nucleus [9]. They may constitute an inhibitory pathway involved in vergence movements.

Branches of the ophthalmic division of the trigeminal nerve join the three nerves innervating the eye muscles at their passage through or along the sinus cavernosus. They probably supply the proprioceptive innervation of the extrinsic eye muscles. Stretch receptors have been found in the extrinsic eye muscles of different species [10]. Their central connections are established through the ophthalmic subdivision of the semilunar ganglion and not through the nucleus of the mesencephalic tract of the trigeminal nerve.

8

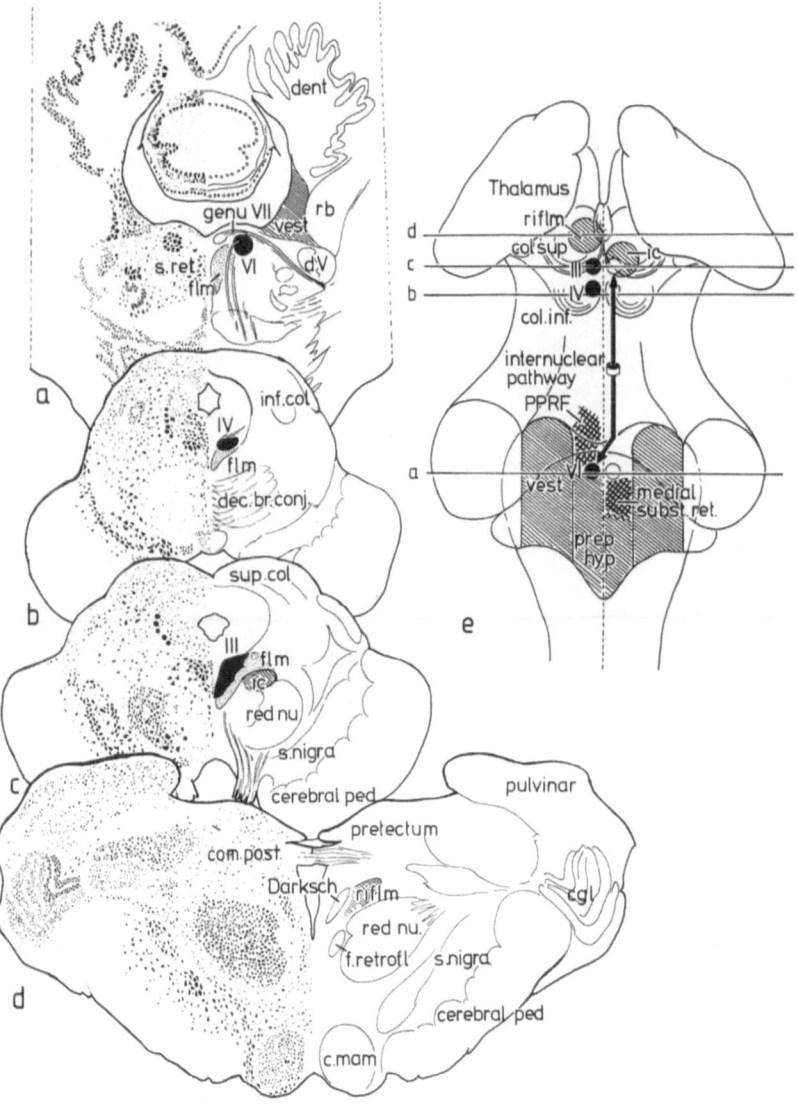

Figure 5. Some structures in the brainstem concerned with eye movement. The level of the sections a–d is indicated in the diagram of the brainstem in e. Drawings of the sections are taken from Nieuwenhuys, Voogd and van Huijzen, The Human Nervous System, Springer Verlag, Berlin, Heidelberg, New York, 1978. c.mam: mamillary body; Darksch: nucleus of Darkschewitsch; dec.br.conj: decussation of the brachium conjunctivum; dent: dentate nucleus; dV: spinal tract of trigeminal nerve and nucleus; flm: medial longitudinal fascicle; ic: interstitial nucleus of Cajal; inf.col: inferior colliculus; PPRF: pontine paramedian reticular formation; prep.hyp: nucleus prepositus hypoglossi; rb: restiform body; riflm: rostral interstitial nucleus of the medial longitudinal fascicle; s.ret: substantia reticularis; sup.col: superior colliculus; vest: vestibular nuclei.

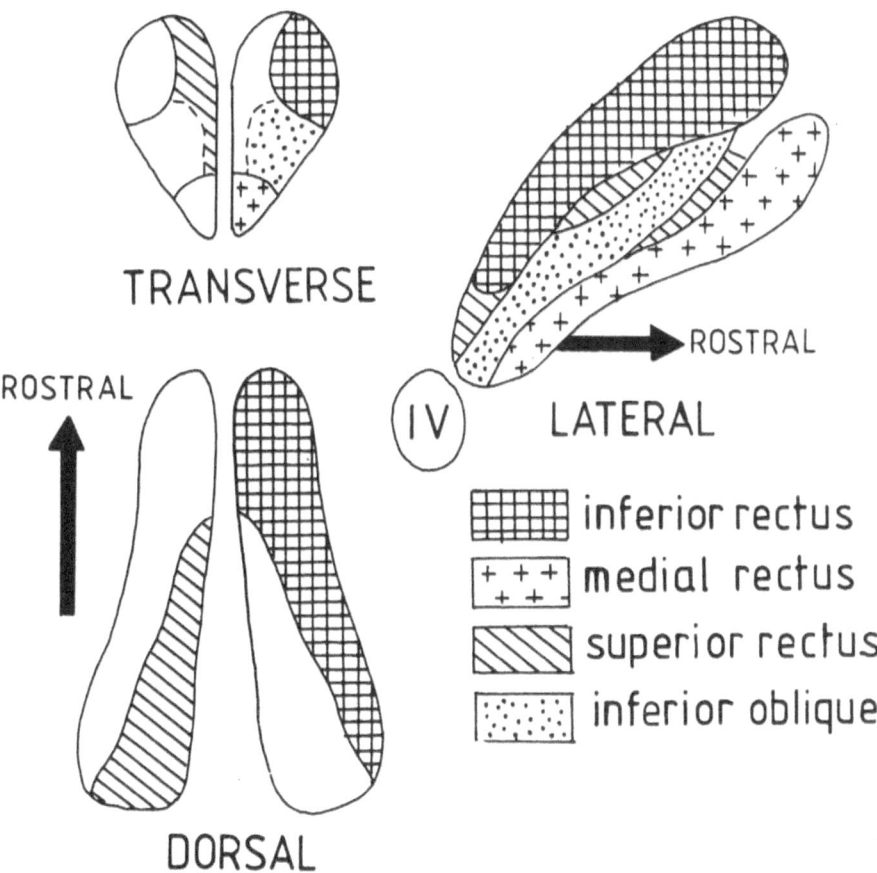

TRANSVERSE

ROSTRAL

DORSAL

ROSTRAL

(IV) LATERAL

⊞⊞ inferior rectus

[+ + +] medial rectus

▨ superior rectus

[∴∴] inferior oblique

Figure 6. Columnar localization of motor neurons innervating the extrinsic eye muscles in the nucleus of the oculomotor nerve of the monkey. Redrawn from Warwick (1953).

3. Afferent connections of the oculomotor nuclei. Gaze centers

The afferent connections of the oculomotor nuclei were investigated with retrograde axonal tracer methods in experimental animals. Injections of the abducens nucleus in monkeys recently were published by Langer et al. [9]. These injections resulted in the retrograde labeling of cells in a number of locations. Labeled cells in the dorsomedial reticular formation of the pons, located just rostral from the injected abducent nucleus, represent the horizontal gaze center. This region is better known as the paramedian pontine reticular formation (PPRF, Fig. 5) and contains the horizontal excitatory burst neurons, which program horizontal saccades (Collewijn, chapter 2). These cells are known to project directly to the ipsilateral lateral rectus motor neurons of the VIth nucleus and, through the internuclear pathway originating from the same nucleus, to the medial rectus motor neurons of the contralateral IIIrd nerve nucleus (Fig. 10a).

Labeled cells are also present caudal to the level of the abducens nucleus in the medullary reticular formation. These cells probably correspond to inhibitory burst neurons [11]. Other labeled cells are found bilaterally in the vestibular nuclei and the adjacent nucleus prepositus hypoglossi, and in the contralateral nucleus of the oculomotor nerve.

Injections with retrograde tracers in the oculomotor and trochlear nuclei [12, 13] result in labeling of cells in the contralateral interstitial nucleus of Cajal and the ipsilateral rostral interstitial nucleus of the medial longitudinal fascicle. The latter nucleus, called rostral iMLF for short, has been shown to contain the vertical burst neurons which program the vertical saccades. The rostral iMLF is located rostral to the interstitial nucleus and ventrolateral to the central grey (Fig. 5). Bilateral lesions of the iMLF cause a vertical gaze paralysis in monkeys. Human cases with vertical gaze paralysis collected from the literature show lesions which are centered upon the same region at the meso-diencephalic junction [14] (Fig. 8).

4. Afferent connections of the gaze centers

Something can be gained from a study of the afferent connections of the gaze centers as outlined in the previous paragraphs. However, the cells which are labeled from injections with retrograde tracers in the oculomotor nuclei, only constitute the final link in a cascade of connections leading to the saccade (Collewijn, chapter 2, for a discussion of the generation of saccades). The existence of afferent connections to the gaze centers from the cerebral cortex, the tectum, and the vestibular and central cerebellar nuclei, therefore does not tell us how these centers use the saccade generating system (Fig. 7).

The superior colliculus has strong connections both with the rostral iMLF and the PPRF (see Holstege and Collewijn [15] for a study of the efferent connections of the superior colliculus in the rabbit). It is known from the work of Robinson [16] (see also McInwain) [17] that stimulation of different points on the superior colliculus leads to saccades in different directions. The saccade generating map in the superior colliculus appears to be in register with the map of the visual field, which on its turn is determined by the regular termination of the fibers of the optic tract in the most superficial layers of the colliculus [18]. The linkage of visual input and saccade generating output of the colliculus is not so simple, because there is no evidence supporting the existence of direct connections between the superficial layers, which receive the direct projection from the retina, and the deep layers which give rise to the main descending efferent systems.

Several parts of the cerebral cortex are connected with the rostral iMLF and the PPRF either by direct connections descending in the internal capsule or through the superior colliculus. The primary visual and visual association cortex and the

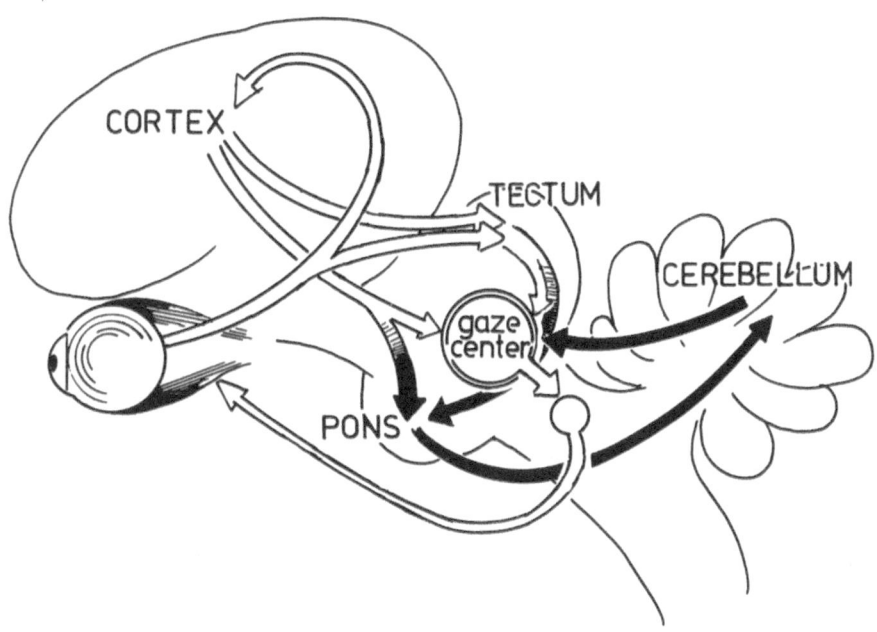

Figure 7. Connections of gaze centers from cerebral cortex and tectum opticum. Both are also connected with the gaze centers through a cerebellar loop.

frontal eye field both have access to the superior colliculus. Visual cortex terminates superficially, frontal cortex in the deep layers of the superior colliculus [19]. Direct connections to the gaze centers in the monkey originate from the frontal but not from the visual cortex [20, 21].

An additional connection of the cerebral cortex and the superior colliculus with the gaze centers involves a cerebellar loop. As is usual for the cerebellum the afferent side of this loops consists of separate climbing fiber (olivo-cerebellar) and mossy fiber paths. The climbing fiber path from the frontal cortex may pass through the accessory oculomotor nuclei in the rostral central grey at the meso-diencephalic junction, the medial and central tegmental tracts and the inferior olive [22]. The superior colliculus has a direct connection with the inferior olive [23]. The mossy fiber pathways from the visual and frontal cortex and the superior colliculus relay in the pontine nuclei. Phylogenetically the tectopontocerebellar system even may be considered as the original pathway involving the pons. The cerebellar afferents involved in saccadic control thus have access to extensive regions of the cerebellar cortex, more extensive than the classical visual area of the cerebellum which comprises the vermal lobules VI and VII, situated behind the primary fissure.

On the efferent side the cerebellar loop would involve the central nuclei, which are known to project to the reticular formation, including the gaze centers. On the other hand the central nuclei, namely the fastigial nuclei are connected with

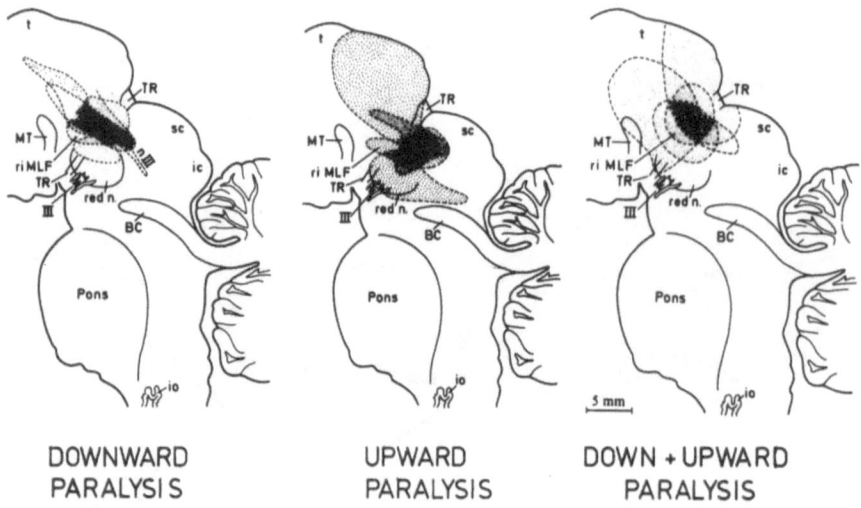

DOWNWARD
PARALYSIS

UPWARD
PARALYSIS

DOWN + UPWARD
PARALYSIS

Figure 8. The localization of lesions in patients with paralysis of vertical gaze. From Büttner-Ennever et al. (1982) bc: brachium conjuctivum; ic: inferior colliculus; io: inferior olive; MT: mamillothalamic tract; riMLF: rostral interstitial nucleus of the medial longitudinal fascicle; sc: superior colliculus; t: thalamus; TR: fasciculus retroflexus.

the vestibular nuclei. The vestibular nuclei are the center for the execution of compensatory eye movements, to be discussed in the next paragraph. The fastigial nucleus may constitute the link between the systems controlling saccades and compensatory eye movements.

6. Connections involving the vestibular nuclei

The vestibular nuclei occupy a central position in the execution of compensatory eye movements. They constitute the final common path for the vestibuloocular and optokinetic reflexes as well as for the compensatory reflexes from the neck muscles. The connections between the vestibular nuclei and the eye muscle nuclei constitute a fast, 'hard-wired' system, which is organized according to the three axis of the semicircular canals and the sets of eye muscles which execute compensatory movements around these same axis. Double, excitatory and inhibitory connections are established between the vestibular nuclei and the eye muscle nuclei. Excitatory connections mainly use the medial longitudinal fascicle and are crossed; inhibitory connections use the ipsilateral medial longitudinal fascicle [24, 25, 26]. Only certain parts of the vestibular nuclei give origin to these direct oculomotor pathways. These are the superior vestibular nucleus and an extension of this nucleus located ventral to the dentate nucleus within the floccular pedun-

13

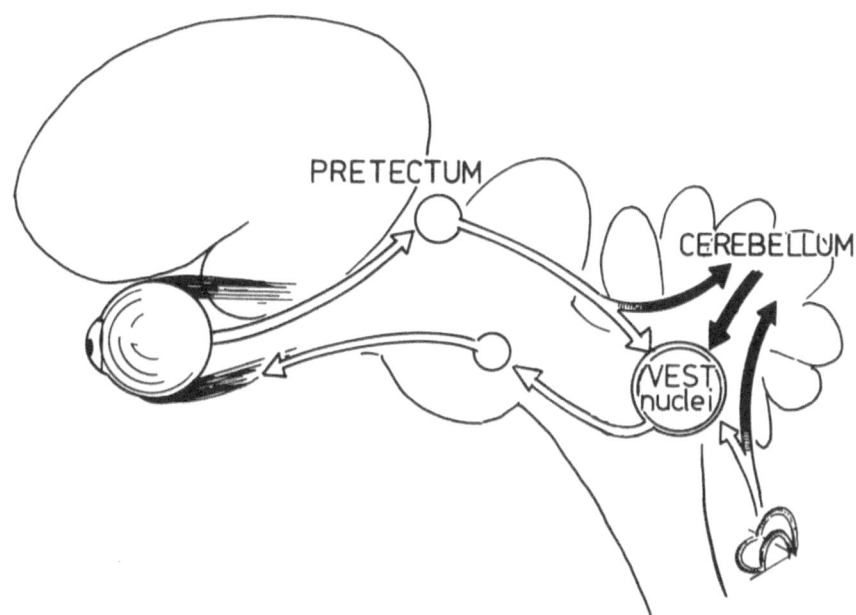

Figure 9. The vestibular nuclei are the final common path for compensatory eye movements, both in the vestibulo-ocular reflex and in the optokinetic reflex. The vestibular labyrinth and the pretectum also feed into the vestibular nuclei through a cerebellar loop.

cle, the so called 'group Y', (in the human brain this group probably is entirely incorporated in the superior vestibular nucleus) and the rostral, magnocellular part of the medial vestibular nucleus (often indicated as the ventral part of the magnocellular lateral vestibular nucleus of Deiters). Other parts of the vestibular nuclei may be involved in oculomotor control through more complicated, intra-nuclear or commissural pathways (Fig. 9).

The data from which the diagrams of the vestibulo-ocular connections (Fig. 10) were drawn were mainly taken from Highstein's studies in the rabbit [27, 28, 29], but they seem to have a general validity for the mamalian nervous system [30]. The adaptations which may become neccessary to provide for species differences in the position of the eyes are usually made by changes in the insertion and the line of traction of the eye muscles and usually do not invoke changes in the wiring of the system [6].

Excitatory connections leading to movements around the horizontal axis are relayed to the lateral and medial recti through the medial vestibular nucleus and the contralateral abducens nucleus and its recrossing internuclear pathway with the IIIrd nerve nucleus [31, 32, 33]. Excitation of the hair cells in the crista of the horizontal semicircular canal is obtained with movement of the endolymphe towards the ampulla (Fig. 10a). The appropriate compensatory eye movement is a rotation of both eyes in the plane of the horizontal canal in the same direction as the movement of the endolymphe. This movement is made by the ipsilateral

14

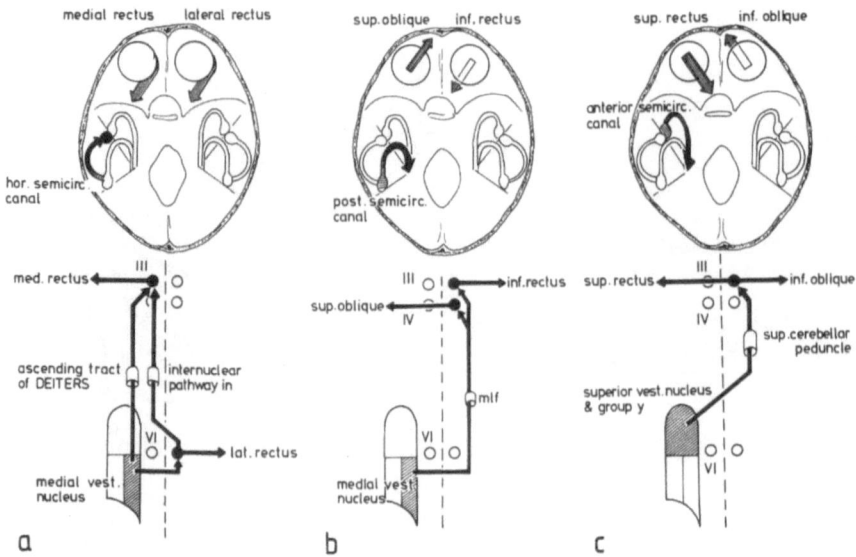

Figure 10. Excitatory connections for compensatory eye movements in the plane of the three semicircular canals. Mainly based upon data from Highstein et al. in the rabbit. mlf: medial longitudinal fascicle.

medial rectus and the contralateral lateral rectus muscles. An additional pathway connecting the medial vestibular nucleus with the motor neurons innervating the medial rectus muscle occupies the lateral part of the medial longitudinal fascicle. This pathway, which is known as the 'ascending tract of Deiters', does not seem to be present in all mammals.

Excitation of the hair cells in the cristae of the vertical canals is obtained by movement of the endolymphe away from the ampullae. Compensatory eye movements from excitation of the posterior vertical canal are executed by the ipsilateral superior oblique and the contralateral inferior rectus muscles (Fig. 10b). These excitatory connections are also relayed through the medial vestibular nucleus and the contralateral medial longitudinal fascicle. Because the fibers of the trochlear nerve cross within the brainstem, excitation of the contralateral medial longitudinal fascicle results in a contraction of the ipsilateral superior oblique. Excitation of the anterior canal leads to a contraction of the ipsilateral superior rectus and the contralateral inferior oblique (Fig. 10c). The appropriate connections are established through the superior vestibular nucleus (or rather the group Y) and the decussating fibers of the superior cerebellar peduncle. Contraction of the ipsilateral superior rectus is obtained because the fibers of the oculomotor nerve innervating this muscle are crossed (Fig. 6).

Inhibitory connections for the eye muscle nuclei originate from the same vestibular nuclei and ascend in the ipsilateral medial longitudinal fascicle. The anatomical analysis of the system is complicated by the presumed intermingling of the excitatory and inhibitory oculomotor connections of the vestibular nuclei and therefore far from complete. Moreover detailed anatomical studies which link the afferents of individual canals to its vestibulo-oculomotor system have not been attempted. What is known of these canal afferents points to a wide spread and a high degree of overlap between the afferents of different canals in all vestibular nuclei.

The connections between the retina and the vestibular nuclei, which subserve the optokinetic reflex, also have remained enigmatic. The first link in these pathways are the nuclei of the accessory optic tract, two or three cellgroups located at the surface of the rostral mesencephalon which receive an offshoot of the optic tract (see 35 and 15 for reviews). The accessory optic system is organized in subsets of neurons which process information related to movement in one of the three rotational axis of the semicircular canals. These nuclei project to the pontine and medullary reticular formation, the nucleus prepositus hypoglossi, the inferior olive and the pons. It is not clear how the connections between the nuclei of the accessory optic system and the vestibular nuclei are established. The nucleus prepositus hypoglossi [36] and the reticular formation are likely candidates, but the most elaborate connection between the accessory optic system and the vestibular nuclei uses the vestibulo cerebellum.

A vestibulo-cerebellar loop with vestibular and visual input and an output to the vestibulo-oculomotor system, has received much attention during the last 15 years, because it was used as a model-system to study the adaptation of the vestibulo-ocular reflex by the cerebellum [30]. The role of the vestibulo cerebellum certainly is not limited to adaptive control of the vestibulo-ocular reflex, but also includes the optokinetic system. More recently it was shown that the vestibulo cerebellum also is essential for the execution of smooth pursuit movements in animals possessing a fovea (Zee, chapter 17). In humans suffering from olivo-ponto-cerebellar atrophy the impairment of smooth pursuit seems to be correlated with the damage to the flocculus [37]. The cerebellar lobules involved in the adaptation of compensatory eye movements (flocculus and nodule) are different from those engaged in the saccade generating system (lobules VI and VII), but the output of both parts of the cerebellum overlaps in certain parts of the vestibular nuclei.

References

1. Wolff E (1968): Anatomy of the eye and orbit. 6th ed. Revised by RJ Last. Lewis, London.
2. Nieuwenhuys R, Voogd J, van Huijzen Chr (1978): Human Central Nervous System Synopsis and Atlas. Springer Verlag, Berlin-New York.
3. Henn VA, Büttner-Ennever JA, Hepp K (1982a): The primate oculomotor system. I. motor neurons. A synthesis of anatomical, physiological and clinical data. Human Neurobiol 1: 77–85.
4. Henn V, Hepp K, Büttner-Ennever JA (1982b): The primate oculomotor system. II. Premotor system. Human Neurobiol 1: 87–95.

5. Leigh RJ, Zee DS (1983): The neurology of eye movement. Davis Cy, Philadelphia.
6. Graf W, Simpson JI (1981): Relations between semicircular canals, the optic axis and the extra-ocular muscles in lateral-eyed and frontal-eyed animals. In: Fuchs AF, Becker W (eds), Progress in oculo-motor research. Elsevier Amsterdam, pp 409–417.
7. Warwick R (1953): Representation of the extra-ocular muscles in the oculomotor nuclei of the monkey. J Comp Neurol 98: 449–504.
8. Büttner-Ennever KA, d'Ascanio P, Gysin R (1982): The localization of large and small motor neurons in the oculomotor nucleus of the monkey. In: Physiological Aspects of Eye Movements, Roucoux A, Crommelinck M (eds), Dr W Junk, Publishers, pp 345–349, The Hague, Boston, London.
9. Langer T, Kaneko CRS, Scudder CA, Fucks AF (1986): Afferents to the abducens nucleus in the monkey and cat. J Comp Neurol 245: 379–400.
10. Daunicht WJ (1983): Proprioception in extraocular muscles of the rat. Brain Res 278: 291–294.
11. Hikosaka O, Igusa Y, Nakao S, Shimazu H (1978): Direct inhibitory synaptic linkage of pontomedullary reticular burst neurons with abducens motor neurons in the cat. Exp Brain Res 33: 337–352.
12. Graybiel AM, Hartweg EA (1974): Some afferent connections of the oculomotor complex in the cat: an experimental study with tracer techniques. Brain Res 81: 543–551.
13. Büttner-Ennever JA, Büttner U (1978): A cell group associated with vertical eye movements in the rostral mesencephalic reticular formation of the monkey. Brain Res 151: 31–47.
14. Büttner-Ennever JA, Büttner U, Cohen B, Baumgartner C (1982): Vertical gaze paralysis and the rostral interstitial nucleus of the medial longitudinal fasciculus (rostral iMLF). Brain 105: 125–149.
15. Holstege G, Collewijn H (1982): The efferent connections of the nucleus of the optic tract and the superior colliculus in the rabbit. J Comp Neurol 209: 139–175.
16. Robinson DA (1972): Eye movements evoked by collicular stimulation in the alert monkey. Vision Res 12: 1795–1808.
17. McIlwain JT (1986): Effects of eye position on saccades evoked electrically from superior colliculus of alert cats. J Neurophysiol 55: 97–113.
18. Huerta M, Harting JK (1984): Connectional organization of the superior colliculus. TINS 7: 286–289.
19. Kuypers HGJM, Lawrence DG (1967): Cortical projection to the red nucleus and the brainstem in the rhesus monkey. Brain Res 4: 151–188.
20. Leichnetz GR, Spencer RF, Smith DJ (1984a): Cortical projections to the nuclei adjacent to the oculomotor complex in the medial dien-mesencephalic tegmentum in the monkey. J Comp Neurol 228: 359–387.
21. Leichnetz GR, Smith DJ, Spencer RF (1984b): Cortical projections to the paramedian tegmental and basilar pons in the monkey. J Comp Neurol 228: 388–408.
22. Onodera S (1984): Olivary projections from the meso-diencephalic structures studied by means of axonal transport of horseradish peroxidase or tritiated aminoacids. J Comp Neurol 227: 37–49.
23. Hess DT (1982): The tecto-olivo-cerebellar pathway in the rat. Brain Res 250: 143–148.
24. Highstein SM (1971): Organization of the inhibitory and excitatory vestibulo-ocular reflex pathways to the third and fourth nuclei in rabbit. Brain Res 32: 218–223.
25. Highstein SM, Ito M (1971): Differential localization within the vestibular complex of the inhibitory and excitatory cells innervating IIIrd nucleus oculomotor neurons in rabbit. Brain Res 29: 358–362.
26. Nakao S, Sasaki S, Schor RH, Shimazu H (1982): Functional organization of premotor neurons in the cat medial vestibular nucleus related to slow and fast phases of nystagmus. Exp Brain Res 45: 371–385.
27. Highstein SM (1973): The organization of the vestibulo-oculomotor and trochlear reflex pathways in the rabbit. Exp Brain Res 17: 285–300.

28. Highstein SM, Reisine H (1979): Synaptic and functional organization of vestibulo-ocular reflex pathways. Progress in Brain Res 50: 431–442.
29. Highstein SM, Ito M, Tsuchiya I (1971): Synaptic linkage in the vestibulo-ocular reflex pathway of the rabbit. Exp Brain Res 13: 306–326.
30. Ito M (1984): The cerebellum and neural control. Raven Press, New York.
31. Highstein SM, Baker R (1978): Excitatory termination of abducens internuclear neurons on medial rectus motor neurons: relationship to syndrome of internuclear ophthalmoplegia. J Neurophysiol 41: 1647–1661.
32. Gacek RR (1977): Location of brainstem neurons projecting to the oculomotor nucleus in the cat. Exp Neurol 57: 725–749.
33. Gacek RR (1979): Location of abducens afferent neurons in the cat. Exp Neurol 64: 342–353.
34. Maciewicz R, Phips BS (1983): The oculomotor internuclear pathway: a double retrograde labeling study. Brain Res 262: 1–8.
36. McCrea RA, Baker R, Delgado-Garcia J (1979): Afferent and efferent organization of the prepositus hypoglossi nucleus. Progress in Brain Res 50: 653–665.
35. Simpson JI (1984): The accessory optic system. Ann Rev Neurosci 7: 13–41.
37. Zee DS, Yee RD, Cogan DG, Robinson DA, Engel WK (1976): Oculomotor abnormalities in hereditary cerebellar ataxia. Brain 99: 207–234.

The physiology of eye movement

H. COLLEWIJN

1. Purpose and types of eye movement

Why do our eyes move? One basic reason is that the visual system functions optimally only under certain constraints of positioning and velocity of the retinal image. Limited slip velocity is a basic requirement: images moving at more than a few deg/sec across the retina are seen blurred. A primary source of such slip is rotation of the head. The vestibulo-ocular reflex (VOR) and optokinetic reflex (OKN) generate a counterrotation of the eye in the head which largely compensate the head movement, with a relatively stable direction of gaze (position of eye in space) as a result. The compensatory eye movement is in principle continuous and smooth, and has a velocity approximating that of the head, with opposite direction. This smooth component is interrupted by discontinuous steps (fast phases or saccades), which rapidly displace the eye in the direction of the head rotation and at the same time prevent mechanical saturation of the eye-in-head motion. A-foveate animals such as the rabbit only generate these combined eye and head movements, in which gaze is kept almost stable or displaced stepwise over rather large angles.

In species with further developed visual systems, a similar repertoire of smooth and saccadic eye movements is used but with a much more differentiated control. A good use of foveal vision (with the sector of maximal acuity subtending less than 1 deg) would be impossible without an exceptionally good guidance system. This has indeed been developed for both types of movement. Voluntary saccades serve to position a target of interest on the fovea (foveation). In man these can be generated independently of head movements (up to a certain amplitude); they are controlled by cognitive processes of selection and decision and not (or only marginally) by the physical attributes of the stimulus. To keep a moving target on the fovea, it can be tracked by the smooth pursuit system. This is primarily a velocity guidance system under cognitive control. A human subject is free to pursue an arbitrary target amidst other moving or stationary targets.

The frontal position of the eyes and the integration of the two monocular images into a single binocular percept, with stereopsis as a special attribute, required in addition the development of vergence movements, i.e. the fine control of the relative position of the two eyes.

2. Mechanics of orbit: eye muscles

Through the ocular muscles and a connective tissue system of septa and ligaments [1, 2] the eye is suspended in such a way that it executes mainly rotatory movements around a relatively stable center of rotation. Linear displacements in all directions do occur, however [3, 4]. The formerly assumed sideways slipping of the rectus muscles during rotation out of the plane of action of the muscle has not been corroborated by recent CT scan investigations [5].

The motions of eye and orbital structures (together often called the 'plant') are affected by mass, elasticity and damping (viscosity). Although a precise simulation of the mechanics requires complicated higher order models, in practice a simple second order description with lumped elasticity and viscosity terms gives a good approximation. Elasticity determines the force required to *keep* the eye statically in an eccentric position; for the horizontal and vertical movements this force is close to 1 gram/deg.

To *move* the eye an additional force of about 0.2 gram per deg/sec velocity is needed. The mechanical time constant of the eye is about 0.2 sec. For a fast displacement of the eye as during a saccade (velocities of up to 700 deg/sec) a large force is needed during the motion, followed by a much smaller force to maintain the deviated position (Robinson [6]). Accordingly, the agonist muscle shows a pulse-step activation; this is paralleled by a pulse-step inhibition in the antagonist. When the pulse component is too small or absent saccades will be slow. Smooth movements with an appreciable velocity also require greater muscle forces than static positions.

It has been attempted to relate the dynamic and static components of muscular force to different types of muscle fibers. Histochemically, 5–6 types have been distinguished; physiologically fast and slow twitch fibers with single innervation and multiply innervated slow fibers have been recognized. The latter type is extremely fatigue-resistant [7]. The slow fiber types are found predominantly in the orbital layers and the fast ones especially in the global layers. Although there is no sharp distinction, there is evidence that the orbital layers are involved mainly in sustained activity, and the global layers mainly in short periods of strong activity [8].

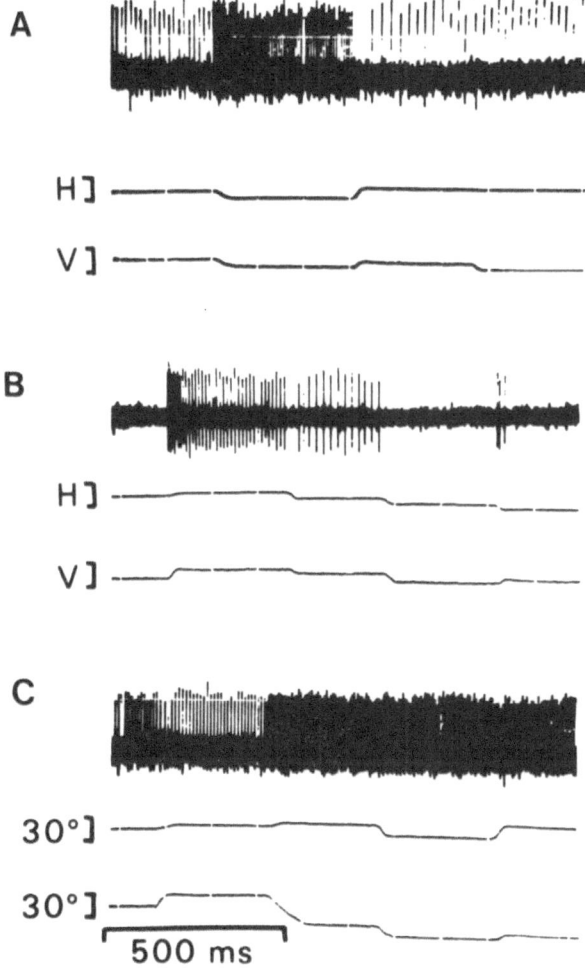

Figure 1. Three different types of oculomotor neurons. Above: neuronal activity; below: horizontal and vertical eye position. A: phasic-tonic neuron; B: predominantly phasic neuron; C: predominantly tonic neuron. From: Henn et al. [9].

3. The motor neurons

These are localized in the motor nuclei III, IV and VI. In addition these nuclei contain interneurons, projecting elsewhere; in the abducens nucleus these amount to 50% of the neuronal population. Motor neuronal activity can be divided similarly to that of eye muscles (Fig. 1). Most motor neurons show a phasic-tonic activity: phasic during an eye movement in the pulling direction of the muscle, tonic during the ensuing fixation. Opposite motions are accompanied by inhibition instead of activation. Other neurons show predominantly either a phasic or tonic activation [9]. Quantitative studies of the relation between motor neuron activity, eye position and velocity have been done e.g. by Robinson [6] who could reasonably account for this relation by summing a position and velocity term each with their own coefficients; furthermore a position threshold has to be exceeded before a neuron shows static activity (Fig. 2). Position sensitivity (in the eye position range where the neuron is active) is highest in phasic-tonic motor neurons (e.g. 55 AP sec $^{-1}$ deg^{-1}); it is much lower in tonic neurons (e.g. 2 AP sec $^{-1}$ deg^{-1}). Phasic motor neurons develop a sustained activity only with extreme eye positions.

4. Premotor circuits involved in saccade generation

Lesions of two circumscript brainstem areas abolish saccades. These are the paramedian pontine reticular formation (PPRF) for horizontal, and the rostral interstitial nucleus of the medial longitudinal fasciculus (riMLF) for vertical saccades.

The PPRF lies between the levels of the trochlear and abducens nuclei. It receives (among others) fibers from the contralateral superior colliculus and cortex (FEF, frontal eye field). Among the many efferent connections are those to the ipsilateral abducens and riMLF nuclei. The connection to the abducens nucleus mediates horizontal gaze through direct projections to abducens motor neurons and interneurons (internuclear neurons) the axons of which ascend through the MLF to the contralateral oculomotor nucleus, particularly the medial rectus division (Fig. 3). The riMLF projects mainly to the superior and inferior rectus and oblique muscles motor neurons in nuclei III and IV [10, 11].

Neurons in the PPRF show a characteristic activity before and during saccades (Fig. 4). They show a burst of activity (bursters) or a short period of inhibition (pause cells). Medium-lead bursters increase their activity 6–12 msec before the start of a saccade. Long-lead bursters fire earlier but with a less marked beginning. Pause neurons are continuously active at 150–200 AP/sec, with brief interruptions starting 8–16 msec before and lasting through the duration of a saccade. They are found mainly near the midplane in the caudal PPRF. Medium-lead bursters are active in relation with horizontal saccades to the ipsilateral side.

The number of action potentials in a burst is positively correlated with the size of the saccade. Burster activity related to vertical saccades is located in the riMLF; oblique saccades require combined activity of both riMLF and PPRF bursters. Pause neurons inhibit the generation of saccades; electrical stimulation of their activity can even suppress saccades completely. Bursters fire only while pause neurons are silent. The medium-lead bursters provide the pulse signal to the motor neurons; it is assumed that the subsequent step necessary to maintain the new eye position is produced by a circuit with (mathematically) integrating properties. This 'neural integrator' is a crucial element in current oculomotor models.

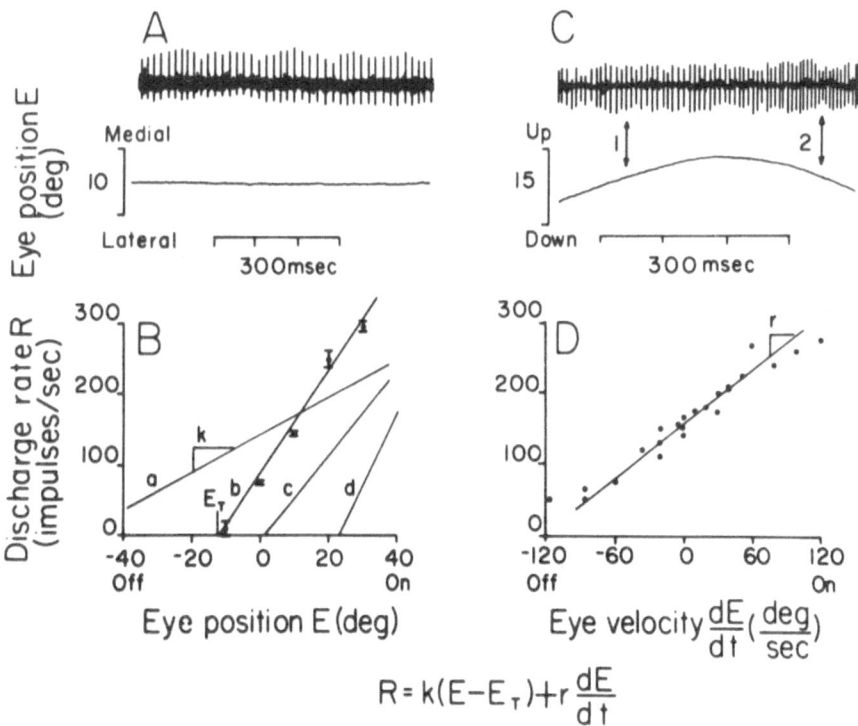

Figure 2. Discharge rate (R) of motor neurons in relation to eye position (E) and velocity (dE/dt). A: steady discharge during fixation. B: discharge rate/eye position curves for four cells showing extremes of threshold (E_T) and slope (k). C: although eye position is similar at times 1 and 2, the discharge rates are different because of the opposite directions of eye velocity. D: discharge rate/eye velocity curve for one motor neuron, with slope (r). The relation between the different parameters is expressed in the equation at the bottom. From Robinson [6].

It is needed in all cases of transformation of velocity-coded signals into position-coded signals. It has not been definitely localized but the prepositus hypoglossi nucleus is a likely candidate [12, 13]. Presumably the long-lead bursters excite the medium-lead bursters. In addition to excitatory burst neurons there are also groups of complementary inhibitory burst neurons. The actual neuroanatomy of the mutual interconnections is now being worked out.

A particularly difficult question concerns the control of saccade generators by visual inputs. An important element is the retinal localization of a target which we want to foveate. This localization specifies the desired ocular displacement in retinal coordinates, which are subsequently transformed into retinotopic localizations in the superior colliculus and cortex, where somehow the commands to the premotor circuits are generated.

Combined, total lesions of superior colliculus and FEF profoundly disable the generation of saccades [14], the defects due to partial lesions are more subtle.

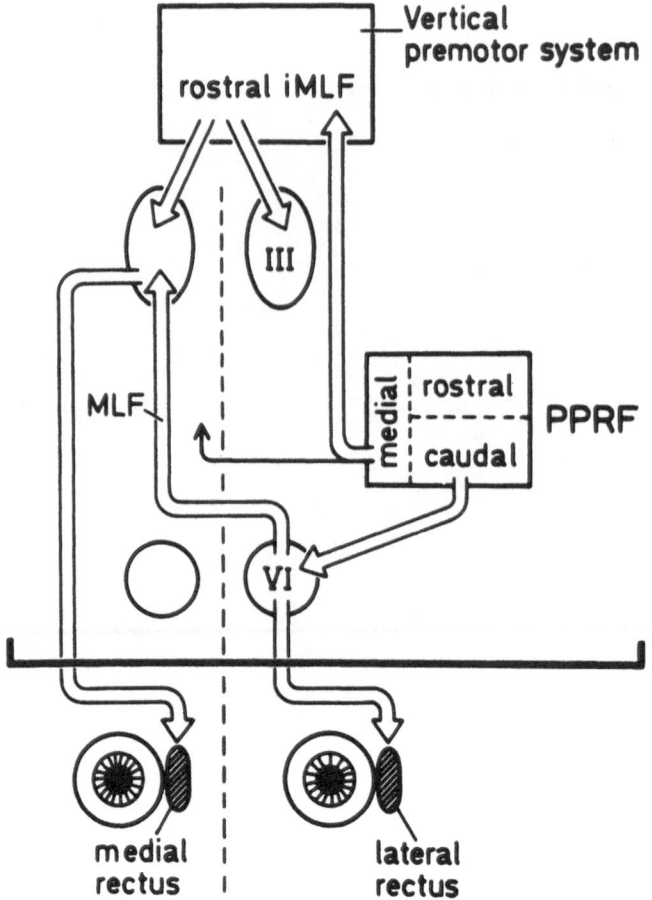

Figure 3. Scheme for the generation of saccadic eye movements. From Henn et al. [10].

The descending pathways from cortex and colliculus decussate at the transition mesencephalon-pons. The retinotopic, sensory projection upon the superior colliculus is paralleled by a motor projection in register. Stimulation of a specific locus of the colliculus leads to a saccade which aims the fovea towards the locally represented point of the visual field. The superficial collicular layers contain purely visual units, whereas cells with 'motor'properties are situated deeper. These latter cells show visual excitation mainly in the case that a saccade will be made towards the visual target ('enhancement'; see Wurtz and Albano [15]). The anatomical relations between superficial and deep collicular layers are still some-what controversial. In addition to the retino-topic localization, true spatial location may be encoded somehow by integrating retinal information with information of eye-in-head and head-on-body position.

Stimulation of the frontal cortical eye field (FEF; area 8; pre-arcuate gyrus in

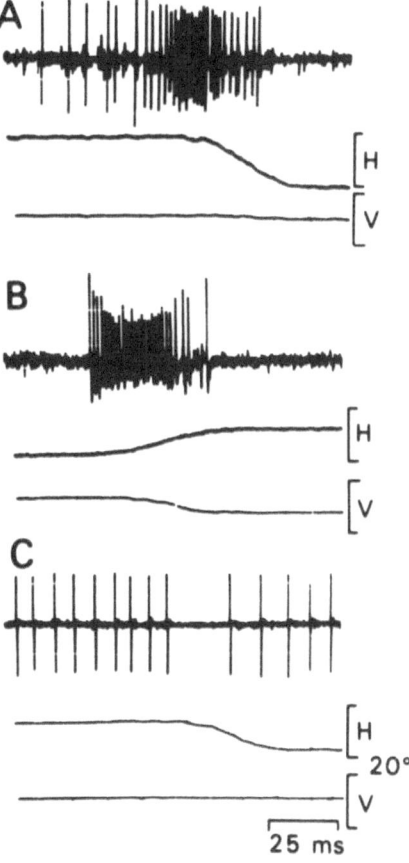

Figure 4. Recordings of single neurons in the PPRF (top traces). A: long-lead burster; B: medium-lead burster; C: pause neuron. Bottom traces: horizontal and vertical eye position. From Henn et al. [10].

monkey) leads to contralaterally directed saccades, often with a vertical component. Purely vertical saccades require a symmetrical, bilateral stimulation. The latency of the elicited saccades is short (about 25 msec). Recently it was established that spontaneous saccades in the monkey are preceded by activity of FEF neurons [16, 17].

The disturbances due to FEF lesions are subtle. Although saccade generation is not permanently disturbed, patients have difficulty in suppressing a saccade when a target is suddenly presented in the periphery (automatism of colliculus?) and also in making saccades to remembered locations of a target [18]. Normal saccades show a characteristic shape with typical values of total duration and maximal velocity for each amplitude (Fig. 5). Duration as well as maximal velocity increase with size, but velocity saturates at about 700 deg/sec. Patients

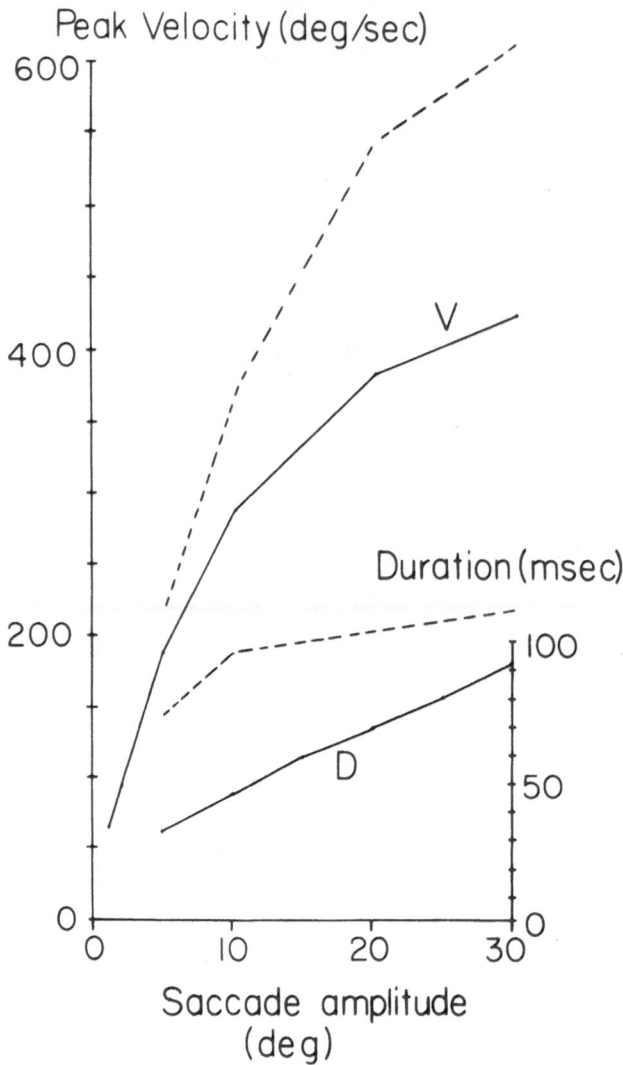

Figure 5. The mean relation between saccadic amplitude, peak velocity (V) and duration (D), for normal subjects. Dashed lines indicate ± 1 standard deviation of velocity (From: Leigh and Zee [19]).

with 'slow saccades' often show a systematic shift of this distribution with increased durations and lowered velocities.

5. Vestibulo-ocular and optokinetic reflexes

The smooth component of these reflexes generates a counterrotation of the eye during head movements. The sensory inputs are derived from the semicircular canals which signal (for short rotations) head angular velocity, and from the visual system. The relevant visual motion detection is processed exclusively subcortically in the rabbit and passes from the retina to the pretectal nucleus of the optic tract (NOT) and from there to (among others) the prepositus hypoglossi nucleus and the medullary reticular formation, from where the vestibular nuclei may be reached secondarily [20]. Furthermore the NOT projects to the cerebellum through the dorsolateral pontine nuclei and the dorsal cap of the inferior olive. In the cat, the NOT receives a strong projection from the visual cortex in addition to direct retinal fibers. Recently, Hoffmann and Distler [21] have shown that in the monkey the NOT has retained its visual direction-selective properties which, however, are almost exclusively derived from indirect descending cortical projections rather than from direct retinal projections. Thus, the more primitive subcortical circuits are heavily controlled by cortical processes in primates.

Macular vestibular inputs exert considerable tonic eye positional control in the rabbit, but such reflexes have become vestigial in man.

The main premotor stations for VOR and OKN are the medial and superior vestibular nuclei. The three-neuronal reflex arc (vestibular hair cell – vestibular nuclear neuron – oculomotor neuron) is the most direct connection in the VOR, but more complex additional circuits are essential, as the canals code for head *velocity*, while the motor neurons have to encode also eye *position*. One, or more, probably several, integrators are used to create the position signal out of the velocity signal and also to lengthen the time constant of the VOR, which is about 20 sec in man, while the canals have a time constant of only 3–4 sec.

For very low frequencies of head rotation and for constant rotational velocities the signals from the canals become unreliable or disappear. In daily life this creates no problems because vestibular information is always supplemented by visual information. The VOR can be investigated in isolation in darkness; the OKN can be isolated by rotating a full-field visual stimulus around the stationary subject. Both are in fact laboratory artifacts. The VOR is very fast (latency about 10 msec) and thus ensures an immediate stabilization of gaze; the OKN is sustained indefinitely long and works also for low velocities, but has a much longer latency (about 100 msec). The two systems acting in synergy stabilize gaze optimally. A function of the OKN alone in normal conditions is the suppression of drift of the eye in the head. In the light, drift velocity is only about 0.1 deg/sec; darkness often causes a tenfold increase.

Virtually all canal-sensitive neurons in the vestibular nuclei are also modulated by large field visual motion stimuli. Thus, the vestibular nuclei are a common interface between the motor neurons and vestibular, visual and probably also somatosensory inputs. The premotor properties are reflected by the finding that many vestibular neurons show activity patterns resembling those of oculomotor neurons.

The complementary nature of VOR and OKN is also seen in after-effects of rotation. Post-rotatory vestibular nystagmus is cancelled by optokinetic after-

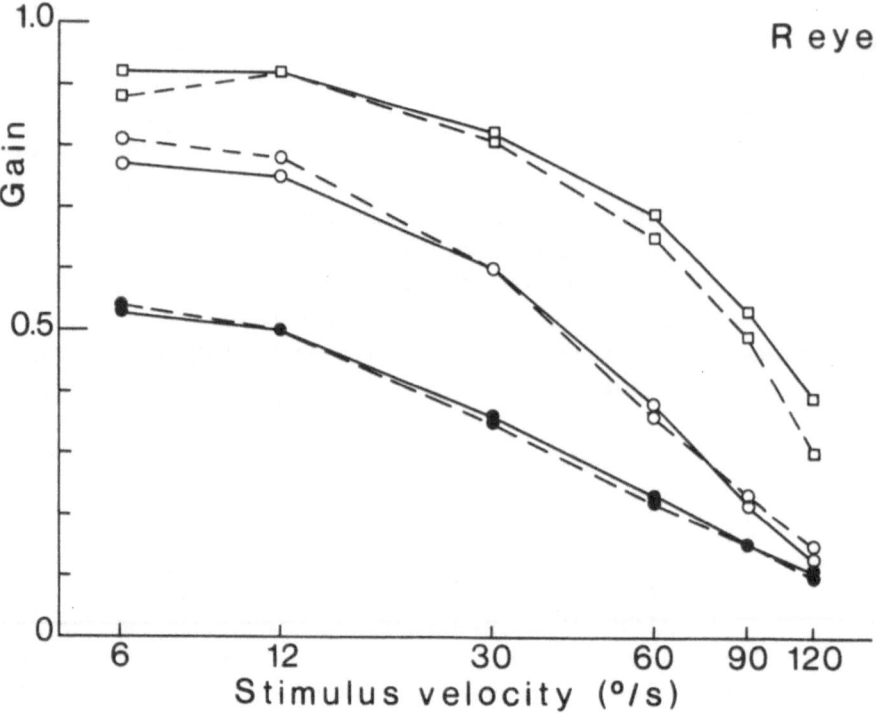

Figure 6. Mean slow phase gain of 'stare' OKN of 5 subjects looking with the right eye only. Continuous lines: rotations to the left; dashed lines: rotation to the right. Squares: stimulation of whole visual field; open circles: stimulation of a central retinal sector (width 20 deg) only; dots: stimulation of periphery only, with occlusion of central sector of 20 deg (from: van Die [23]).

nystagmus so that after continued rotation of a subject *in the light* virtually no postrotational nystagmus is observed.

6. Input-output relations of OKN and VOR

In recent years, performance of VOR and OKN has been evaluated with scleral search coil techniques [22] in normal human subjects. Some results on human OKN [23, 24] are shown in Fig. 6. Horizontal motion of a full-field stimulus was presented to normal subjects with the instruction to look at the pattern but not to pursue any detail ('stare' OKN). Gain (the ratio slow phase eye velocity/stimulus velocity) was about 0.9 for stimulus velocities of 6 and 12 deg/sec. In the range 30–120 deg/sec, gain decreased progressively with the increase of stimulus velocity (Fig. 6, squares).

The role of the central and peripheral parts of the retina in eliciting OKN was assessed by selective masking. Either a central sector (total width 20 deg) or the

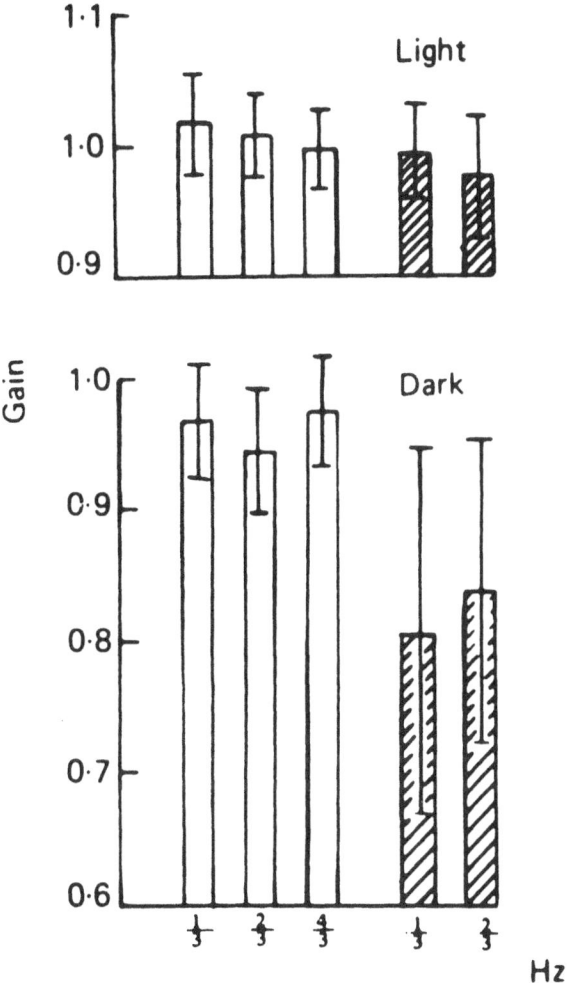

Figure 7. Average velocity gain of compensatory eye movements of 5 subjects in the light (top) and in the dark (bottom) and for active (open columns) and passive (hatched columns) head motion at frequencies of 1/3, 2/3 and 4/3 Hz. The error bars (± 1 S.D.) indicate the variation between subjects and eyes (from: Collewijn, Martins and Steinman [25]).

complementary periphery was occluded by masks, the edges of which were stabilized on the retina. As shown in Fig. 6, occlusion of the center (dots) caused a much larger reduction in OKN gain than occlusion of the periphery (open circles). Thus, human OKN seems to be predominantly controlled by the central retina. This predominance was unaffected by the velocity or spatial frequency of the stimulus pattern.

Some important aspects of compensatory eye movements during head movements are illustrated in Fig. 7. Head oscillations in the range 0.33–1.33 Hz were

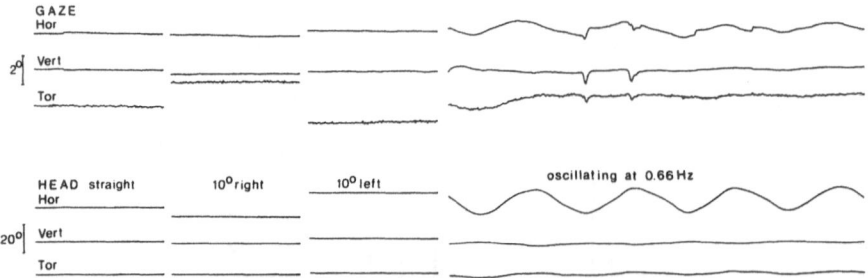

Figure 8. Stability of horizontal, vertical and torsional gaze positions (upper three traces) during static (left 3 panels) and dynamic (right panel) horizontal head displacements. Head movements are shown in the lower 3 traces, subjects fixated a point target at optical infinity. Notice the difference in calibration (by a factor 10) between gaze and head traces. Gaze represents eye position in space, not in the head.

produced either actively by the subject, or passively by oscillation of the chair [25]. This was done in the dark (VOR) as well as in the light (VOR + OKN). Subjects were instructed to fixate a stationary target and to continue trying to do this also in the dark. The effect of frequency on gain was negligible in the range used. In the light, gain was close to, but never exactly equal to unity. In te dark, gain of compensatory eye movements was lower and also much more variable with passive motion than during active head oscillation. In agreement with earlier work [26] it has to be concluded that passive oscillation in the dark, as used in many routine tests, is unlikely to yield reliable or even reproducible values for VOR gain. In view of the physiological synergy of OKN, VOR and motor activity the most realistic estimates of the gain of compensatory eye movements are obtained in subjects making active head movements while looking at a visual target. A representative recording of gaze stability during horizontal head oscillation is shown in Fig. 8. Eye and head motions were recorded in three dimensions (horizontal, vertical and torsion). A consistent finding is that during dynamic head motion (but not during static deviations) gaze is fluctuating slightly with the head due to imperfect compensation. Gaze instabilities in horizontal and vertical directions can be characterized by standard deviations of gaze position of about 7 min arc with the head held stationary and about 16 min arc during head movement. Gaze velocities remain usually lower than 1 deg/sec. Gain of VOR + OKN is about 0.98.

In the torsional direction, static gain (counterroll) is very low (of the order of 0.10), as has been known for a century. However, we could recently establish [27] that during dynamic head oscillation around the sagittal axis substantial counterroll of the eyes occurs, which is entirely transient in nature. Gain of this dynamic counterroll increases with frequency and amounts to about 0.4 at 0.16 Hz and 0.6 at 0.66 Hz. Thus, torsional stability of the eye is grossly inferior to horizontal and vertical stability. This applies to fixation with the head stationary as well.

7. Smooth pursuit

In addition to the global OKN, humans possess a smooth pursuit system to selectively follow moving targets of interest. Probably the same system is used to maintain fixation of a stationary target.

The most important stimulus for smooth pursuit is a moving target projected on the central retina. However, this stimulus is only effective once the subject makes the voluntary decision to look and keep looking towards this target. Thus, perceptual and cognitive processes are essential in the control of smooth pursuit.

Smooth pursuit is often supplemented by saccades; the saccadic component increases whenever the smooth component fails to track the target correctly. This is especially the case when the target moves fast or follows an irregular (unpredictable) trajectory. Smooth pursuit gain tends to fall rapidly when the stimulus velocity is increased, as shown in Fig. 9, for a point target moving according to a triangular wave form [28]. However, the absolute gain values have only a limited validity. They can be affected by such factors as the extent and structure of the target and its trajectory. Of major importance is the decision of the subject to follow one or another target; subjects can even effectively select among identical target configurations which overlap each other totally and can be distinguished only by motion contrast [29].

Under some conditions even illusory targets can be followed, which have no direct retinal parallel. An example is the pursuit of the imaginary center of a rolling wheel, of which only two single points on the circumference are shown. Some people can pursue motion of their own finger in darkness, probably using proprioceptive signals or copies of their motor commands (efference copy). So called 'sigma pursuit' (pursuit of the illusionary motion of a row of stroboscopically illuminated targets) may be largely controlled by efference-copy signals [30].

Cortical control is essential in smooth pursuit. Insight in the trajectory of the target (predictability) may lead to extremely effective pursuit with no time delay and small spatial errors; in this case the subject has built some kind of 'internal model' of the target motion which he uses to generate pursuit. Pursuit is often even generated in anticipation, before the target really moves [31, 32], can continue during transient disappearance of a target [33] and can reach very high velocities (> 150 deg/sec) when self-generated target motions are pursued [34].

This summary will make it clear that smooth pursuit can not be modelled satisfactorily as a simple negative feedback system with retinal slip velocity as the only input. The pathways used in pursuit are only partially understood. Bilateral destruction of the visual cortex leads – not surprisingly – to complete loss of pursuit and (according to most authors) also of OKN. Unilateral hemispherectomy leads to deficient (but not absent) pursuit to the ipsilateral side. This is probably not due to the unilateral loss of the area striata, which by itself does not induce a clear defect, but to the loss of parietal cortex. Lesions in parietal area 7, which receives visual input by way of the peristriate cortex and the superior

A

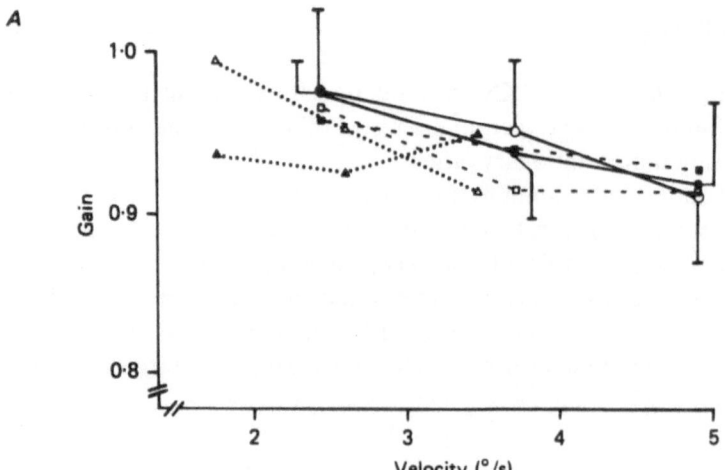

Velocity (°/s)

B

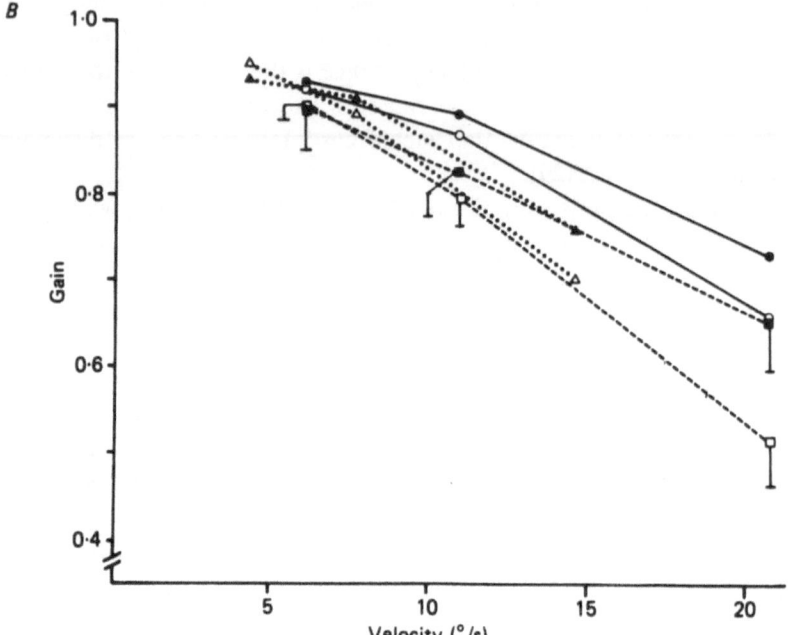

Velocity (°/s)

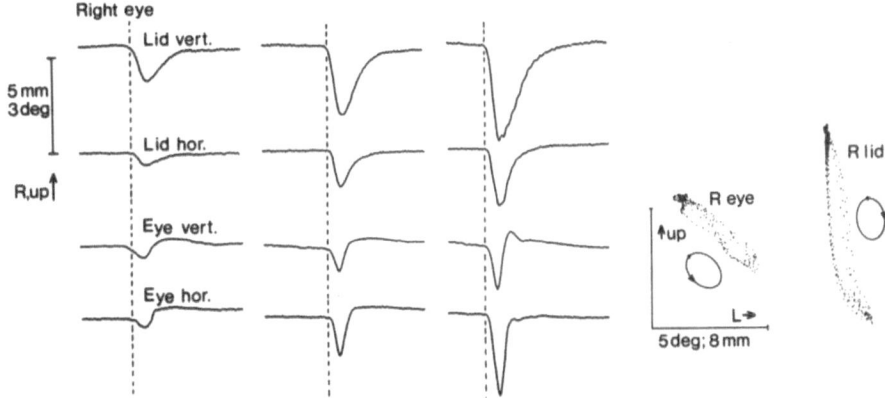

Figure 10. Vertical and horizontal lid and eye positions as a function of time, for blinks of different size (left 3 panels) and two-dimensional trajectories of upper lid and eye during 3 successive large blinks (right 2 panels). Ellipses and arrows show the direction in which the trajectory was followed. Recordings from right eye and lid; trajectories shown as seen by observer facing the subject (adapted from Collewijn, van der Steen and Steinman [37]).

temporal gyrus cause deficits in smooth pursuit. Area 7 projects heavily to the FEF and to the pontine nuclei. The latter connection may be significant, as the pontine nuclei in turn project to the cerebellar flocculus, a structure which appears to be crucial to smooth pursuit. Floccular lesions induce profound, permanent defects of smooth pursuit in monkey and man.

Some Purkinje cells in the flocculus of the monkey seem to encode the direction of gaze in space. During smooth pursuit with the head stationary they encode eye velocity; during fixation of a stationary target while the head moves their activity remains unchanged. Possibly these cells summate vestibular signals (with eye velocity signals into gaze velocity signals [35, 36]. Further summation with retinal slip could lead to representation of target motion in space.

8. Eye movements during blinks

With the search coil it is also possible to measure reliably the eye movements associated with lid closure [37]. These eye movements proved to be consistently down and nasalward during voluntary and reflex blinks (Fig. 10) and had amplitudes of 1–5 deg. These motions can not be recorded with the EOG due to very large lid movement artifacts. Prolonged, voluntary lid closure was followed by a slow, tonic ocular deviation; in contrast to classical notions this was consistently upward in only half of the subjects. Tonic downward deviation occurred in the other half. However, a tendency was observed for this downward deviation to be converted in an upward deviation when the closure of the lids was mechanically impeded. Thus, any interference with lid movement during attempted closure may provoke the classical ocular elevation as described by Bell.

References

1. Koornneef L (1977): New insights in the human orbital connective tissue. Arch Ophthal 95: 1269–1273.
2. Koornneef L (1977): Spatial aspects of orbital musculo-fibrous tissue in man. Thesis, University of Amsterdam.
3. Evinger C, Shaw MD, Peck CK, Manning KA and Baker R (1984): Blinking and the associated eye movements in humans, guinea pigs and rabbits. J Neurophysiol 52: 323–339.
4. Enright JT (1984): Saccadic anomalies: vergence induces large departures from ball-and-socket behavior. Vision Res 24: 301–308.
5. Simonsz HJ (1984): Investigations of ocular counterrolling and Bielschowsky head-tilt test, stiffness in passive ocular rolling and displacement of recti eye muscles. Thesis, University of Amsterdam.
6. Robinson DA (1978): The functional behavior of the peripheral oculomotor apparatus: a review. In: G Kommerell (ed) Disorders of ocular motility. Bergmann Verlag, München, pp 43–61.
7. Lennerstrand G (1981): Postnatal development of eye muscle function. In: G Lennerstrand, DS Zee, EL Keller (eds) Functional basis of ocular motility disorders. Pergamon Press, Oxford, pp 39–47.
8. Collins CC (1975): The human oculomotor control system. In: G Lennerstrand and P Bach-y-Rita (eds) Basic mechanisms of ocular motility and their clinical implications. Pergamon Press, Oxford, pp 145–180.
9. Henn V, Büttner-Ennever JA, Hepp K (1982): The primate oculomotor system. I. Motor neurons. Human Neurobiol 1: 77–85.
10. Henn V, Hepp K, Büttner-Ennever JA (1982): The primate oculomotor system. II. Premotor system. Human Neurobiol 1: 87–95.
11. Büttner-Ennever JA, Büttner U, Cohen B, Baumgartner G (1982): Vertical gaze paralysis and the rostral interstitial nucleus of the medial longitudinal fasciculus (rostral iMLF). Brain 105: 125–149.
12. Cheron G, Godaux E, Laune JM, Vanderkelen B (1986): Lesions in the cat prepositus complex: effects on the vestibulo-ocular reflex and saccades. J Physiol (London) 372: 75–94.
13. Cheron G, Gillis P, Godaux E (1986): Lesions in the cat prepositus complex: effects on the optokinetic system. J Physiol (London) 372: 95–111.
14. Schiller PH, True SD, Conway JL (1979). Effects of frontal eye field and superior colliculus ablations on eye movements. Science 206: 590–592.
15. Wurtz RH, Albano JE (1980): Visual-motor function of the primate superior colliculus. Ann Rev Neurosci 3: 189–226.
16. Bruce CJ, Goldberg ME (1985): Primate frontal eye fields. I. Single neurons discharging before saccades. J Neurophysiol 53: 603–635.
17. Bruce CJ, Goldberg ME, Bushnell MC, Stanton GB (1985): Primate frontal eye fields. II. Physiological and anatomical correlates of electrically evoked eye movements. J Neurophysiol 54: 714–734.
18. Guitton D, Buchtel HA, Douglas RM (1982). Disturbances of voluntary saccadic eye movement mechanisms following discrete unilateral frontal lobe removals. In: G Lennerstrand, DS Zee, EL Keller (eds) Functional basis of ocular motility disorders. Pergamon Press, Oxford. pp 497–499.
19. Leigh RJ, Zee DS (1983): The neurology of eye movement. Davis, Philadelphia.
20. Holstege G, Collewijn H (1982): The efferent connections of the nucleus of the optic tract and the

superior colliculus in the rabbit. J Comp Neurol 209: 139–175.

21. Hoffmann KP, Distler C (1986): The role of direction selective cells in the nucleus of the optic tract of cat and monkey during optokinetic nystagmus. In: EL Keller and DS Zee (eds) Adaptive processes in visual and oculomotor systems. Pergamon Press, Oxford.

22. Collewijn H, Van der Mark F, Jansen TC (1975): Precise recordings of human eye movements. Vision Res 15: 447–450.

23. van Die GC (1983): Stimulus respons relaties van de optokinetische nystagmus van de mens. Thesis, Erasmus University Rotterdam.

24. van Die GC, Collewijn H (1982): Optokinetic nystagmus in man. Human Neurobiol 1: 111–119.

25. Collewijn H, Martins AJ, Steinman RM (1983): Compensatory eye movements during active and passive head movements: fast adaptation to changes in visual magnification. J Physiol 340: 259–286.

26. Barr CC, Schultheis LW, Robinson DA (1976): Voluntary, non-visual control of the human vestibulo-ocular reflex. Acta Otolaryngol 81: 365–375.

27. Collewijn H, van der Steen J, Ferman L, Jansen TC (1985): Human ocular counterroll: assessment of static and dynamic properties from electromagnetic scleral coil recordings. Exp Brain Res 59: 185–196.

28. Collewijn H, Tamminga EP (1984): Human smooth and saccadic eye movements during voluntary pursuit of different target motions on different backgrounds. J Physiol 351: 217–250.

29. Kowler E, Van der Steen J, Tamminga EP, Collewijn H (1984): Voluntary selection of the target for smooth eye movement in the presence of superimposed, full-field stationary and moving stimuli. Vision Res 24: 1789–1798.

30. van der Steen J, Tamminga EP, Collewijn H (1983): A comparison of oculomotor pursuit of a target in circular, real, beta or sigma motion. Vision Res 23: 1655–1661.

31. Kowler E, Steinman RM (1979): The effect of expectations on slow oculomotor control-I. Periodic target steps. Vision Res 19: 619–632.

32. Kowler E, Steinman RM (1979): The effect of expectations on slow oculomotor control-II. Single target displacements. Vision Res 19: 633–646.

33. Becker W, Fuchs AF (1985): Prediction in the oculomotor system: smooth pursuit during transient disappearance of a visual target. Exp Brain Res 57: 562–575.

34. Collewijn H, Steinman RM, van der Steen J (1985): The performance of the smooth pursuit eye movements system during passive and self-generated stimulus motion. J Physiol (Lond.) 366, 19P.

35. Lisberger SC, Fuchs AF (1978): Role of primate flocculus during rapid behavioural modification of vestibulo-ocular reflex. I. Purkinje cell activity during visually guided horizontal smooth pursuit eye movements and passive head rotation. J Neurophysiol 41: 733–763.

36. Lisberger SG, Fuchs AF (1978): Role of primate flocculus during rapid behavioural modification of vestibulo-ocular reflex. II. Mossy fiber firing patterns during horizontal head rotation and eye movement. J Neurophysiol 41: 764–777.

37. Collewijn H, Van der Steen J, Steinman RM (1985): Human eye movements associated with blinks and prolonged eyelid closure. J Neurophysiol 54: 11–27.

Pathophysiology of horizontal and vertical eye movement disorders

U. BÜTTNER and J.A. BÜTTNER-ENNEVER

Analysis of the oculomotor system has shown, that five different types of eye movements can be clearly distinguished: saccades, the vestibulo-ocular reflex (VOR), smooth pursuit eye movements, optokinetic nystagmus (OKN) and convergence movements.

Each type of eye movement is generated by different premotor structures, which are to a large extent anatomically separate. It is only at the extra-ocular motor neurons, that the signals from these various premotor circuits converge and form a final common pathway. Thus the precise knowledge of the anatomy and the function of these premotor structures often makes it possible to exactly localize lesions which are causing specific oculomotor deficits. The main premotor areas of the oculomotor system lie in the brainstem and the cerebellum. Since the anatomy and the eye movements are similar in man and monkey, most experimental studies have been performed in these animals.

Up to now the premotor structures for *saccade* generation in the brainstem have been most extensively studied with regard to functional properties, anatomical pathways and correlation with clinical and experimental findings. The following chapter will summarize some of these results. It should be kept in mind that saccade generation in the brain is under the influence of cortical areas [1, 2], superior colliculus [3] and cerebellar structures [4].

1. Saccades

Saccades are fast conjugate eye movements, which occur spontaneously or voluntarily to (stationary) visual targets. Basically the fast phases of vestibular and optokinetic nystagmus are also saccades and utilize saccadic premotor pathways in the brainstem.

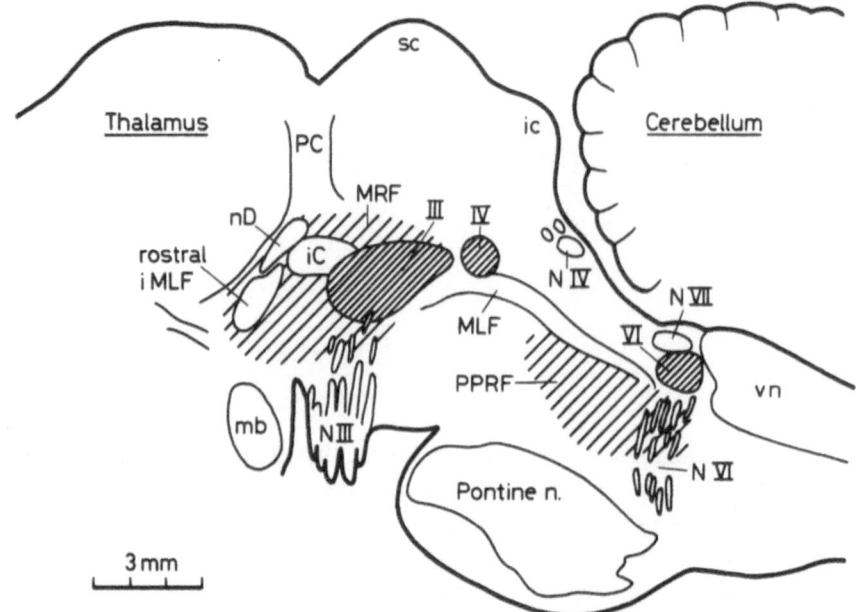

Figure 1. Parasagittal view of the brainstem (Rhesus monkey). The paramedian pontine reticular formation (PPRF) is the immediate premotor structure for horizontal saccades; the mesencephalic reticular formation (MRF) contains nuclei for the generation of vertical saccades. Abbreviations: ic – inferior colliculus; iC – interstitial nucleus of Cajal; mb – mamillary body; MLF – medial longitudinal fasciculus; N III – oculomotor nerve; N IV – trochlear nerve; N VI – abducens nerve; N VII – facial nerve, nD – nucleus Darkschewitsch, PC – posterior commissure; sc – superior colliculus; vn – vestibular nuclei; III – oculomotor nucleus, IV – trochlear nucleus, VI – abducens nucleus.

2. The paramedian pontine reticular formation (PPRF)

The immediate premotor structure for saccades in the horizontal plane lies in the paramedian zone of the pontine reticular formation rostrally and ventrally to the abducens nucleus (VI) (Fig. 1). Lesions here lead to a horizontal gaze palsy with the following main features: 1.) No saccades or fast phases of nystagmus can be elicited to the ipsilateral side, even when the eyes are in the contralateral hemifield. 2.) During the VOR the eyes can be driven across the midline into the ipsilateral hemifield. 3.) At rest the eyes can be held in midposition [5, 6].

Electrical stimulation in the PPRF evokes saccades to the ipsilateral side [7]. Single unit recordings in alert behaving monkeys have distinguished several types of neurons related to saccades [8] (Fig. 2). *Long-lead burst neurons* start to increase their activity up to 150 msec before saccade-onset. *Short-lead burst neurons* have latencies of 6–15 msec before saccade-onset. For most burst neurons the 'preferred' direction for activity increase is horizontal and ipsilateral. However, also burst neurons with a contralateral and a vertical preferred direction

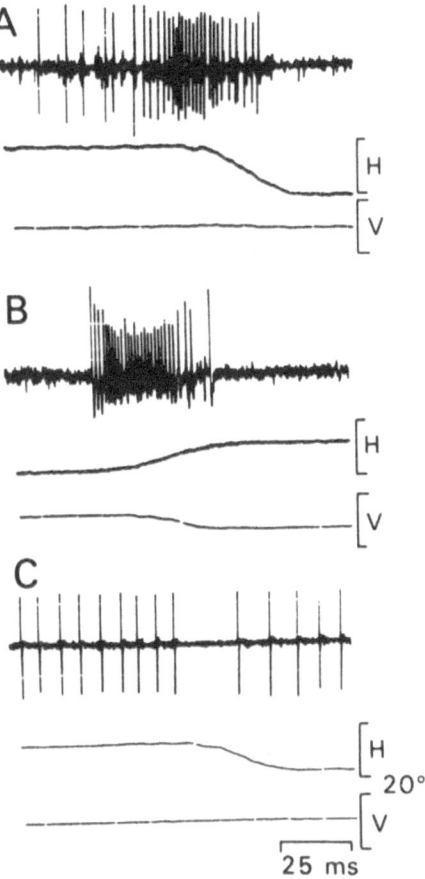

Figure 2. Different types of premotor neurons involved in the generation of saccades. A: long-lead burst neuron; B: short-lead burst neuron; C: pause neuron. Beside neuronal activity horizontal (H) and vertical (V) eye position are shown [25].

have been found [9]. Burst neurons only encode parameters (size and direction) of saccades or fast phases of nystagmus; their activity shows no relation to slow conjugate eye movements. It is assumed that long lead burst neurons provide an input to short lead burst neurons. *Pause neurons* have a high, constant firing rate, which only is interrupted shortly before and during saccades. One type of these are *omnipause neurons* which pause with all saccades and lie in a cluster along the midline below the abducens nucleus (Fig. 3). They lie within the recently outlined nucleus raphe interpositus (rip) [10]. Omnipause neurons are considered to provide a trigger or gating function in the generation of saccades.

The premotor signals from the PPRF eventually activate the abducens motor neurons on the same side and the medial rectus motor neurons on the con-tralateral side. It is now established, that there is *no* direct anatomical connection

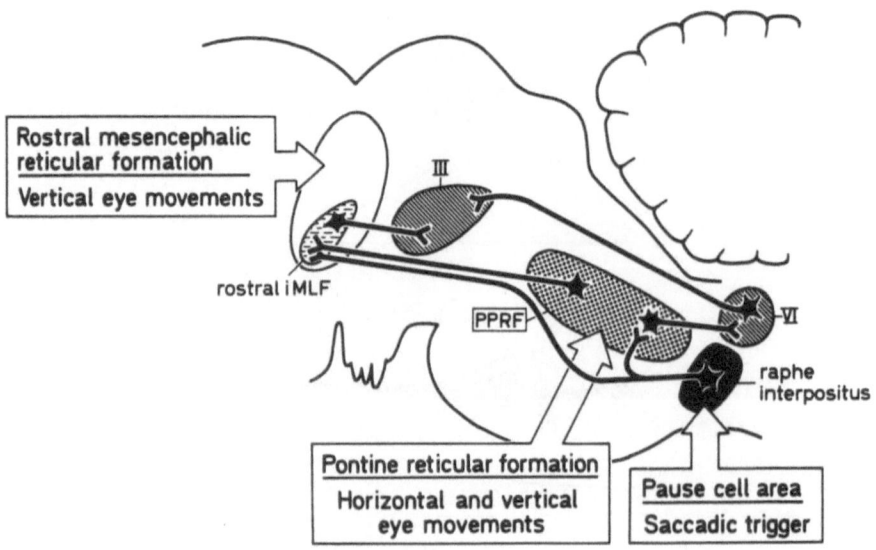

Figure 3. Summary diagram of major pathways involved in horizontal and vertical saccade generation.

between the PPRF and the contralateral medial rectus division of the oculomotor nucleus. Thus, all information for ipsilateral horizontal saccades is first transferred from PPRF to the ipsilateral abducens nucleus.

3. Abducens nucleus

The abducens nucleus not only contains motor neurons, whose axons innervate the lateral rectus muscle, but about 40% of the neurons within the abducens nucleus are so called 'internuclear neurons'. They are intermingled with the motor neurons [11]. Their axons cross the midline at the abducens level and ascend within the contralateral MLF to the medial rectus division of III. Single unit recordings in alert monkeys demonstrate a burst-tonic activity pattern, which can be related to the saccade (burst) and the eye position (tonic). The activity pattern of the 'internuclear neurons' is similar to that of the motor neurons [12]. Thus, the information for horizontal saccades reaches the oculomotor nucleus via the abducens nucleus.

Accordingly a lesion of the abducens *nucleus* leads to a horizontal gaze palsy to the ipsilateral side, and can be clearly distinguished from the monocular deficit after an abducens *nerve* lesion. With an abducens nucleus lesion, in contrast to a PPRF lesion, the eyes cannot be driven into the ipsilateral hemifield during the VOR. This reflects that all saccadic as well as vestibular premotor signals are integrated at the abducens nuclear level.

4. Mesencephalic Reticular Formation (MRF)

A vertical gaze paralysis, that is absence of vertical saccades, can be either upward, downward or combined up- and downward. It indicates a lesion in the mesencephalic reticular formation (MRF), which lies immediately rostral to the oculomotor nucleus. For all vertical eye movement deficits the lesion has to be bilateral or at the midline [13]. Anatomically the MRF is an illdefined structure. It is bordered medially by the nucleus interstitialis of Cajal (iC) and nucleus Dark-schewitsch (nD); dorsally by the nuclei of the posterior commissure (npc) and the posterior commissure. Recently an additional structure within the rostral MRF related to vertical saccades was delineated in monkey [14] and man [15] and was named rostral interstitial nucleus of the medial longitudinal fasciculus (rostral iMLF).

5. Rostral interstitial nucleus of the MLF (rostral iMLF)

The cells of *rostral iMLF* lie within the most rostral extension of the MLF immediately rostral to iC. The border between rostral iMLF and iC is roughly at the level where tractus retroflexus passes through the region. The rostral iMLF is situated as a wingshaped structure dorsomedial to the red nucleus (Fig. 4). A useful landmark is the posterior thalamo-subthalamic artery at the dorsal border of rostral iMLF.

The following findings support the assumption that rostral iMLF is an immediate premotor structure in the generation of vertical saccades.

1. Anatomy. Rostral iMLF receives a strong input from the PPRF on the same side. This includes a definite projection from the nucleus raphe interpositus, the area containing 'omnipause' neurons [10]. The fibers from the PPRF ascend close to, but outside, the fascicles of MLF. In turn the rostral iMLF projects directly to the vertical motoneuron divisions of the oculomotor nucleus and the trochlear nucleus on the *same side* as shown in Figs. 5 and 6 [16].

2. Physiology. Neurons in the rostral iMLF encode parameters of either up- or downward saccades [17]. Neurons with a preferred up- or downward direction for activity changes are found intermingled with each other. The neurons are generally short-lead burst neurons (Fig. 2). No long-lead burst or pause neurons and also no neurons which encode parameters of horizontal saccades have been encountered there.

42

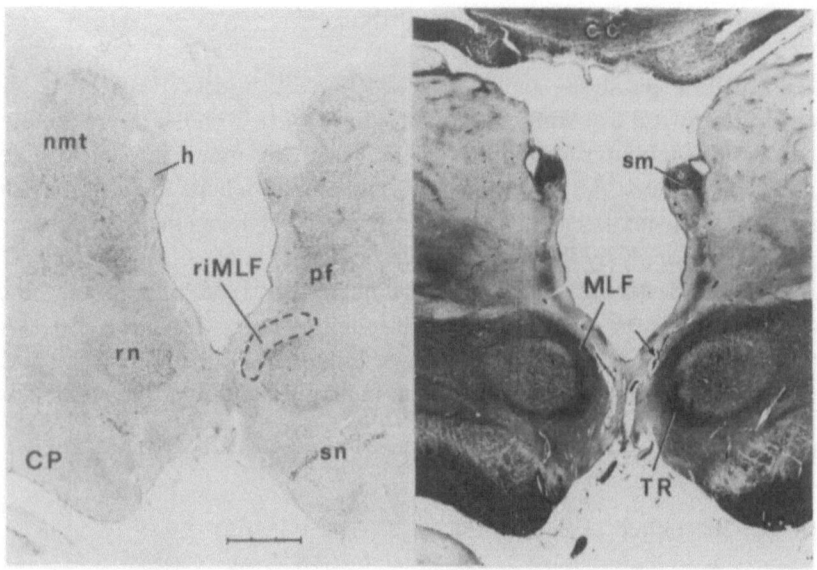

Figure 4. Transverse sections of the human mesencephalon stained with cresyl violet (left) and Weigert myelin stain (right) to demonstrate the location of rostral iMLF dorsomedially to the red nucleus (rn). The arrow at the right side points at the posterior thalamo-subthalamic paramedian artery. Abbreviations: CC: corpus callosum; CP: cerebral peduncle; h: habenular complex; MLF: medial longitudinal fasciculus; nmt: nucleus medialis thalami; pf: parafascicular nucleus; sm: stria medullaris; sn: substantia nigra; TR: tractus retroflexus.

6. Functional comparison of rostral iMLF, iC and nD

In the earlier literature iC and nD were considered as main structures in eye movement control. With the new knowledge about rostral iMLF and its connections a critical reevaluation about the function of iC and nD is mandatory.

There is no evidence for a premotor role of *nD* in eye movement control. There are no connections with the PPRF, the vestibular or the oculomotor nuclei. It is known to receive a projection from the limb region of the premotor cortex [18] and projects to the inferior olive [19]. However, *fibers* from the adjacent rostral iMLF and iC to the oculomotor nucleus pass close to and around nD. This provides an explanation why nD is often involved in lesions causing a vertical gaze paralysis.

However, iC is definitely involved in eye movement control, although the precise function has yet to be determined. In contrast to rostral iMLF, iC does not receive an input from PPRF. The vestibular nuclei have a strong projection to iC compared to the weak projection to the caudomedial division of rostral iMLF. The course of the efferents differs for rostral iMLF and iC. Rostral iMLF projects ipsilaterally to iC and the oculomotor (III) and trochlear (IV) nucleus (Fig. 5).

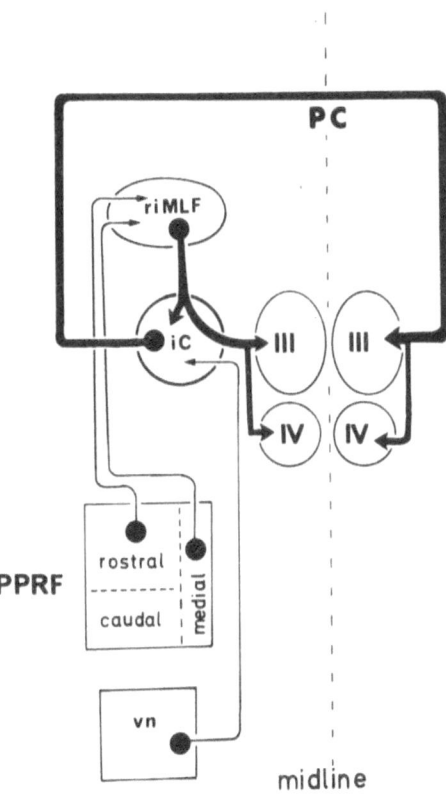

Figure 5. Comparison of some afferent and efferent connections of iC and riMLF. Whereas riMLF receives its main input from PPRF, the vestibular nuclei are a major input to iC, riMLF projects mainly to iC and the vertical motoneurons on the *ipsilateral* side and iC via the posterior commissure (PC) to the *contralateral* vertical motor neurons.

Recently, it could be shown with intracellular staining and autoradiographic tract tracing methods that rostral iMLF neurons give rise to collaterals to the ipsilateral iC as well as the oculomotor nucleus (Büttner-Ennever, Highstein, Holstege, unpublished results). The vertical motor neurons contacted by rostral iMLF move both eyes in one plane (Fig. 6). These are the inferior oblique and the inferior rectus muscle for the ipsilateral eye and the superior rectus and superior oblique muscle of the contralateral eye. The motor neurons for all 4 muscles are localized on one side of the brainstem, iC projects contralaterally via the posterior commissure (PC) to the oculomotor and trochlear nucleus.

Thus, iC receives a major input from the vestibular nuclei and rostral iMLF and projects to the contralateral oculomotor nucleus. This strategic location would allow iC to play a major role in coordinating the vertical premotor oculomotor signals. Both nuclei have descending axons running in MLF, which supply among other structures the vestibular nuclei and spinal cord.

ri MLF

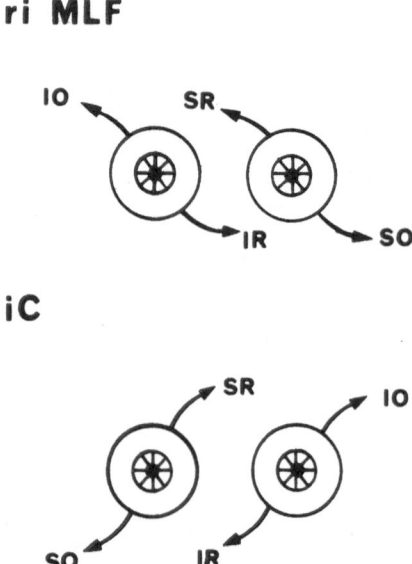

iC

Figure 6. riMLF and iC innervate motor neurons, whose pulling direction is in one 'off-vertical' plane. The innervation pattern for the left riMLF and left iC is shown. Together they have access to all vertical eye muscle motor neurons.

7. Lesions causing a vertical gaze paralysis

In the monkey bilateral lesions of rostral iMLF cause an isolated downward gaze paralysis [20]. Clinically the rostral iMLF is involved bilaterally in all patients with either a downward gaze paralysis, or a combined up- and downward gaze paralysis [15]. As discussed above, the involvement of nD probably reflects the damage of passing fibers and not a genuine involvement of nD in eye movement control. The difference between lesions causing a downward gaze paralysis or a combined up- and downward gaze paralysis, is not yet clear. It is, however, remarkable that all cases with a downward gaze paralysis are usually the result of two separate lesions, one on each side [15, 21]. Whereas an up- and downward gaze paralysis can be caused by a single lesion extending on both sides of the midline. This might also provide an explanation for the fact that an isolated downward gaze paralysis is clinically a very rare event compared to the much more common combined up- and downward gaze paralysis.

An isolated upward gaze paralysis can be produced by lesions of the posterior commissure, npc or in the mesencephalic reticular formation caudal to rostral iMLF.

8. The coordination of horizontal and vertical saccades

Since most saccades are not purely horizontal or vertical, but rather oblique, the two components have to be coordinated. All evidence suggests that the PPRF plays a major role in this coordinating process. The PPRF contains neuronal elements which not only encode parameters of horizontal but also of vertical saccades. Furthermore long-lead burst and pause neurons are only found in the PPRF. It could be shown that electrical stimulation in the omnipause area, the nucleus raphe interpositus, not only interrupts the horizontal but also the vertical component of saccades [22]. It was described that this pontine area projects to the rostral iMLF [14, 23]. That the PPRF is not only a premotor structure for horizontal but for all saccades is further demonstrated by lesion studies. Bilateral lesions of the PPRF can lead to a gaze paralysis in all directions, if the lesions are in the caudal PPRF. In the rostral PPRF bilateral lesions cause a complete horizontal gaze paralysis but preserve vertical saccades [24].

Acknowledgements

Supported by Deutsche Forschungsgemeinschaft SFB 220 D7, D8. The authors are grateful to B. Liebold and B. Pfreundner for typing the manuscript.

References

1. Bruce ChJ, Goldberg ME (1985): Primate frontal eye fields. I Single neurons discharging before saccades. J Neurophysiol 53: 603–635.
2. Schiller PH, Sandell JH (1983): Interactions between visually and electrically elicited saccades before and after superior colliculus and frontal eye field ablations in the rhesus monkey. Exp Brain Res 49: 381–392.
3. Raybourn MS, Keller EL (1977): Colliculoreticular organization in primate oculomotor system. J Neurophysiol 40: 861–878.
4. Hepp K, Henn V, Jaeger J (1982): Eye movement related neurons in the cerebellar nuclei of the altert monkey. Exp Brain Res 45: 253–261.
5. Bender MB, Shanzer S (1964): Oculomotor pathways defined by electrical stimulation and lesions in the brainstem of monkeys. In: MB Bender (Ed), The Oculomotor System, Harper and Row, New York, pp: 81–140.
6. Henn V, Büttner U (1982): Disorders of horizontal gaze. In: Functional Basis of Oculomotor Motility Disorders. Eds: G Lennerstrand, D Zee, E Keller. Oxford, Pergamon Press, 431–439.
7. Cohen B, Komatsuzaki A (1972): Eye movements induced by stimulation of the pontine reticular formation: evidence for integration in oculomotor pathways. Exp Neurol 36: 101–117.
8. Fuchs AF, Kaneko CRS, Scudder CA (1985): Brainstem control of saccadic eye movements. Ann Rev Neurosci 8: 307–337.
9. Luschei ES, Fuchs AF (1972): Activity of brain stem neurons during eye movements of alert monkey. J Neurophysiol 35: 445–461.
10. Büttner-Ennever JA, Pause M (1985): Neuroanatomic identification of a raphe nucleus in the

pons associated with omnipause neurons of the oculomotor system in the monkey. Soc Neurosci Abstr 11: 1042.

11. Steiger HJ, Büttner-Ennever JA (1978): Relationship between motor neurons and internuclear neurons in the abducens nucleus: A double retrograde tracer study in the cat. Brain Res 148: 181–188.

12. McCrea RA, Strassman A, Highstein SM (1986): Morphology and physiology of abducens motor neurons and internuclear neurons intracellularly injected with horseradish peroxidase in alert squirrel monkeys. J Comp Neurol 243: 291–308.

13. Bender MB (1980): Brain control of conjugate horizontal and vertical eye movements. A survey of the structural and functional correlates. Brain 103: 23–69.

14. Büttner-Ennever JA, Büttner U (1978): A cell group associated with vertical eye movements in the rostral mesencephalic reticular formation of the monkey. Brain Res 151: 31–47.

15. Büttner-Ennever JA, Büttner U, Cohen B, Baumgartner G (1982): Vertical gaze paralysis and the rostral interstitial nucleus of the medial longitudinal fasciculus. Brain 105: 125–149.

16. Nakao Sh, Shiraishi Y (1983): Direct projection of cat mesodiencephalic neurons to the inferior rectus subdivision of the oculomotor nucleus. Neurosc Lett 39: 243–248.

17. Büttner U, Büttner-Ennever JA, Henn V (1977): Vertical eye movement related activity in the rostral mesencephalic reticular formation of the alert monkey. Brain Res 130: 239–252.

18. Hartman-v. Monakow K, Akert K, Künzle H (1979): Projections of precentral and premotor cortex to the red nucleus and other midbrain areas in Macaca fascicularis. Exp Brain Res 23: 91–105.

19. Bürgi SM (1952): Some observations on the fiber connections of the di- and mesencephalon in the cat. II. Fiber connections of the pretectal region and the posterior commissure. J Comp Neurol 96: 139–177.

20. Kömpf D, Pasik T, Pasik P, Bender MB (1979): Downward gaze in monkeys. Stimulation and lesion studies. Brain 102: 527–558.

21. Pierrot-Deseilligny Ch, Chain F, Gray F, Serdaru M, Escourrolle R, Lhermitte F (1982): Parinaud's syndrome. Electrooculographic and anatomical analyses of six vascular cases with deductions about vertical gaze organization in the premotor structures. Brain 105: 667–696.

22. King WM, Fuchs AF (1977): Neuronal activity in the mesencephalon related to vertical eye movements. In: Control of Gaze by Brain Stem Neurons, Developments in Neuroscience, 1, Eds: Baker R, Berthoz A: 319–326. New York: Elsevier/North Holland.

23. Langer T, Kaneko CRS (1983): Efferent projections of the cat oculomotor reticular omnipause neuron region: an autoradiographic study. J Comp Neurol 217: 288–306.

24. Henn V, Lang W, Hepp K, Reisine H (1984): Experimental gaze palsies in monkeys and their relation to human pathology. Brain 107: 619–636.

25. Henn V, Hepp K, Büttner-Ennever JA (1982): The primate oculomotor system. II. Premotor system. Human Neurobiol 1: 87–95.

Section II

Clinical and paraclinical examination

Bedside examination

A.G.M. VAN VLIET

1. Definitions of types of eye movement

There are two principal types of eye movement: those that bring images to the fovea, and those which hold images steady on the retina.

Simultaneous eye movement in the same direction is called conjugate and in opposite direction disjunctive. When moving between two points, eyes usually move conjugately, provided the two points do not lie on a line bisecting the angle formed by visual axes (bisector). Pure disjunctive movement occurs along this bisector. In the horizontal plane, terms used are convergence and divergence.

On the basis of differences in velocity, fast (saccades) and slow eye movement is distinguished. The latter includes pursuit, vestibular and optokinetic systems. Vergence eye movement is characteristically slow.

Table 1 represents a summary of the main functional classes of eye movement, in usual order of examination.

2. Examination of eye movements

Examination of eye movement can be subdivided as follows: 1. general impression; 2. eye position and spontaneous movement; 3. voluntary eye movement; 4.

Table 1. Functional classes of eye-movement.

Class of eye movements	Main function
Saccade	brings images onto the fovea; these are referred to as 'voluntary movements'
Smooth pursuit	holds an image on the fovea
Optokinetic-vestibular	holds images steady on the retina during brief (vestibular) or sustained (optokinetic) head rotation
Vergence	brings images of a single object onto both foveae

pursuit eye movement; 5. optokinetic nystagmus; 6. eye movement upon passive head movement; 7. caloric testing; 8. (con)vergence; 9. tests for diplopia and strabismus.

2.1. General impression

General impression describes the disability examing a patient. Important features are head-tilt and/or nodding or thrusting movement of the head. Altered head position may indicate an oculomotor dysfunction e.g. in patients with squint. Head thrust to the side replaces saccades in oculomotor apraxia. Patients with latter condition are unable to make horizontal saccades. A diminished palpebral fissure may point to ptosis; if otherwise larger than usual, this may be indicative for proptosis or lid retraction.

Conjugate deviation of eyes, any obvious lack of parallelism between visual axes and gross nystagmus on direct forward gaze, often congenital, gives a general indication of the disorder.

2.2. Eye position and spontaneous movement

The first step in examining eye movement is to inspect eye position at rest, and in relation to the head position (deviation to one side?) or to each other (squint? skew deviation?). Eyes (and sometimes the head) persistently deviating to one side is the result of a destructive lesion ipsilateral or an irritative focus (epileptic) contralateral to the deviation. Such a supranuclear disorder of eye movement is called a gaze palsy. Although there may be no rest deviation of eyes, spastic paresis of gaze can be demonstrated in a patient with a destructive lesion only if he is sufficiently alert to close eyes voluntarily. Passive opening of the forcibly closed eyes may demonstrate lateral (and upward) deviation of eyes in a direction away from the side of the lesion.

Examination of squint will be done in tests for diplopia and strabismus.

Any regular (or irregular) rhythmic eye movement (nystagmus and other oscillations) should be described. Interpretation of nystagmus will be further discussed in chapter 15.

2.3. Voluntary eye movement

Voluntary eye movement is examined by instructing the patient to look in *nine* positions of gaze. This results in 'command movements'. Saccades are examined without offering a fixation point, and then with a target. The examiner observes whether eye movement is conjugate or dissociate or no movement at all. Lesions

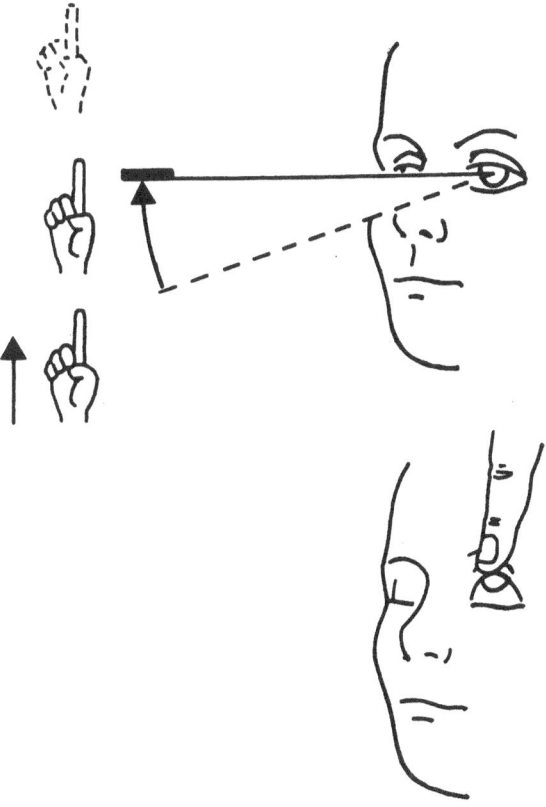

Figure 1. Bell's phenomenon in supranuclear palsy.

of the medial longitudinal fasciculus (MLF) disturb synchrony of eye movement. The complete MLF syndrome includes paralysis of the medial rectus in the adducting eye and causes horizontal nystagmus of the abducting eye. Subtle forms will demonstrate unequal movement of eyes; i.e. sluggish movement of the adducting eye and (sometimes) overshoot of the abducting eye (chapter 18).

If paralysis of upward gaze exists, it is important to determine, with the Bell's phenomenon (test), whether there is a supranuclear or infranuclear palsy. Bell's phenomenon is an upward rolling of the eyeballs via a subcortical reflex on closing eyes. This can be observed when attempts are made to close eyelids against resistance. In patients who cannot elevate eyes on command, presence of a Bell's phenomenon indicates that upward gaze palsy is due to a supranuclear lesion (Fig. 1).

2.4. Pursuit eye movement

While examining pursuit eye movement the patient is asked to fixate the examiner's thumb moving in front (at a distance of about one meter, in horizontal or vertical plane, over an angle of excursion of about 60° with a frequency of 0.3 Hz).

2.5. Optokinetic nystagmus

Eliciting optokinetic nystagmus, the patient is asked to look at ordinary tape measure, which the examiner moves in front horizontally and then vertically. A better stimulus is the presentation of a series of pictures, fitted to a rotating drum. The normal response consists of a regular nystagmus: slow pursuit movement interrupted by quick phases in opposite direction. Optokinetic nystagmus is disturbed in deep hemispheric lesions, congenital nystagmus and internuclear ophthalmoplegia. In the latter, optokinetic nystagmus testing demonstrates sluggish movement of the medial rectus.

2.6. Eye movement in passive head movement

If eye movement is found to be paralysed both on command and on testing pursuit eye movement, it is important to determine, by means of reaction to passive head movement, whether there is a supra- or infranuclear palsy. The patient is asked to fixe a stable object and his head is passively turned in the plane of gaze paralysis. Normally, a rapid passive head rotation elicits an initial contraverse deviation of eyes (oculocephalic reflex or doll's head manoeuvre) followed by a prompt recentering (Fig. 2). At a high frequency, this reaction is almost exclusively a vestibulo-ocular reflex. The doll's head manoeuvre only tests pursuit systems at a low frequency. In pursuit palsy, a normal response to doll's head manoeuvre indicates that brainstem pathways in the caudal part of pons and third nerve nuclear complex are unimpaired. This does not occur in nuclear or infranuclear paralysis.

The doll's head manoeuvre is of great help in comatose patients. It is elicited by holding the eyelids open and rapidly rotate the head to one side and then to the other. If eyes are observed to move conjugately opposite to head movement, the reflex is intact (Fig. 3).

In non-comatose patients, oculo-cephalic reflex can be examined by using Frenzel glasses positive lenses of 20 diopters with a small light at each external canthus. In this way, visual fixation is abolished and the nystagmus during the doll's head manoeuvre is not suppressed. The doll's head manoeuvre may be a useful test in relation to the cerebellar function in the non comatose patient. The vestibulo-ocular reflex is inhibited by fixation of an object that moves together

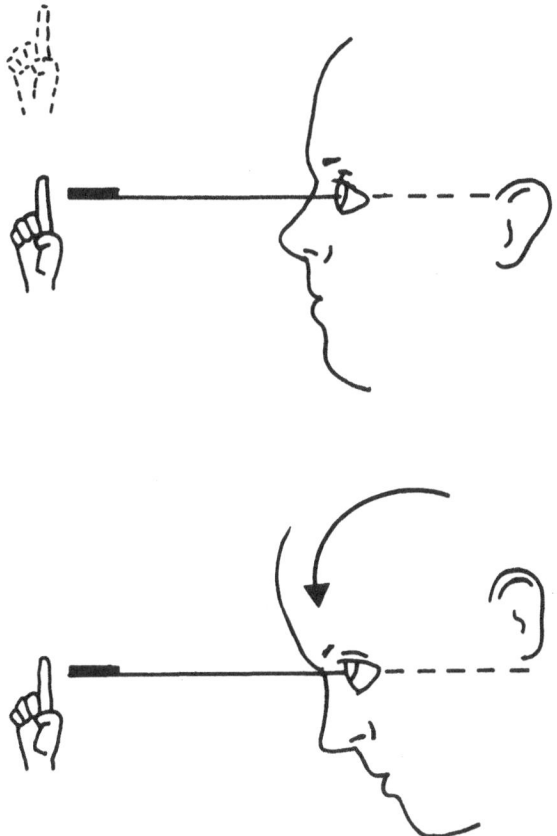

Figure 2. Oculocephalic reflex.

with the head; i.e. a spatula set between the teeth. The patient is asked to fixate a point at the end of the spatula. This suppression is effective up to 1 Hz. At higher frequency the vestibulo-ocular reflex breaks through and eyes deviate with interrupting saccades. The ability to cancel or suppress the vestibulo-ocular reflex using visual fixation is a function of pursuit system; impairment of fixation suppression is usually accompanied by a deficit of smooth pursuit eye movement. In patients with cerebellar disorders, suppression may be disturbed or absent and corrective saccades will already be present at a lower frequency of oscillation (Fig. 3).

2.7. Caloric testing

Ice-water caloric responses should be carried out in patients who have no eye movement, tested for doll's head manoeuvre, or in situations in which rapid head

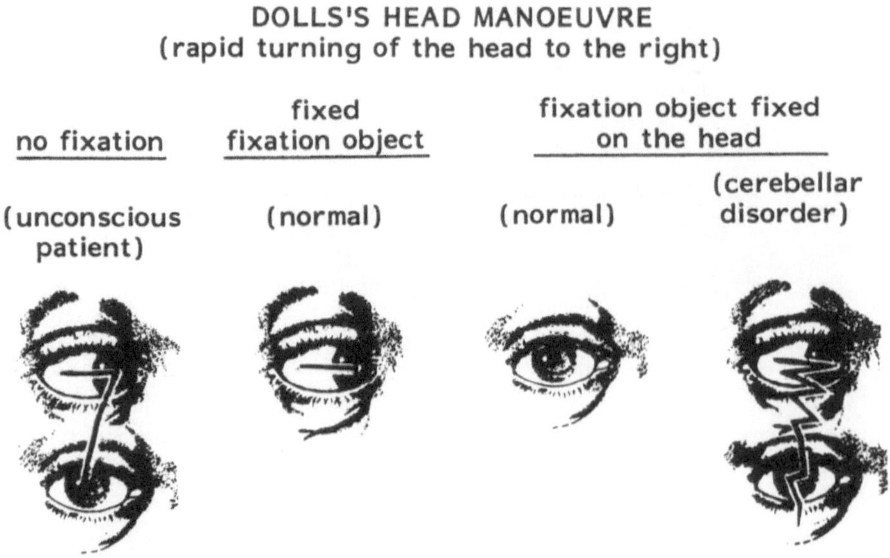

DOLLS'S HEAD MANOEUVRE
(rapid turning of the head to the right)

no fixation	fixed fixation object	fixation object fixed on the head	
(unconscious patient)	(normal)	(normal)	(cerebellar disorder)

Figure 3. (From Leigh & Zee, The Neurology of Eye Movement).

movement is inadvisable. At bedside, 10 ml to 20 ml of ice water is flushed into the ear canal with the head tilted 30° above the horizontal plane. Pontine oculogyric pathways are intact if a slow eye movement towards the side of ice water infusion occurs. If this is disjunctive or absent, a brainstem lesion is suspected.

2.8. Convergence

The near reflex (convergence) is linked neurophysiologically with accommodation and pupillary constriction and is tested by asking the patient to look at his own finger as it moves towards his nose. Convergence paralysis as a component of various neurological syndromes can be distinguished from functional convergence weakness by the associated constriction of the pupil, which accompanies efforts of convergence in case of an organic disorder.

2.9. Tests for diplopia and strabismus

The primary eye position is that while looking straight ahead. Eye position in adduction, abduction, elevation or depression is called secondary position, and that after combined horizontal and vertical movement; tertiary position. If there is a misalignment or deviation of the visual axis, strabismus or heterotropia exists. Strabismus is latent if abnormal position becomes apparent only after disruption of fusion. If latent condition is referred to suffix '-tropia' is replaced by '-phoria', e.g. heterophoria. In concomitant strabismus, the angle of squint remains constant in various positions of gaze, which occurs not in non-concomitant strabismus.

Double vision reflects ocular misalignment and usually indicates an infranuclear disorder of eye movement. The lesion may be located in: the cranial nerves, or in the eye muscles or the nuclear cell complex within the brainstem.

In clinical practice it is advised to limit to two possibilities. One should ask whether signs could be due to a lesion of one of the three cranial nerves: oculomotor nerve (III), trochlear nerve (IV) or abducens nerve (VI). If not, the lesion is likely to be located in eye muscles or in the nuclear cell complex in the brainstem.

The clinical test for diplopia and strabismus is composed of four parts: a. inspection; b. assessment of eye movement; c. diplopia testing, consisting of objective and subjective diplopia and d. if necessary, in each of the three above-mentioned steps, head-tilt test of Bielschowsky.

2.9.1. Inspection

Examination usually starts with inspection. One should note if there is any head-tilt or -turn, exophthalmus, ptosis, strabismus or skew deviation.

Ocular motility defects frequently give rise to abnormal posture of the head. In the majority of cases, ocular torticollis is a manner of achieving binocular single vision and may be observed in all types of non-concomitant strabismus. In congenital strabismus, the head is tilted principally towards the shoulder on that side where the fixating eye is situated. There is no satisfactory explanation for this type of torticollis.

To evaluate the degree of ptosis, auxiliary action of frontalis muscle, causing wrinkling of the forehead, must be eliminated. The examiner pushes the frontal muscle down and asks to look upwards. The extent to which the eyelid can be raised indicates the strength of the levator palpebrae muscle. If ptosis is psychogenic, there is no wrinkling of the forehead.

Examination of strabismus in primary position should extend to secondary position and even in diagonal directions, and will therefore be discussed in the next section on assessment of range of eye movement.

Skew deviation refers to any vertical misalignment of the visual axes secondary to acquired supranuclear or vestibulo-ocular disruption. This sign implicates brainstem disease but has no specific localizing value.

2.9.2. Assessment of range of eye movements

The patient is asked to follow a small target through the full range of the nine cardinal positions of gaze. The corneal reflection of Hirschberg is a simple method for diagnosing ocular alignment. If the patient is instructed to follow a pen-light, position of corneal reflection cardinal gaze directions can be observed. This is most easily achieved by causing the patient to gaze steadily at a fixation

ALTERNATE COVER TEST

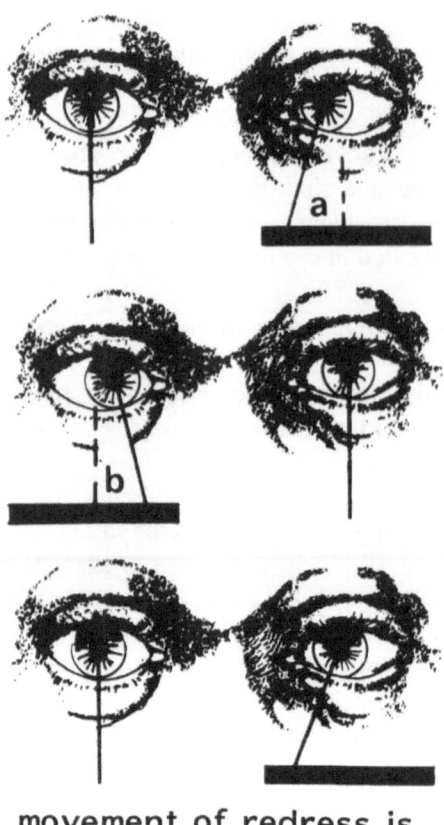

movement of redress is
the same in both eyes

Figure 4. (From Leigh & Zee, The Neurology of Eye Movement).

light and studying the corneal reflexes while the head is held in various postures, including when the head is tilted towards the left and right shoulders. If corneal reflections in both eyes appear in the centre of the pupils, the optical axes are correctly aligned. This method is particularly valuable when facial asymmetries such as epicanthic folds, hypertelorism or ptosis create the false impression of strabismus.

If strabismus exists, the best is to start with an alternate cover test in order to establish whether strabismus is concomitant. If occlusion is quickly transferred from one eye to the other in a way that binocular viewing is prevented, refixation will be noted. With concomitant strabismus movement of refixation is equal in both eyes (Fig. 4).

Then the patient is asked to follow a small target into the nine cardinal positions

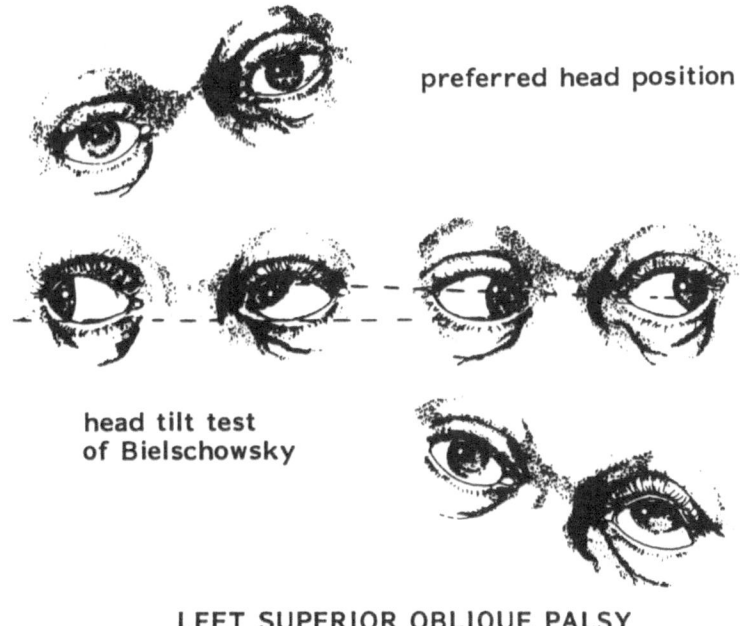

preferred head position

head tilt test
of Bielschowsky

LEFT SUPERIOR OBLIQUE PALSY

Figure 5. (From Leigh & Zee, The Neurology of Eye Movement).

of gaze. The examiner must be on the lookout for any restriction of movement in either or both eyes in particular directions of gaze. The 6th nerve innervates the lateral rectus muscle, and it follows that if an eye cannot be deviated laterally, a lesion of the 6th nerve can be inferred. The 3rd nerve is involved in eye movement in any other direction; thus a failure of movement in any other direction allows an inference of a lesion in the 3rd nerve. In clinical practice it comes down to the following: If there is a horizontal restriction, one should check whether abduction of one eye is restricted, or whether there is a restriction in all (other) directions of gaze, this in order to point to an abduction palsy or an oculomotor palsy.

If there is no horizontal restriction, the paretic eye follows a diagonal line then a slight vertical deviation in primary position becomes worse on gazing to the right. Whether it is a restriction of an elevator or of a depressor, the vertical deviation is strongest for a rectus in abduction and for an oblique muscle in adduction. In Fig. 5, this implies weakness of right superior rectus or left superior oblique muscle. If vertical deviation is more marked on downward gaze, there is a weakness of the left superior oblique muscle. If at the same time, there is an obvious tilt, in our case to the right shoulder, i.e. contralateral to the upward-deviating adducting left eye, then there is a left trochlear nerve palsy (Fig. 5).

Using the head-tilt test of Bielschowsky the diagnosis can be ascertained. If vertical deviation increases when the head is tilted to the same side as the upward-deviated eye (in our case an increase of the upward deviation of the left eye), then the test is positive and diagnosis of left trochlear palsy is established.

2.9.3. Diplopia testing

The best way of exactly examining strabismus is the 'cover' test. The patient fixates a distant target, firstly with eyes in primary position, and then, if necessary, in each of the four other cardinal gaze directions, which are easily attained by passively head turning during continuous fixation. In primary position, one eye is covered and then uncovered. If a nonfixating eye is covered, nothing will happen. If there is strabismus and the fixating eye is covered, refixation will occur. Uncovering, the previously covered eye will refixate, unless there is no preferred fixation (alternating preferred fixation). The amplitude of deviation of the normal eye (secondary deviation) if covered is larger than of the covered paretic eye (primary deviation) (Fig. 6).

A frequently occurring diagnostic problem is the differentiation between paralytic and non-paralytic strabismus. Sometimes a history of strabismus since childhood solves the problem. The absence of diplopia in such patients is due to suppression, amblyopia or abnormal retinal correspondence. In the case of a superior oblique paralysis, the family photo album may prove that a head-tilt was already present in childhood.

If there is no history of longstanding strabismus, examination is crucial. Most non-paralytic horizontal deviations of the eye axes are concomitant, i.e. have a fixed angle of strabismus. A non-concomitant, non-paralytic form of vertical deviation is the so-called hyperactivity of the inferior oblique muscle. This causes a hyperdeviation in adduction, but no deviation in primary position.

This is more difficult if eyes appear to move normally, although the patient still complains of diplopia. In order to solve this problem one has to recall: (a) If the patient looks in the direction of action of the paretic muscle, the two images are maximally separated, and (b) the target seen by the paretic eye is projected more peripherally.

In order to prevent fusion and to enlarge the difference between the double images, Maddox rods are used. Maddox rods are series of cylindrical bars which transform a point into a red line, so that the examiner knows which image belongs to which eye.

If there is horizontal diplopia the patient is asked to report the direction of ocular deviation that produces the largest separation of images, and which eye, according to the cover test, appears to correspond with the most peripheral image. In uncrossed diplopia there is external rectus paresis of the abducting eye, and in crossed diplopia there is internal rectus paresis of the adducted eye (Fig. 7).

In vertical diplopia the patient is asked to report whether upward or downward gaze produces the widest separation of images; this direction identifies the paretic muscles, namely the superior rectus or inferior oblique of one eye, or the inferior rectus or superior oblique of the other eye; the most peripherally appearing image

ALTERNATE COVER TEST

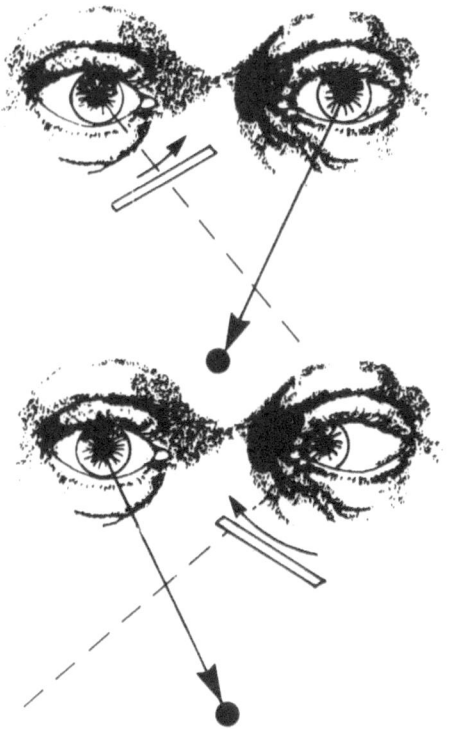

deviation of the sound
eye is greater than that
of the paretic eye

Figure 6. (From Leigh & Zee, The Neurology of Eye Movement).

belongs to the paretic eye. Next, the patient is asked to report whether the vertical deviation of the paretic eye is greater in adduction or in abduction, thus differentiating between an obliques or a rectus paresis. Here, too, the head-tilt test of Bielschowsky may be applied to confirm the diagnosis of superior oblique palsy.

For any puzzling acquired disorder of eye movement with or without ptosis but with normal pupils, myasthenia gravis is suspected. Myasthenia is the classic example used by neuro-ophthalmologists to show how to establish a diagnosis by means of subtle extra-ocular muscle signs.

Myasthenia ranks very high on the list of missed diagnoses, because many physicians are unaware of the variations in presentation. Ocular muscle involvement occurs in 90% of myasthenias and accounts for the initial complaint in 75%.

60

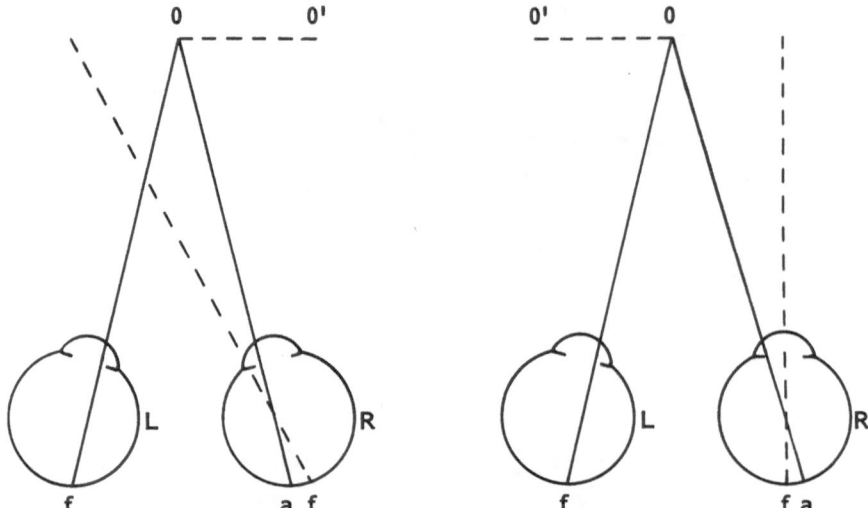

uncrossed diplopia right-sided sixth nerve palsy   crossed diplopia right-sided medial rectus palsy

Figure 7.

Clinically, ptosis may be more apparent during sustained upward gaze. In cases of unilateral ptosis, the contralateral upper lid may be retracted but will assume a normal position if the ptotic side is occluded. Cogan has described a 'lid twitch' sign, which is elicited by having the patient rapidly redirect his gaze from the downward to the primary position. The lid will then be seen to twitch upwards or slowly resettle to the ptotic position. The combination 'lid twitch' with increase in ptosis during sustained upward gaze confirms myasthenia gravis, even if the Tensilon test is negative. A characteristic sign in asymmetric ptosis is the 'see-saw ptosis'. If the ptotic eyelid is lifted up, the other eyelid drops; letting it go, the contralateral eyelid moves upwards again.

References

Daroff RB, Troost BT (1978): Supranuclear disorders of eye movements. In: Glaser JS: Neuro-ophthalmology. Harper & Row, Hagerstown, Maryland, U.S.A., pp 201–218.

Glaser JS (1978): Infranuclear disorders of eye movements. In: Glaser JS: Neuro-ophthalmology. Harper & Row, Hagerstown, Maryland, U.S.A., pp 245–284.

Leigh RJ, Zee DS (1983): The neurology of eye movement. FA Davis Company, Philadelphia.

Orthoptic investigation of ocular motor disturbances

J.J.M. BIERLAAGH

The orthoptic investigation of ocular motility disturbances in this chapter is limited to the following five subjects: 1. ocular torticollis; 2. diplopia; 3. eye movements; 4. synoptophore; 5. hess-screen test.

1. Ocular torticollis

An ocular torticollis consists of three components: a. face turn towards the right or left side; b. head-tilt to the right or left shoulder; c. chin held up or down.

ad a. A face turn can be caused by: a deviation in the horizontal plane to avoid a limitation of adduction or abduction; a deviation in a vertical plane to avoid a vertical deviation, which is maximal looking sidewards; nystagmus, when the fixing eye is held in adduction.

ad b. A head-tilt to the right or left shoulder is seen particularly in torsional deviations, usually when an oblique muscle is involved; for example, in superior oblique palsy the head tilt will be towards the unaffected side.

ad c. The chin may be held up or down to compensate for a vertical eye deviation.

A torticollis is usually adopted to avoid diplopia and to obtain comfortable binocular vision. The position of the head is directed towards the position of maximum deviation in a way that the eyes are in a position of minimal deviation .

When analysing an ocular torticollis one has first to observe the position of the eyes in the orbit; the deviation of the head will be in the opposite direction. For example: when the eyes are directed towards the right the deviation will be on laevoversion, so either the right medial rectus or the left lateral rectus has to be affected (Fig. 1).

When the eyes are placed in dextro elevation, the deviation should be found in laevo depression. In other words, the cause may be found in either the right superior oblique or the left inferior rectus (Fig. 2).

Description of the ocular torticollis is very important. Of the three compo-

62

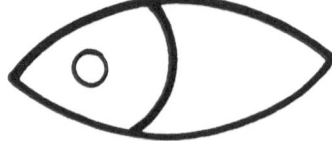 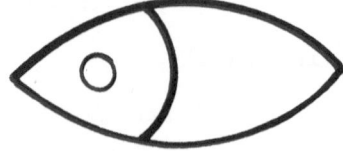

Figure 1. Torticollis – face turn left: eyes in dextroversion.

nents, one may be more obvious and all three components are therefore graded,
e.g.:

– marked face turn right		face turn right +++
– slight tilt towards the left]	or [	head tilt left ++
– chin slightly elevated		chin up +

2. Diplopia

When analysing diplopia there may be three components: horizontal, vertical,
torsional.

A torsional component is least frequent and is usually only present in acquired
superior oblique palsies. In congenital superior oblique palsies the localisation of
the images has been subjectively adjusted and may give an incorrect picture.

In order to analyse and differentiate the horizontal and vertical component in
double vision a Maddox Rod is used. This is a red coloured glass with parallel
running glass cylinders, which transform a spot of light into a line (Fig. 3).

The glass, with the rods horizontal, is held in front of one eye and the patient is
asked to fix a spot of light. The eye covered by the Maddox glass will see a vertical
red line and thus we can examine the extent of horizontal diplopia. First the
situation in the primary position is examined: are the images seen crossed (exo) or
uncrossed (aeso). Next the distance between line and light in dextro- and laevoversion will be compared. An increase in the separation of the images indicates a
limitation of movement in that particular direction.

For example: in the primary position there is uncrossed diplopia and the
separation of the images increases in dextroversion, this is indicative of limited

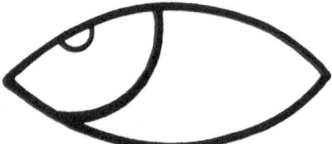 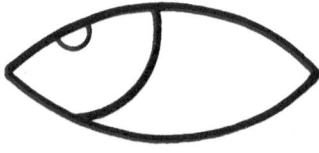

Figure 2. Torticollis: face turn left, chin held down, tilt towards left shoulder. The eyes will be in a
position of dextro elevation.

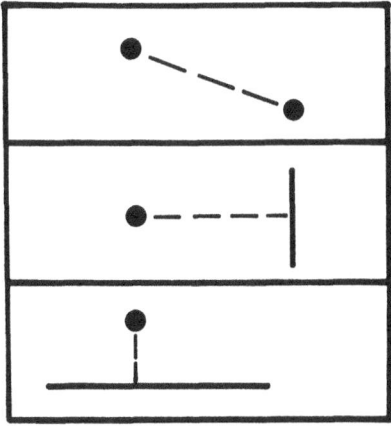

Figure 3. Diplopia test: a. using a light only, b. using a maddox rod, with a vertical line for the horizontal deviation, c. using a maddox rod, with a horizontal line to examine the vertical deviation.

abduction of the right eye. If on the other hand crossed images in the primary position appear and the separation increases in dextroversion, it indicates a limited adduction of the left eye.

In evaluation of the vertical component of diplopia the axis of the Maddox Rod is held vertical, giving a horizontal line in the covered eye. Examination starts in the primary position and the patient is asked, whether the line is seen above, under or through the light. The images are crossed; if there is a hypertropia the line seen by the affected eye will be located under the light. We then compare the distance between the images in various directions (for example: do they further separate in dextro- or laevoversion?; is the separation of images maximal in upward or downward gaze?).

For instance: Maddox Rod in front of the right eye. In the primary position the patient sees the line under the spot of light, in other words the right eye is deviated in an upward direction. If we then compare the separation of images in dextro- and laevoversion and if the distance increases in laevoversion, maximum deviation will be found in laevoversion. The eye muscles, responsible for a deviation in this direction are the oblique muscles of the right eye or the vertical recti of the left eye. Comparing the situation in elevation and depression, we can exclude the relevant elevators or depressors. Suppose the separation increases in depression, only one muscle can be at fault; in laevo depression the right superior oblique and the left inferior rectus are involved. A right hypertropia can only be caused by a limitation of the superior oblique.

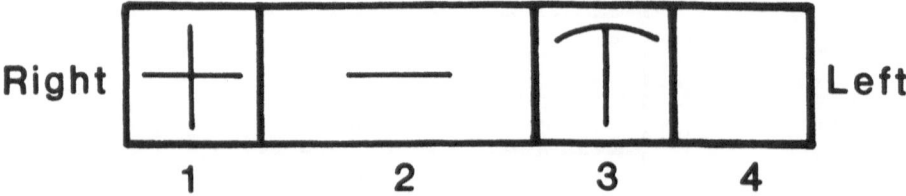

Figure 4. Scheme to record ocular movements.

3. Ocular movements

To describe deviations of ocular movement we use a scheme in our orthoptic department, in which we note diagonal, vertical, torsional and horizontal incomitances (Fig. 4).

1. The diagonal incomitances (compartment 1): Diagonal incomitances are investigated in the oblique directions of gaze, i.e. dextro and laevo elevation and dextro and laevo depression. The abducting eye is made the fixing eye and the position of the adducted eye will be described and an alternating covertest has to be performed. In the upper field of gaze we assess the action of the inferior obliques, in the lower field the superior obliques. This will be recorded in compartment 1.

If it is filled in as in Fig. 5, it means an overaction of both inferior obliques, but right more than left and a hypoaction of both superior obliques, right and left equally.

2. With vertical incomitances the changes are described, which occur in the vertical deviation when the patient looks away from the primary position. These incomitances are recorded in compartment 2. Example: in primary position we find a right hypertropia (R/L). Comparing the vertical deviation looking to the right and to the left and looking up or down will reveal, where the deviation is greatest: looking up or down and looking right or left. This is noted as in Fig. 6.

3. In compartment 3 the results of the head-tilting test of Bielschowsky are scored. This test is always carried out when a vertical deviation is present to see, whether a superior oblique palsy may be the cause. The test is called positive

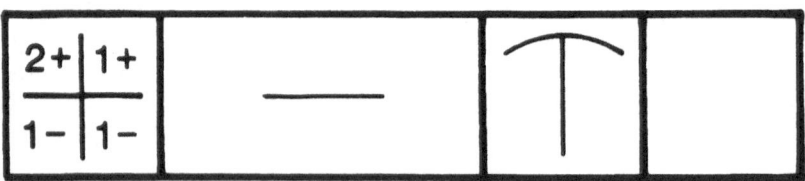

Figure 5. Overacting inferior obliques; underacting superior obliques.

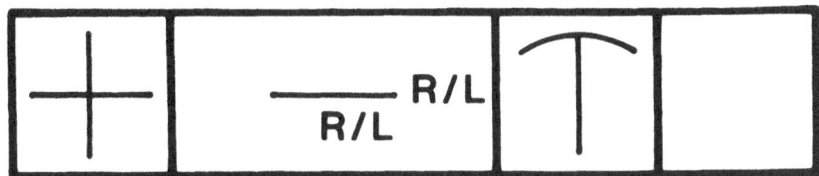

Figure 6. R/L (right hypertropia) maximum in laevoversion and depression.

when a right hypertropia (R/L) increases by tilting the head towards the right shoulder.

The same holds true when a left hypertropia (L/R) is present; when the deviation increases by tilting the head towards the left, the test is positive and is noted as in Figs. 7 and 8.

4. Horizontal incomitances are defined as:

a. A, V, X and Y variations in the horizontal angle of deviation, findings, which are not so important in neuro-ophthalmological conditions. This variation is recorded in compartment 4. For example: An aesodeviation is a convergent deviation which increases on looking up and decreases on looking down.

b. Adduction or abduction limitations. These are important in neuro-ophthalmology patients. For example: when the right eye has an abduction limitation, there will be a marked aesodeviation on looking towards the right. This we also record in compartment 2, together with a possible variation in the vertical deviation (Fig. 9).

4. The synoptophore

The synoptophore is used to obtain the angle of deviation in a horizontal, vertical and torsional way. Usually this will only be done in the primary position, but if necessary can be carried out in various positions of gaze.

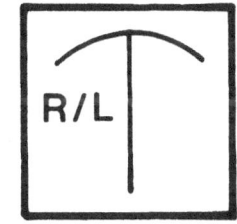

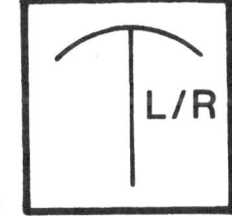

Figure 7. Positive Bielschowsky test towards the right.

Figure 8. Positive Bielschowsky test towards the left.

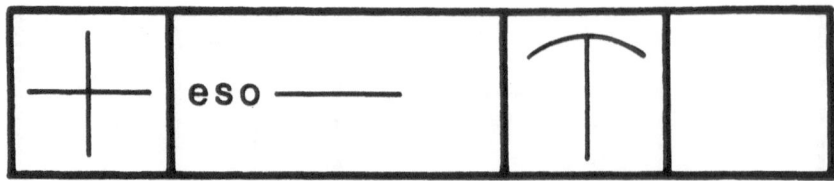

Figure 9. Aesodeviation due to abduction limitation of RE.

When there is a horizontal deviation as well as a vertical one, it is difficult to measure the correct vertical deviation, especially when the horizontal deviation is large. In order to measure the vertical deviation correctly we have to divide the horizontal angle equally between the two eyes, in other words instead of placing the fixing eye at the nought position when the horizontal angle is +20, the fixing eye is placed at +10. In this way we measure the correct vertical deviation, which is called real vertical deviation (RVD).

The synoptophore is used to examine the state of binocular vision. If suppression is found, this indicates a congenital or a long standing condition.

Monocular eye movements (ductions) may also be examined on the synoptophore, especially when a Hess test cannot be carried out.

5. The Hess-screen test

The Hess-screen test is used to record hyper- or hypo-actions of the ocular muscles, while the eyes are dissociated by means of red and green goggles. One eye can only see the red image, the other eye green only (so that patient should not be colourblind). Besides the red and green goggles, we use red and green lights also of complementary colours. The patient holds one light, which projects a line of light and has to place this through the examiner's line at right angles. The examination starts in primary position and then continues in a radius of 15° around the primary position. If necessary, a radius of 30° can also be used. The test is carried out fixing right and fixing left and recorded on Hess recording charts. Fixing right the deviation of the left eye is recorded and fixing left we obtain the deviation of the right eye. In case of a paresis the field of the affected eye is smaller, when fixing with the sound eye and this is based on the laws of innervation of Hering and Sherrington.

To interpret a Hess-screen the size of the fields of the two eyes are compared. The smaller field belongs to the affected eye and gives the primary deviation, the larger field belongs to the unaffected eye (secondary deviation). A limitation of movement in one eye will cause an overaction of the synergist in the other eye. Examining the smaller field we look for the direction of maximum limitation and compare this with the overaction in the other field. Fig. 10 gives an example of a

NAME .... No.

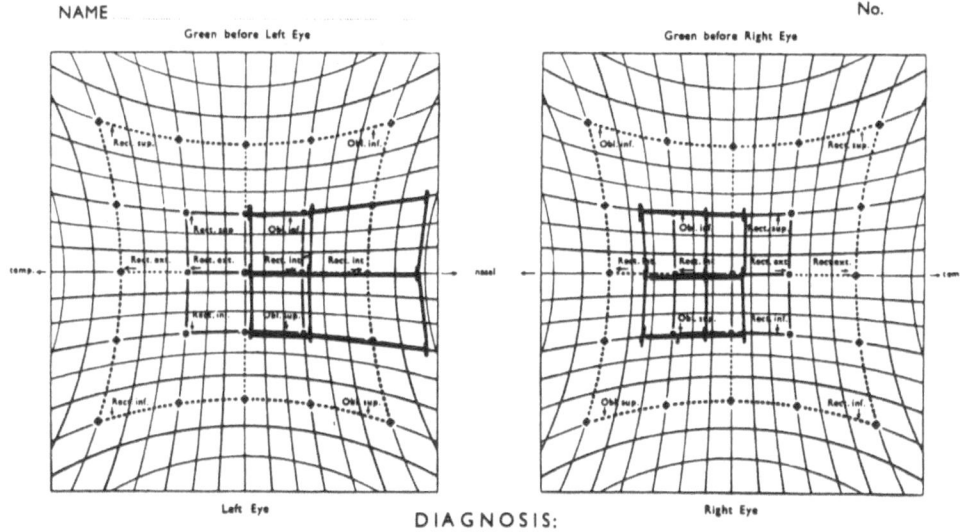

Figure 10. Hess scheme of a right VI nerve palsy.

right six nerve palsy. Fixing with the left eye the angle of deviation is +7 (primary deviation). Fixing with the right eye the angle increases to +15 (secondary deviation). Because the maximum angle appears by fixation with the right eye the latter has to be the affected one. The deviation is maximal in dextroversion and the left medial rectus shows a marked overaction. Whether the condition improves or deteriorates will be clearly visible on repeated Hess examination to

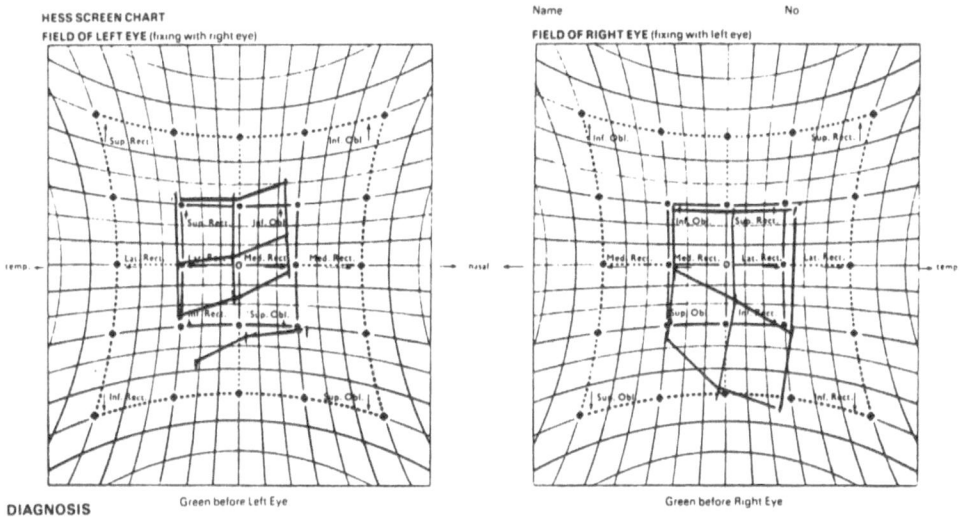

Figure 11. Hess chart showing left IVth nerve palsy.

68

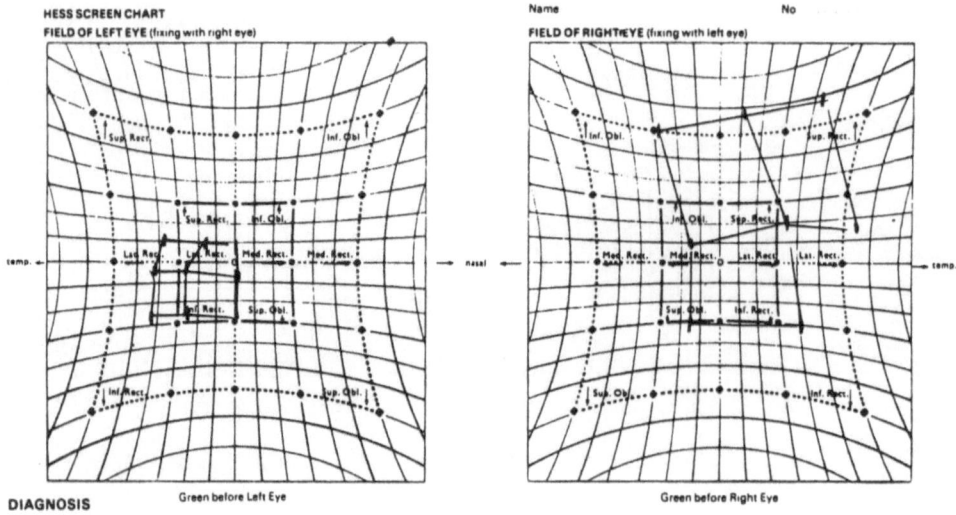

Figure 12. Hess chart showing left IIIrd nerve palsy.

examiner as well as patient. Figs. 11 and 12 represent left fourth nerve palsy and left third nerve palsy respectively.

References

Cashell GTW, Durran IM: Handbook of Orthoptic Principles. Churchill Livingstone, Edinburgh, London, Melbourne and New York.

Fundamentals and basic properties of clinical eye movement recording techniques

J.P.H. REULEN

Over the past years, the neuro-ophthalmological clinic has benefitted from fundamental research into the oculomotor system. In particular, the introduction of noninvasive methods for the recording, analysis and quantification of subclinical abnormalities of the oculomotor system has permitted systematic studies of normal and abnormal eye movement parameters.

There are several kinds of oculomotor subsystems. The various kinds of eye movements can be classified into fast saccades, slow smooth pursuit movements, optokinetic nystagmus (OKN), vestibulo-ocular reflexes (VOR) and vergence eye movements. It is not clear whether eye movements during fixation of a stationary target, i.e. microsaccades (amplitude 2–20'), microdrift and tremor (amplitude 20–40", frequency 70–90 Hz) can be regarded as separate oculomotor subsystems.

Objective recordings of the aforementioned eye movement systems have shown that many disorders can be characterised by specific patterns of oculomotor abnormalities [1, 2, 3]. The main aim here is briefly to describe the general principles and properties of those recording techniques, which are most commonly used in clinical research and diagnostics.

1. General aspects

As the differences between the aforementioned types of eye movements are characteristic, quantification of a particular kind of oculomotor subsystem sets different criteria for the optimum recording technique. Consequently, in addition to many of the existing methods, a growth in the development of new methods can be observed, in particular, rather expensive computerised and TV camera-equipped systems [4, 5, 6].

An ideal technique for recording the various types of eye movements, both for fundamental research and for clinical diagnostics, should meet the following demands.

1. Easy, nontraumatic application in the case of subjects without former experience or special motivation.
2. High resolution, as well as a sufficiently wide dynamic measuring range (frequency bandwidth).
3. An ample linear range for the relation between signal and eye rotation.
4. Flexible, adjustable measuring range for the different applications.
5. Good stability, no signal drift.
6. No interference with normal vision and a sufficiently large field of view.
7. Insensitive to slight translations of the head. No need for a rigid head stabilisation.
8. Simultaneous measurement of horizontal and vertical eye movements and eventually rotatory movements.
9. Insensitive to ambient illumination, eyelid artefacts and insensitive to electromyographic and/or electromagnetic noise.

As can be expected, no existing method satisfies all listed criteria. In practice, it is found that the three most commonly used methods in clinical practice are: a. electronystagmography (ENG); b. methods based on the reflection of infrared light (IR); c. methods based on magnetic induction (MI).

Nowadays, ENG is the most commonly applied clinical technique for the measurement of eye movements. Because of this, its properties will be discussed in great detail in this chapter. Furthermore, general aspects of the infrared reflection (IR) and magnetic induction (MI) methods will be presented. For more details concerning the two last-named category of methods, relevant references are listed.

2. Description of the methods

2.1. Electronystagmography (ENG)

2.1.1. Principle
ENG is the most commonly applied technique for recording eye movements in humans and is a relatively simple, nontraumatic method. It has been a valuable tool in the study of physiology and pathophysiology of horizontal eye movements. Its usefulness in studying vertical eye movements, however is rather limited, as will be discussed later.

The ENG method is based on the existence of a cornea-retinal difference in electrical potential of about 1 mV. To avoid confusion in nomenclature with the term EOG: electro-oculography (EOG) is the quantification of the cornea-retinal potential in the light and in the dark.

Miniature Ag-AgCl skin electrodes are placed at the outer canthi of each eye to record horizontal eye movements (Fig. 1).

To record vertical eye movements, skin electrodes are placed immediately

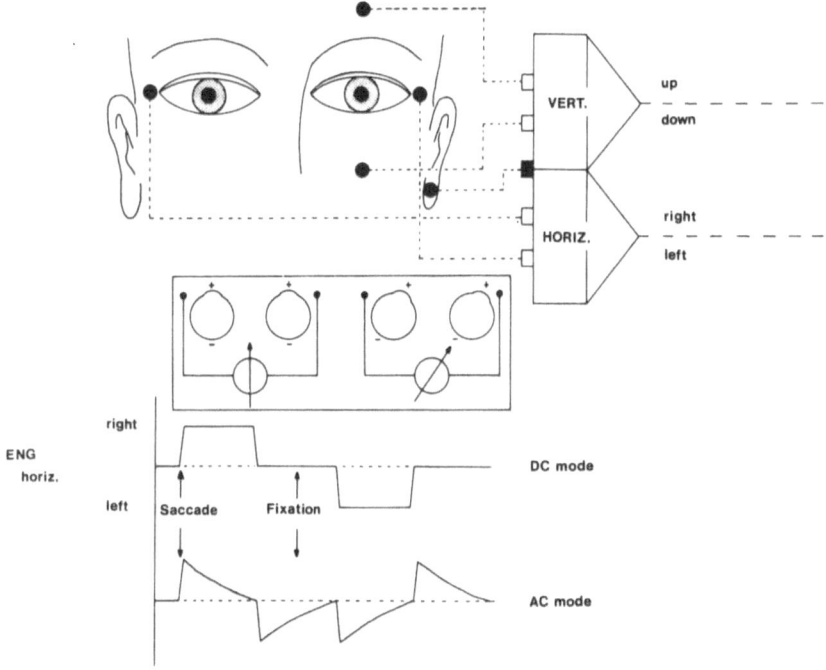

Figure 1. Principle of the ENG method. Electrodes are positioned for binocular horizontal and monocular vertical recording. The influence of DC or AC recording on the trajectories of horizontal refixation saccades are shown (source Brandt and Büchele [1]).

above the eyebrow and below the inferior rim of the orbit. Upon eye movement into the direction of either electrode, this electrode will raise its electrical potential while the contralateral electrode will lower its potential. Amplification of the potential difference between both electrodes results in a signal representing eye movement. In practice, 1 degree of eye movement evokes an average potential of 10–20 microvolt. In this way it is possible to record horizontal and vertical eye movements of both eyes, simultaneously or apart.

2.1.2. General properties

The ENG method requires relatively inexpensive equipment and is fairly rather comfortable in use, so that it can be rather easily applied. The ENG signal is independent of slight head movements. For head stabilisation, a chin rest combined with a support at the back of the head is adequate. The field of view is not limited by the positioning of the electrodes and patients wearing spectacles can be measured without problems. Moreover, eye movements can be recorded when the eyes are closed, as is important for the recording of caloric or vestibular nystagmus.

The measuring range is large (horizontal 70–80 degrees; vertical 50 degrees) with a linear relation between signal and horizontal eye rotation up to 30 degrees, and 20 degrees for vertical eye rotation. Such a large linear measuring range is necessary for the reliable recording of optokinetic or vestibular nystagmus. The rather high noise level of the ENG position signal limits resolution to about 1–2 degrees with a frequency bandwidth from DC to 60 Hz (−3 dB down).

The fact that the cornea-retinal potential is altered when changes occur in the level of ambient illumination, does not interfere with the clinical application of the ENG method, provided the patient has adapted for 10–15 minutes to the level of illumination of the oculomotor laboratory.

2.1.3. Sources and prevention of disturbances

The ENG signal is not free of disturbances. The major sources are: a) electromagnetic interference (50 or 60 Hz); b) high-frequency electromyographic signals; c) low-frequency drift; d) eyelid artefacts.

sub a) The mains supply may give rise to substantial electromagnetic interference with a fixed frequency (50 or 60 Hz) and a sinusoidally varying amplitude. To reduce the sinusoidal component, differential amplifiers with a high common-mode rejection ratio (> 100.000) should be used. Furthermore, cables connecting the electrodes to the amplifiers should be short twisted and shielded, of course in combination with proper earthing of the patient. With regard to this last, for reasons of electrical safety, it may be desirable to use optically or magnetically coupled differential amplifiers [7].

To reduce 50 Hz interference, the electrical resistance between each electrode and the skin should be less than 5 kOhms. This can be accomplished by proper cleaning and abrasion of the skin with petroleum ether and rubbing the electrode paste into the skin before adjusting the electrode. Use of so-called collars is advised to ensure rigid mechanical application of the electrodes to the skin.

sub b) Muscle activity, resulting in high-frequency electromyographic signals may give rise to a lower ENG signal-to-noise ratio. In general, high frequency noise can be reduced by the application of low-pass analog electronic filters (LP). Of course, the choice of the bandwidth of the LP filter should obviate significant disturbance of the eye movements under study. Practically, this means that for the reliable study of saccadic or nystagmoid quick-phase eye movements, a bandwidth of up to 60 Hz should be selected while, for reliable study of maximal saccadic or quick-phase velocity, a bandwidth of up to 80 Hz is advised [8]. A much lower bandwidth (up to 20 Hz) can be used for the study of slow phase velocity of OKN, vestibular or caloric nystagmus. If other cut-off frequencies are used, particularly in the study of abnormality of maximal saccadic velocity, each laboratory should of course determine its own reference values.

sub c) Drift can be described as a slow change of the ENG signal without movement of the eyes. In particular, the study of smooth pursuit eye movements and slow phase nystagmus velocity can be obscured by the presence of drift. Moreover, in the case of drift, eye position cannot be accurately determined. To reduce the influence of drift, most commercially available ENG systems are provided with an AC mode of measurement (Fig. 1): the eye-position signal is fed through a high-pass analog electronic filter causing an amplitude reduction of the low-frequency signal components. However, the application of an AC mode makes accurate measurement of eye position impossible, as is illustrated in Fig. 1. The exponential decline of the eye position signal is characterised by a so-called AC time constant. In daily practice, a compromise must be found between the value for the AC time constant selected and the maximum tolerable drift of the ENG signal. An AC time constant of 20 seconds (high-pass cut-off frequency 0.01 Hz) is a good compromise. A technical aid is an offset-reset mechanism, which permits temporary switching of the AC time constant to a lower value (0.5 sec) to compensate for an (electrode) offset potential caused by signal drift. An other piece of advice for the reduction of electrode offset is to keep the electrodes, if not applied short-circuited, in a physiological salt solution.

sub d) Eyelid artefacts may have major effects on trajectories and peak velocities of vertical saccades particularly [9, 10]. When the eyes move in the vertical direction the eyelids also move. Gaze up causes an elevation of the eyelid and gaze down a lowering of the eyelid. The eyelid movements cause a change in tissue resistance between the corneoretinal dipole and the electrode opposite to the change in ENG potential due to vertical eye movement. The extent of the artefact varies between subjects and also somewhat between saccades of similar size in one and the same subject. Up saccades with ENG have peaked, overshooting trajectories that are probably produced by movement of the eyelids (Fig. 2) [9]. Furthermore, the peak velocities of up and down saccades are exaggerated. The immobilization of the eyelids does not adequately decrease the effects of the artefact [10].

As lid movements are associated with all vertical eye movements, this implies that all vertical ENG recordings, even without blinks, are highly contaminated by changes in lid position and therefore essentially unreliable as an eye-position monitor [10].

Eye blinks are consistently accompanied by transient downward and nasalward movements of both eyes with amplitudes of 1–5 deg [9].

The horizontal ENG-recordings may also not be free of artefacts due to eye blinks. In particular, if the eyes are deviated in a lateral position (> 20 deg), eye blinks may cause eye movement-like signals. This is particularly important for the diagnosis of gaze-evoked nystagmus, since eye blinks may induce artefacts resembling gaze-evoked nystagmus. Also, correct diagnosis of internuclear ophthalmoplegia (INO) may be obscured, since the simultaneous occurrence of a horizontal saccade together with an eye blink may result in ENG signals that mimic an INO-like pattern of eye movements. For this reason, the diagnosis of INO with an ENG technique should always include a vertical electrode lead to control for eye blinks.

2.1.4. Monocular versus binocular ENG registrations

Since the orientation of the nasally and temporally positioned electrodes with respect to the electrical dipole is not symmetrical, there is a difference in amplitude for eye movements in the nasal or temporal direction. Also the tissue inhomogeneity of the surrounding media, as well as the cross-talk of the electric dipole of the other eye into the ENG signal of the fellow eye may contribute to this, in particular as regards the nasally positioned electrodes. In the summated binocular electrode derivation (Fig. 1), which is normally used for the measurement of nondissociated conjugate eye movements, no problems due to crosstalk are present. However, the study of dissociated (for example INO, muscle paresis, myasthenia gravis or strabismus) or nonconjugate eye movements such as vergence eye movements demands a monocular ENG registration for each eye separately.

To summarize, despite serious drawbacks, the ENG method has proved to be of great value in the clinical study and diagnosis of vestibular and neurological eye-movement disorders. However, ophthalmological interest in the oculomotor system in particular concerns vergence eye movements, eye-position maintenance, miniature eye movements and eye movements induced by cover tests. From the foregoing it can be concluded that for these applications the ENG method is not suitable.

3. Methods based on the reflection of infrared light

3.1. Principles

The principle of reflection of infrared light (IR) by the eye has led to the development of many techniques which may be divided into three major classes: a) corneal reflection methods (CR); b) pupil-scanning methods (PS); c) iris-scleral reflection methods (IRIS). The major principles of these three categories of methods are briefly described below.

Corneal reflection methods

Reflections of a bright object from the front surface of the cornea form a virtual image behind the surface which can be recorded. Light is also reflected from each surface of the eye at which there is a change in refractive index (back surface cornea, front and rear surface of the lens). These reflections are referred to as the Purkinje images. Measurement of the relative displacements of the Purkinje images represent a technique for measuring the orientation of the eye in space since the position of the corneal reflection is a function of eye position. This principle has led to the development of a class of eye-movement instruments known as corneal reflection systems [5, 11–14].

A major drawback of these methods is the need for rigid head stabilization and a limited measuring range. Generally, the slight translations of the eye occurring during eye rotation degrade the accuracy of CR methods. Head-mounted corneal reflection techniques measure eye position with respect to head position although with a poor resolution (about 2 deg.). Eizenman [14] has recently proposed technical solutions for some of the problems mentioned.

Pupil scanning methods

The pupil is easily distinguished from the surrounding iris by its difference in reflectance of light. Movement of the eye causes an eccentric pupil image, which can serve as a basis for eye angle measurement. Systems based on the scanning of the pupil area by infrared light sources mostly use infrared-sensitive TV cameras in combination with a digital computer [4, 15–17]. The pupil scanning methods allow free head movements and are in principle well adapted to clinical examinations. However, apart from being rather expensive, the measuring range and temporal resolution of these methods are rather limited. Furthermore, unless the system is made in duplo, it is not possible to measure the movements of both eyes simultaneously. Because of the computerized and rather complicated apparatus, these methods have not yet become tools for general clinical application. What is more, calibration and alignment of the systems is far from simple and demand well trained personnel.

From the foregoing it is clear that simultaneous binocular eye-movement recording using corneal reflection or pupil scanning methods is rather complicated and expensive since practically the complete measuring system would have to be duplicated.

Iris-scleral reflection methods

The sharp boundary between the iris and the sclera, the limbus, contributes to a difference in reflectance of IR light [5, 18–20]. Part of the reflected light is detected by infrared-sensitive detectors. To measure horizontal eye movements, detectors are positioned in front of the eye so that their 'receptive' fields match the iris-sclera transition both on the nasal and on the temporal side. The sharp border between the iris and the sclera contributes to a difference in reflectance of the IR light. Upon movement of the eye, for example in the case of abduction, the nasally positioned detector will measure an increased scleral IR reflection while the temporally placed detector measures a decreased iris reflection. Subtraction of the nasal and temporal detector signals gives eye position with respect to head position.

The IRIS technique can be extended to measurement of vertical eye movement by the proper positioning of the illumination areas of the emitters and the viewing areas of the detectors.

IRIS systems are likely candidates for clinical application. Because of this, the general properties of these systems will now be discussed in more detail.

3.2. General properties

A major advantage of IRIS systems is the low noise level permitting a high resolution of some minutes of arc with a sufficiently high bandwidth (100 Hz, −3 dB). In principle the recording of eye movement is free of drift, permitting DC mode of operation, which is important in particular for disconjugate eye-movement registration and for the measurement of eye position. Since IRIS methods are noncontacting to the eye they are almost ideal as far as clinical application and versatility are concerned.

The IRIS method allows for simultaneous recording of the movements of both eyes, which is particularly valuable for a reliable diagnosis of disconjugate eye-movement disorders, such as (internuclear) ophthalmoplegia, myasthenia gravis and muscle paresis. Compared with the costs of other systems based on the principle of IR reflection, IRIS systems are fairly inexpensive. The application, set-up and alignment of IRIS systems is not complicated and does not require experienced personnel. It is also possible to measure eye movements with closed eyes, as during active eye movements the cornea displaces the eyelid towards the detection array, causing a change in the amount of reflected IR light [21]. Calibration of these signals is complicated, so that, for example only the presence of vestibular nystagmus of peripheral origin occurring only with closed eyes, can be detected. This, however, satisfies most clinical demands for the testing of the vestibular functions.

A major drawback of existing IRIS methods is a limited measuring range of 30 degrees horizontal and 20 degrees vertical. The range of linearity is limited (horizontal 15 deg) with IRIS, especially in the upward direction (vertical 10 deg.). However, such a measuring range is adequate for reliable measurement of fixation eye movements, for horizontal and vertical saccades and for smooth pursuit eye movements with an amplitude not exceeding 30 deg horizontally or 20 deg vertically.

Measurement of the vertical position by the IRIS method is difficult. In vertical recordings, the eyelid margins can obscure the limbus in the superior and inferior positions. In this method the velocity and the amplitude of up saccades are underestimated [9]. Moreover, asymmetry of amplitudes of up and down saccades may be prominent, as illustrated in Fig. 2. With mechanical retraction or taping up of the eyelids, IRIS methods might become more accurate for vertical eye-movement recording.

Since the IR emitters and detectors are positioned in front of the eyes, the field of view is somewhat limited (horizontal 70 deg; vertical 25 deg). Notwithstanding this limited field of view, proper stimulation of optokinetic nystagmus is still possible.

The interference due to any changes in ambient illumination is overcome by illuminating the eye with chopped IR light and then demodulating at the same frequency.

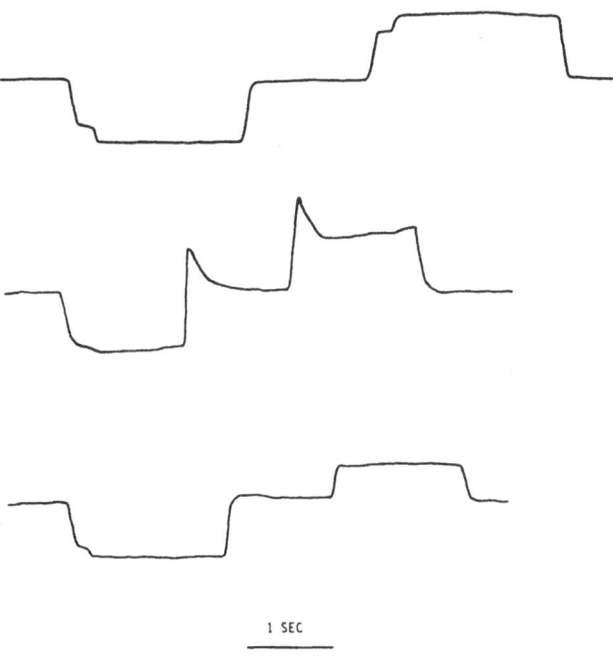

1 SEC

Figure 2. Trajectories of vertical saccades. Refixations were between fixed targets at centre, 15 deg down and 15 deg up. Deflections up are upward. Top: MI method. Centre: ENG method. Note peaked waveform of up saccades. Bottom: IRIS method. Note asymmetry of amplitudes of up and down saccades (source Yee [9]).

Another problem linked to IRIS methods is the crosstalk between the horizontal and the vertical recording channel and vice versa. To put it another way, vertical eye movements may induce a signal in the horizontally positioned IR detectors. Thus, horizontal eye movements may induce a similar signal in the vertically positioned detectors. The crosstalk of a newly developed IRIS system [20] is about ten, which means that a vertical eye movement of 10 degrees causes a virtually horizontal eye rotation of 1 degree. Because of the crosstalk phenomenon, IRIS systems are not suitable for the reliable recording of oblique eye movements. Separate recordings of horizontal or vertical eye movements are possible, while another option is the measurement of the horizontal movements of one eye and the vertical movements of the fellow eye.

Optical methods using small mirrors mounted in contact lenses are excellent methods, in the hands of experts and applied on motivated subjects or patients, in particular for the precise study of fixational eye movements, but are not suitable for general clinical application.

78

3.3 ENG versus IRIS

The most relevant properties of a newly developed IRIS system [20] are listed in Table 1. This system was used to compare simultaneous records of horizontal eye movements obtained by the ENG method and the IRIS technique. Fig. 3 shows refixation saccades between a central position and a peripheral target at 15 degrees left and right of the central spot. Apart from the lower signal-to-noise ratio of the ENG signal, it is clear that the IRIS signal is free of drift. This while the ENG signal shows considerable drift of the signal corresponding to gaze at the central position straight ahead. The influence of the selecfed ENG AC time constant of 20 s [22] can be seen in the ENG signal drifting towards the zero level while gaze is directed at 15 deg. left or right of the central position.

The high resolution of the IRIS method is illustrated in Fig. 4 showing spontaneous small eye movements measured in darkness. The IRIS signal is contaminated by a blink artefact while the horizontal ENG trace remains undisturbed. Furthermore, as indicated by the arrow in Fig. 4, the ENG signal may

Table 1. Major properties of the ENG, IRIS and MI methods

Method	ENG	IRIS	MI
– resolution	1–2 deg	3′	3′
with bandwidth up to	60 Hz	100 Hz	100 Hz
– linear (in deg)			
horizontal	30	25	20
vertical	20	20	20
– measuring range (deg)			
horizontal	70–80	30	50–60
vertical	40–50	25	50–60
– field of view			
hor-vert in deg	unlimited	60×40	90×90
– signal drift	severe	no	no
– spectacle wearing	yes	yes	difficult
– independent of			
ambient illumination?	no	yes	yes
– easy to apply?	yes	yes	no
– expensive?	no	no	yes
– horizontal registration	yes	yes	yes
vertical registration	no	yes	yes
– measurement of torsion	no	no	yes
– horizontal and			
vertical registration			
simultaneously on one eye	no	difficult	yes
– measurement of			
both eyes simultaneously?	yes	yes	difficult
– measurement with			
closed eyes?	yes	difficult	yes

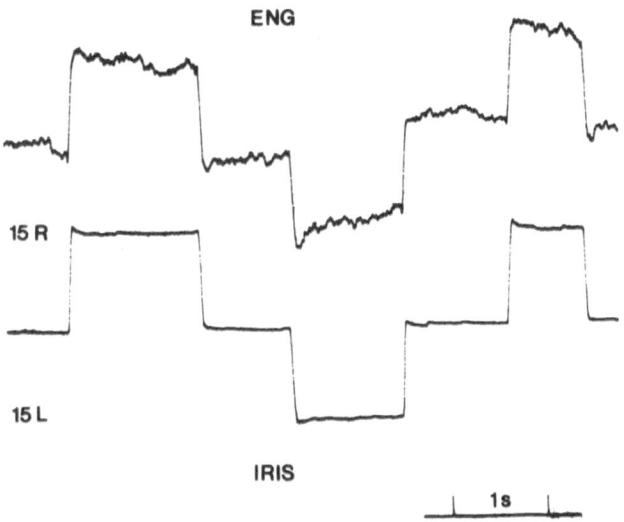

Figure 3. Trajectories of horizontal saccades. Refixations were between fixed targets at centre, 15 deg right and 15 deg left. Top: ENG signal. Bottom: IRIS signal. Note higher noise level and drift of the ENG signal.

vary considerably, so that pendular eye movements with a frequency of about 10 Hz are suggested. However, as may be seen in the IRIS signal the eye does not move. This phenomenon may be caused by crosstalk of EEG signals into the electrodes picking up the ENG signal.

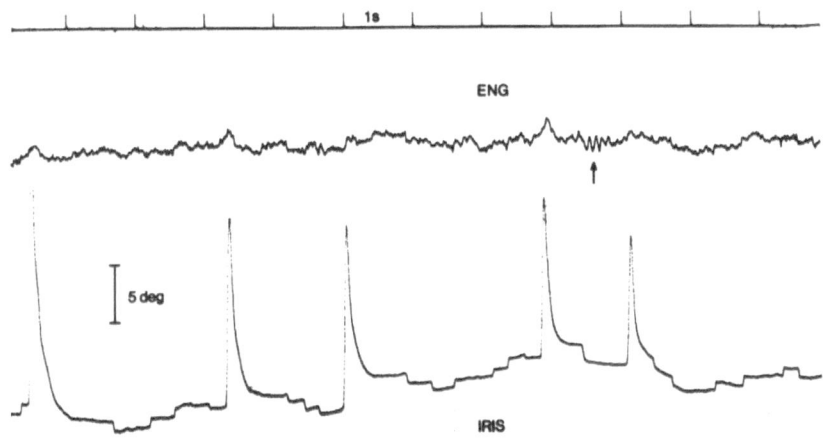

Figure 4. Eye movements recorded in darkness with an ENG and an IRIS technique, showing the high-amplitude resolution of the IRIS method. Note prominent eye blink artefacts in the IRIS trace. Pendular variations of the ENG signal (see arrow) suggest fast oscillatory eye movements while the eye, according to the IRIS signal, does not move.

4. Methods based on magnetic induction (MI)

4.1 Principle

The method that best satisfies the requirements of an ideal technique has been developed by Robinson [23]. In that method, called the MI method, a search coil is mounted in a scleral contact lens which is held to the anaesthetized eye by suction. The coil is subjected to a time-varying magnetic field and a voltage is induced in the coil proportional to the sine of the angle between the eye and the direction of the magnetic field. By phase-sensitive detection of the induction voltage, precise and accurate measurement of horizontal, vertical and torsional eye movements is possible.

4.2. General properties

The MI method is probably the most accurate technique for recording horizontal and vertical eye movements simultaneously, but is not widely used in clinical oculomotor laboratories [24]. It allows for a resolution of some minutes of arc and the linear range of this system is about 20 deg. Detailed properties of the MI method are listed in Table 1.

For a versatile application, Collewijn [25] developed a special flexible ring made of silicone rubber which can be fitted on the limbic area of the eye. The search coil is embedded in the ring. Despite the vast improvement due to the introduction of the silicone rubber ring, the MI method has the drawbacks of being expensive, causing (slight) irritation of the eye and requiring serious cooperation on the part of the subject. Eye irritation may even become prominent, although temporary, as reduction of visual acuity during the period of wearing the contact lens. Since the scleral contact lens can blur vision, relatively large visual targets (diameter 2 deg) are regularly used.

Simultaneous measurement of both eyes requires, apart from a second recording system, a silicone ring in each eye, thus increasing the problems of eye irritation and lead breakage.

A further improvement of the MI technique is the development of a soft contact-lens search coil [26]. Using this sensor, no topical anaesthetic need be applied. Furthermore, this sensor is inexpensive and simple to construct.

Another modification, called the double magnetic-induction method (DMI), of the search coil system was the elimination of the lead wires from the search coil [27, 28]. This, since these wires have proved to be a serious source of eye irritation and frequently break. Although the use of a coil without a lead has distinct advantages, such as increased comfort and elimination of malfunction due to broken leads, other problems are introduced in particular sensitivity to head translation. Several modifications and improvements in the magnetic-field generation and signal-detection electronics have been suggested [29–31]. Recently, a less expensive electronic system has been designed [32]. Undoubtedly further improvements of the MI and the DMI methods will take place in the near future, which will benefit the clinical applicability. Whatever the improvements will be, an eye-contacting device will always be necessary when using this method.

5. Summary

The following guidelines may be used in the selection and application of a suitable clinical eye-movement registration technique.

Method	Application in the measurement of:
ENG	conjugate horizontal saccadic eye movements (>10 deg) vestibular and caloric nystagmus optokinetic nystagmus
IRIS	all types of conjugate and disconjugate horizontal (<40 deg) and vertical eye movements (<25 deg), including smooth pursuit, vergence and fixation eye movements
MI–DMI	all types of oblique and rotatory eye movements (<30 deg)

References

1. Brandt T, Büchele W (1983): Augenbewegungsstörungen. Klink und elektronystagmographie. Gustav Fischer Verlag. Stuttgart. New York.
2. Leigh JR, Zee DS (1983): The neurology of eye movement. Philadelphia: FA Davis.
3. Yee RD (1983): Eye movement recording as a clinical tool. Ophthalmology, Vol 90(3): 211–22.
4. Levine JL (1984): Performance of an eyetracker for office use. Comput Biol Med, Vol 14(1): 77–89.
5. Young LR, Sheena D (1975): Survey of eye-movement recording methods. Behavior Research Methods and Instrumentation, Vol 7(5): 397–429.
6. Jones R (1973): Two-dimensional eye movement recording using a photo-electric matrix method. Vision Res, Vol 13: 425–431.
7. Heuningen van R, Goovaerts HG, de Vries FR (1984): A low-noise isolated amplifier system for electrophysiological measurements: basic considerations and design. Med Biol Eng Comput, 22: 77–85.
8. Bahill AT, McDonald JD (1983): Frequency limitations and optimal step size for the two-point central difference derivate algorithm with applications to human eye movement data. IEEE Trans Biomed Eng, Vol BME-30, 3: 191–194.
9. Yee RD, Schiller VL, Lim V, Baloh FG, Baloh RW, Honrubia V (1985): Velocities of vertical saccades with different eye-movement recording methods. Invest Ophthal, Vol 26: 938–944.
10. Collewijn H, van der Steen J, Steinman RM (1985): Human eye movements associated with

blinks and prolonged eyelid closure. J Neurophysiol, Vol 54, No 1: 11–27.

11. Cornsweet TN, Crane HD (1973): An accurate eye tracker using first and fourth Purkinje images. J Opt Soc Am, 63: 921–928.

12. Crane HD, Steele CM (1978): Accurate three-dimensional eyetracker. Applied Optics, Vol 17, 5: 691–704.

13. Bach M, Bouis D, Fischer B (1983): An accurate and linear infrared oculometer. J Neurosci Methods, 9: 9–14.

14. Eizenman M, Frecker RC, Hallett PE (1984): Precise non-contacting measurement of eye movements using the corneal reflex, Vision Res, Vol 24: 167–174.

15. Merchant J, Morrisette R, Porterfield JL (1974): Remote measurement of eye direction allowing subject motion over one cubic foot of space. IEEE Trans Biomed Eng, Vol BME-21, 4: 309–317.

16. Charlier JR, Hache JC (1982): New instrument for monitoring eye fixation and pupil size during the visual field examination. Med Biol Eng Comput, 20: 23–28.

17. Krueger H (1982): Gerat zur simultanen Registrierung von Blickrichtung, Vergenz und Pupillenweite. Biomedizinische Technik, Bd 27: 59–63.

18. Gauthier GM, Volle M (1975): Two-dimensional eye movement monitor for clinical and laboratory recordings. Electroenceph Clin Neurophysiol, 39: 285–291.

19. Bahill AT, Clark MR, Stark L (1975): Dynamic overshoot in the saccadic eye movements is caused by neurological control signal reversals. Exp Neurol, 48: 107–122.

20. Reulen JPH, Marcus JT, Koops D, de Vries F, Tiesinga G, Boshuizen K (1987): Precise recording of eye movement and pupillary reflex in man. To be published.

21. Comet B (1983): An eye movement recording method operating with a closed eye. Med Biol Eng Comput, 21: 628–631.

22. Reulen JPH, van Heuningen R, Tiesinga G, Bos JE (1986): A computerized eye-movement processor for clinical application: basic considerations and design. Med Biol Eng Comput, 24, 2: 309–315.

23. Robinson DA (1963): A method of measuring eye movement using a scleral search coil in a magnetic field. IEEE Trans Biomed Eng, Vol 10: 137–45.

24. Schlag J, Merker B, Schlag-Rey M (1983): Comparison of EOG and search-coil techniques in long-term measurements of eye position in alert monkey and cat. Vision Res, Vol 23, 10: 1025–1030.

25. Collewijn H, van der Mark F, Jansen TC (1975): Precise recording of human eye movements. Vision Res, Vol 15: 447–450.

26. Kenyon RV (1985): A soft contact-lens search coil for measuring eye movements. Vision Res, Vol 11: 1629–1633.

27. Reulen JPH, Bakker L (1982): The measurement of eye movement using double magnetic induction. IEEE Trans Biomed Eng, Vol BME-29, 11: 740–744.

28. Bour LJ, van Gisbergen JAM, Bruijns J, Ottes FP (1984): The double magnetic induction method for measuring eye movement: results in monkey and man. IEEE Trans Biomed Eng, Vol BME-31, 5: 419–427.

29. McElligott JG, Loughnane MH, Mays LE (1979): The use of synchronous demodulation for the measurement of eye movements by means of an ocular magnetic search coil. IEEE Trans Biomed Eng, Vol BME-26, 6: 370–374.

30. Optican LM, Frank DE, Smith BM, Colburn TR (1982): An amplitude and phase-regulating magnetic-field generator for an eye-movement monitor. IEEE Trans Biomed Eng, Vol BME-29, 3: 206–209.

31. Becker W, Renner A (1985): Measuring eye movements with a search coil: nonlinear filter allows simultaneous recording of horizontal and vertical eye position by means of the phase modulation method. Vision Res, Vol 11: 1755–1758.

32. Remmel RS (1984): An inexpensive eye movement monitor using the scleral search coil technique. IEEE Trans Biomed Eng, Vol BME-31, 4: 388–390.

Section III

Ophthalmic causes of diplopia

Intraocular causes of diplopia

J.A. OOSTERHUIS

A number of intraocular disturbances and diseases may cause diplopia.

The history of the patient is of utmost importance, especially the statement that diplopia is present when one of the eyes is occluded or is only present on binocular vision. *Binocular* diplopia may have an intraocular cause but as a rule the cause is located outside the eye in the ocular muscles, the innervation, or a more central part of the visual pathway. On the other hand, *monocular* diplopia as a rule is caused by an intraocular lesion.

1. Physiological versus pathological diplopia

When examining the patients one must in the first place differentiate between *physiological* and *pathological* diplopia. Physiological diplopia can easily be provoked by fixating an object at some distance and introducing another object nearby in the line of fixation; the latter object elicits diplopia. This type of diplopia is always present but as a rule is not observed in daily life owing to suppression. Diplopia develops when retinal images can not be fused any more and disparate retinal points are stimulated. On sudden awareness of physiological diplopia this may be considered to be an abnormal condition by the patient, who for this reason consults an ophthalmologist. When abnormal causes of diplopia have been excluded and the condition is considered to be of physiological nature, only explanation of the condition to the patient is required.

2. True and pseudo-diplopia

Secondly, one has to differentiate between *true* diplopia and *pseudo*-diplopia. There are two types of *pseudo*-diplopia: diplopia caused by astigmatism and diplopia caused by badly printed text giving the patient the impression of di-plopia. The latter is of no importance but the pseudo-diplopia due to astigmatism is quite a frequent finding in refractive ophthalmology. Some intellectual level of the patient is required to describe the pseudo-diplopia due to astigmatism: complaints of seeing double contours especially in vertical or horizontal direction corresponding with the axis of the astigmatism. Sometimes the remarks of the patient, which letters or what part of the letters are most blurred, are strongly indicative of this diagnosis and of the direction of the axis of the correcting cylindrical lens needed. There is a predisposition of those patients who draw linear designs for developing pseudo-diplopia even by a small degree of astigmatism; in these patients cylindrical refraction has to be carried out with care. Pseudo-diplopia diminishes when looking through a pinhole.

3. Monocular diplopia

In *monocular diplopia* the lesions may be located at different levels of the eye:

Corneal lesions, even when the cornea is completely clear such as in keratoconus and keratoglobus, may lead to a diminished visual acuity, but as a rule without complaints of diplopia. Contact lenses with too small a diameter combined with a large pupil at low level of illumination may lead to complaints of diplopia. A lens with high dioptric value, such as in aphakia, with a strong mobility in vertical direction may cause a vertical diplopia varying with blinking of the eyelids, which is not monocular but binocular.

Abnormal size and configuration of the *pupil*, such as in large peripheral iridectomies or iridodialysis after a blunt trauma, may cause complaints of monocular diplopia.

Complaints of monocular diplopia are common in incipient *cataract*. The diplopia is caused by a prismatic light shifting, which is caused by the clear normal lens structures, 'Wasserspalten', rather than by the cataractous structures. Monocular diplopia may even be the first complaint of the patient in the pre-stage of cataract. Visual acuity may still be normal. Retinoscopy clearly reveals the radial irregular pattern of the lens. Looking through a pinhole should diminish the complaints of diplopia and should improve vision, if decreased. Another pre-stage of cataract is the lens swelling associated with steadily increasing myopia; in this condition the central part of the lens is more myopic than the peripheral part; the different refractive conditions of cortex and nucleus of the lens may cause diplopia with the complaint of unsharp, double contours of all objects. *Subluxation of the lens*, either caused by a trauma or as part of Marfan's syndrome or Marchesani's syndrome, may cause monocular diplopia.

Abnormal conditions in the ocular fundus may cause an elevation or folding of the retina by many causes of great variety, such as subretinal exudation in senile maculopathy or central serous choriopathy, pigment-epithelial detachment, subretinal haemorrhages, or choroidal tumours such as melanoma or metastasis. Generally, the image of the patient is distorted irregularly in all directions, but in

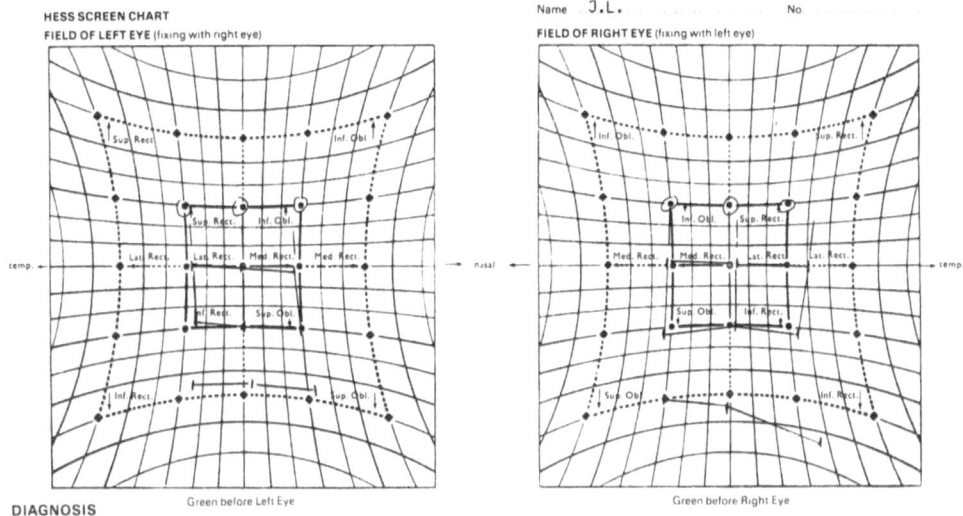

Figure 1.

some cases the distortion may be more or less unidirectional, for instance when retinal traction folds are running more or less parallel, which might be interpreted as diplopia. Vitreous cells and floaters and lesions of the optic disc and optic nerve as a rule do not induce complaints of diplopia.

Monocular diplopia and polyopia may be caused by lesions located in the central optical system or in the occipital lobe.

4. Binocular diplopia

Binocular diplopia may occur after extensive extra-ocular surgery, for instance after several retinal detachment operations. An example is given in the figure showing the Hess chart of a patient. Vertical diplopia occurred after two retinal detachment operations of the left eye in this patient with bilateral aphakia and corrected visual acuity of 1.0 of the right eye and 0.6 of the left eye. With prismatic correction the diplopia disappeared. Scar tissue resulting from the operations had restricted motility of the eye and caused diplopia. Similar conditions are found in symblepharon, for instance after chemical injury, and after surgery for recidivating pterygium.

Motility disturbances may also be caused by *periocular* inflammatory *conditions*, such as (epi-)scleritis, posterior scleritis, tenonitis and myositis, and other orbital processes. Orbital cellulitis complicating sinusitis may cause protrusion of the eye with complete immobility of the eye. Orbital tumours may restrict motility but it is remarkable that even a high degree exophthalmos, caused by a gradually increasing orbital tumour, does not necessarily lead to diplopia. Diplopia caused by motility disturbance after orbital trauma and diplopia in endocrine ophthalmopathy are discussed elsewhere (chapter 9).

Finally, we should not forget the *hysterical type* of monocular and sometimes binocular diplopia, which is not uncommon. However, one should not assume a psychological or psychiatrical background unless by thorough examination other causes of diplopia have been excluded.

Diplopia in concomitant strabismus and other disturbances of fusion

A.Th.M. VAN BALEN

The first and major symptom of many ocular motor disturbances is diplopia. This chapter describes causes of double vision, which can occur in *normal* eye movement.

1. Changes of suppression in concomitant squint due to treatment

Diplopia is generally not found in congenital strabismus because of the sensory adaptation i.e. suppression, amblyopia and/or abnormal retinal correspondence.

In adult life diplopia may occur in concomitant strabismus spontaneously or after orthoptic and surgical treatment. The following aetiological possibilities should be considered.

Suppression decreases spontaneously with time, but will most often decrease under the influence of orthoptic treatment especially during so called anti-suppression treatment, which is initially intended to provoke diplopia. Intensive treatment of amblyopia can also cause decrease of suppression, which in amblyopia, always exists in the binocular situation. This causes annoying diplopia of the peripheral visual fields [1].

Postoperative diplopia after strabismus convergens concomitans can be sensory, motor or sensory-motor origin [2].

According to Haase [3] in patients of more than 9 years of age, we may expect diplopia in 5% in the 6 months following operation. Haase describes diplopia especially in amblyopia with excentric fixation and consecutive exotropia. Todter [4] has seen short term diplopia in 9% of patients over the age of 18 with lasting diplopia in 1%.

Abnormal retinal correspondence is a risk factor and the chance of postoperative diplopia is also higher in exotropia than in esotropia and especially alternating exotropia [5]. Preoperative assessment of suppression in the amblyoscope or by wearing prisms does not give sufficient information to predict postoperative outcome. Postoperative incomitance causes diplopia because the image moves

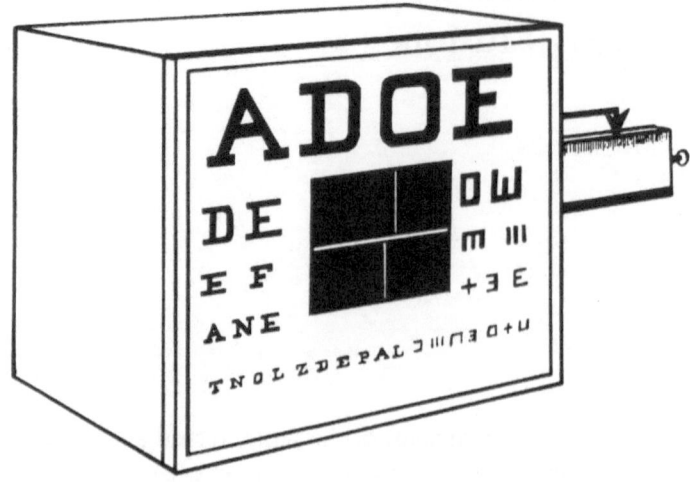

Figure 1. Crone's version of Ogle's apparatus (after Crone, Diplopia 1973).

over the retina. Postoperative overcorrection gives more diplopia than undercorrection, because the image falls far beyond the field of suppression. Postoperative diplopia gives an incentive to fusion and some surgeons prefer overcorrection for that reason. However, the line between postoperative binocular vision and diplopia is very small.

2. Disruption of abnormal and normal fusion

2.1. Latent strabism or heterophoria

An unexpected diplopia occurs in latent strabismus or heterophoria. This is usually a very annoying intermittant diplopia. It concerns the so called primary heterophoria; a concept introduced by Crone [6], distinct from other heterophorias and based on the existence of an abnormal fixation disparity curve, indicating abnormal fusion. The fusional eye movement in response to a retinal disparity is somewhat smaller than the disparity stimulus, especially in the extremes of forced convergence and divergence just before diplopia occurs. The residual disparity, which is called fixation disparity, is so small that there is no diplopia although the bifixation is not completely intact. The occurence of fixation disparity under the influence of 'base out prims' and 'base in prims' is easy to record with help of Crone's version of the instrument of Ogle (Fig. 1).

Identical images (optotypes) are presented to both eyes for peripheral fusion. The centre of these images contains no fusional contours, but two haploscopically visible lines mounted one above the other and capable of being moved horizon-

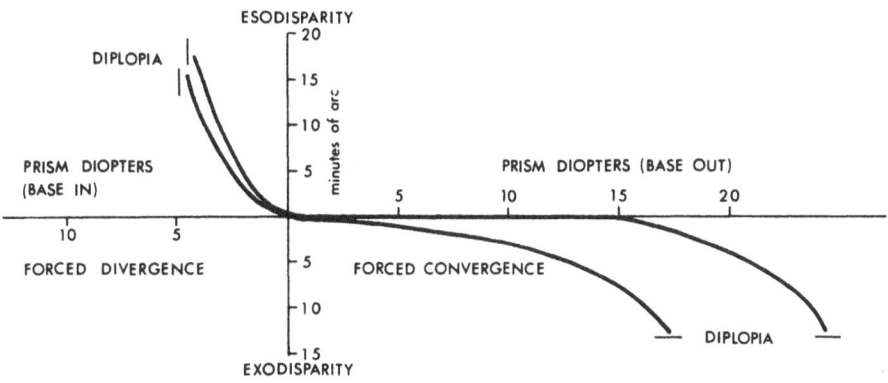

Figure 2. Normal curves and disparity curves at the extremes of convergence (after Crone, Diplopia 1973).

tally towards or away from each other. The upper line is illuminated by polarized light and is visible through a polaroid plate to the right eye only; the lower line is visible to the left eye only. When the lines are positioned in a way so that they appear subjectively to be continuous they are imaged on a row of corresponding points. If they do not objectively form a continuous line this indicates that peripheral fusion has occured between two slightly moving points.

Fixation disparity usually occurs at the limits of horizontal fusion and is the retinal stimulus to sustained fusional convergence and fusional divergence (Fig. 2).

In case of heterophoria, fixation disparity is already observed in the primary position and is then referred to as pathological fixation disparity. In these cases normal correspondence is present in only one position of the eyes, i.e. facultative micro anomaly or not at all, i.e. obligate micro anomaly (Figs. 3 and 4).

In the examination of a case of symptomatic heterophoria, especially a case of heterophoria with intermittent diplopia, the registration of the fixation disparity under the influence of prism loading is of prime importance. This applies to esophoria as well as to exophoria. It should be noted that esophoria is more often symptomatic in the sense of asthenopia. Suppression, if present, is mostly confined to the foveal area. In exophoria suppression is stronger and diplopia is only transiently present during the change from binocular vision to suppression in the deviated position. A typical example of diplopia in heterophoria is the esophoric patient in which the complaints can not be related to the degree of heterophoria; slight esophoria, normal amplitude of fusion and slight decrease of stereoscopic vision can only be invoked as the cause of diplopia on the basis of anomaly of fusion and micro-anomalous correspondence.

Strabismus convergens acutus of Bielschowsky in myopia and of Franceschetti in hypermetropia have both to be categorized in the same group [7]. Strabismus

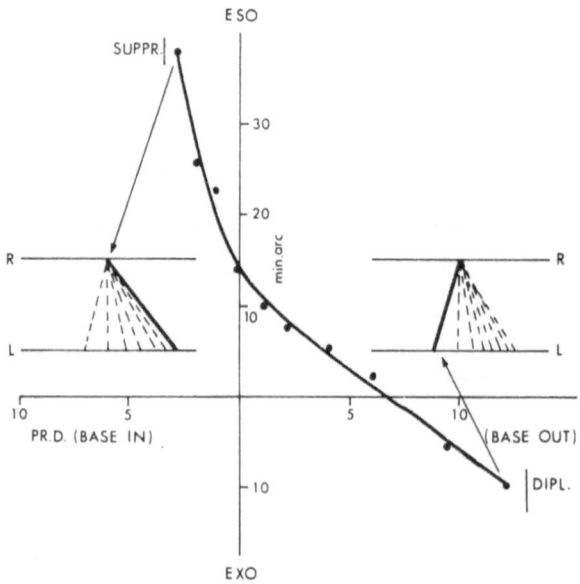

Figure 3. Facultative esodisparity curve (after Crone, Diplopia 1973).

acutus is found in older children and young adults and has to be considered as acute decompensation of pre-existent primary esophoria. The angle usually is great, as can be expected in large heterophoria.

2.2. Congenital or early infantile paralysis with suppression or binocular vision

In most congenital or early infantile paralysis, suppression or binocular vision are both present.

Binocular vision is present when fusion is strong enough to compensate, at least in certain gaze directions. This usually results in torticollis. Congenital paralysis, especially those of vertical muscles can be kept latent for years in this way. When fusion decreases the deviation can become manifest. Characteristic features of those cases are intermittent diplopia and a large amplitude of fusion in one vertical direction. Congenital obliquus superior paralysis is an example. The mean deviation angle of congenital trochlearis paralysis is 5° more than that of acquired trochlearis paralysis. This experimental fact allows us to test the hypothesis that congenital trochlearis paralysis is not paralysis alone, but a combination of paralysis and primary heterophoria. The abnormal fusion in vertical fixation disparity is easily disrupted in later years, which results in intermittant diplopia.

Patients with the Stilling Turck Duane syndrome sometimes have zones of suppression, fusion and diplopia, or a combination in their visual field. Some-

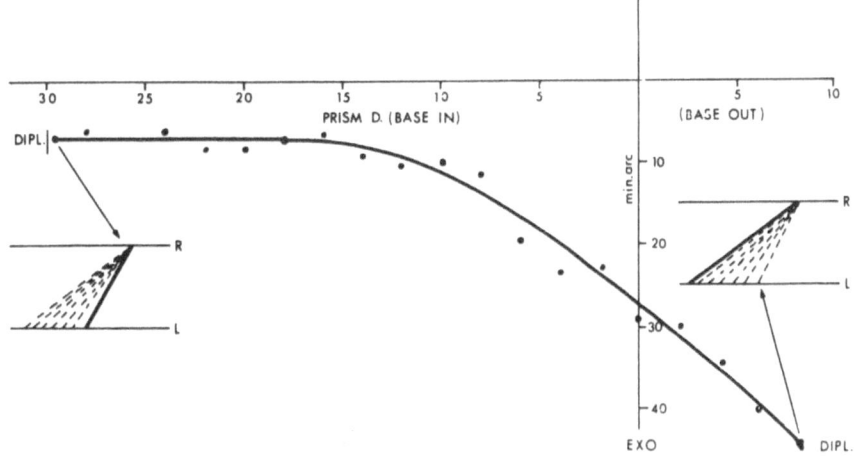

Figure 4. Obligate exodisparity curve (after Crone, Diplopia 1973).

times the diplopia field lies between fusion on one side and binoculair vision on the other side. The complaints are not correlated with the orthoptic findings, even when using the phase difference haploscope of Aulhorn.

2.3. Disturbances of disjunctive eye movements

Disturbances of the disjunctive eye movements nearly always lead to diplopia. The convergence insufficiency of older people causes diplopia while reading. Diplopia can also be caused by convergence spasm. This spasm, recognizable by concomitant miosis and accommodation, is a functional disturbance that is often superposed on esophoria, intermittent exophoria, paresis of the superior oblique, paresis of other muscles or latent nystagmus. A characteristic of this convergent spasm is that the angle of convergence decreases when the fixating eye is in abduction.

2.4. Acquired disturbances of fusion

Important in general ophthalmological practice is the diplopia occurring as a result of acquired disturbance of fusion; i.g. due to head trauma [8] or caused by fever, intoxication, exhaustion, etc. Pre-existent anomalous fusion, as expressed by a fixation disparity, can more easily be disrupted by the above mentioned factors.

Postcommotional and postcontusional fusion disturbances can lead to protracted headache, asthenopia or clear cut diplopia, which needs prism corrections.

94

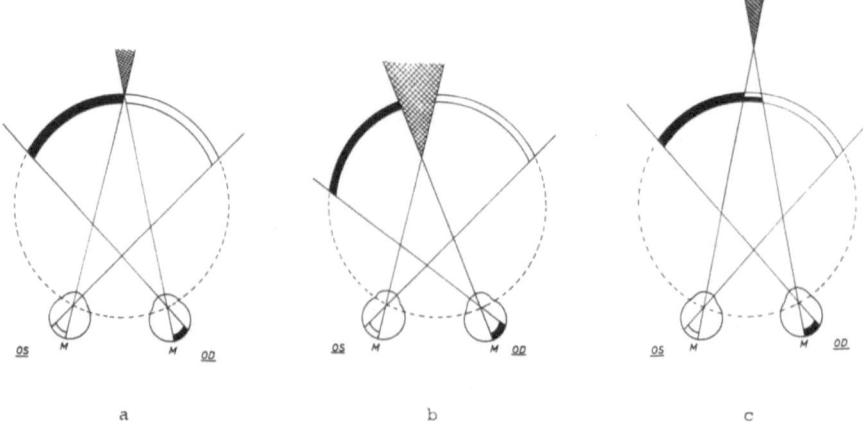

a   b   c

Figure 5. The binocular visual field in bitemporal hemianopia. a. Orthophoria; b. Esophoria; c. Exophoria.

3. Fusion deficiencies by visual field defects

The importance of peripheral visual fields for fusion is manifest in the disturbances that can occur with visual field defects. In bilateral central scotomas fusion may not be disturbed, but in concentric narrowing of the fields and bitemporal hemianopia fusion defects can be found. There is often poor apposition of the hemi-fields in patients with bitemporal hemianopia (Fig. 5a). In the convergent position disjunction of the ocular axes occurs, troubling the reading process (Fig. 5b). In the divergent position of the eye axes [9] diplopia of the center field occurs (Fig. 5c). Elkington [10] found diplopia in 98 out of 250 patients with pituitary adenoma. Fusion can be disturbed by metamorphopsia and foveal diplopia can exist in cases with peripheral fusion. In aniseikonia and cyclotropia the reverse is the case: normal bifoveal fixation with disparity in the periphery. Foveal fusion alone is not sufficient to maintain orthophoria.

4. Summary

In concomitant squint the causes of diplopia usually are shift in the mutual position of normal cooperating eyes, decrease and/or shift of suppression, and disruption of fusion, which is often abnormal.

References

1. Crone RA, Bosch van den JG (1970): The sweet and bitter fruits of orthoptic exercises. In: Winkelman JE, Crone RA, red. Perspectives in Ophthalmology, Amsterdam: Excerpta Medica, 171–8.
2. Pigassou (1963): Diplopie post-operatoire durable dans le strabisme convergent concomitant. Etude clinique. Traitement. Bull Soc Ophthal France, 9–10: 1–10.
3. Haase W, Ehlers P, Sautter H (1979): Die Diplopie-Haufigkeit im Rahmen der operativen Behandlung des Begleitschielens. Klin Mbl Augenheilk, 175: 375–84.
4. Todter F (1981): Diplopie nach Schieloperation bei Erwachsenen. Klin Mbl Augenheilk, 179: 496–500.
5. Schlossman A, Muchnick RS, Stern KS (1983): The surgical management of intermittent exotropia in adults. Ophthalmology, 90:.1166–71.
6. Crone RA (1973): Diplopia. Amsterdam: Excerpta Medica.
7. Thomas MCh (1955): Le traitement de la diplopie. Bull Soc Ophthal France, 18: 1–23.
8. Pratt-Johnson JA (1979): Acquired central disruption of fusional amplitude. Ophthalmology 86: 2140–2.
9. Nachtigaller H, Hoyt WF (1970): Storungen des Seheindruckes bei bitemporale hemianopsie und Verschiebung der Sehachsen. Klin Mbl Augenheilk 156: 8321–36.
10. Elkington SG (1968): Pituitary adenoma. Preoperative symptomatology in a series of 260 patients. Brit J Ophthal 52: 322–8.

Diplopia resulting from mechanical causes in the orbit

L. KOORNNEEF

Intraorbital mechanical causes of diplopia may be classified into five groups: 1. orbital tumours, 2. Graves ophthalmopathy; 3. orbital fractures; 4. myositis; 5. foreign bodies.

1. Orbital tumours

Eye motility disturbances and complaints of double vision in intra-orbital tumours mainly depend on their location and nature. Slowly progressive, noninvasive, benign retrobulbar tumours usually do not induce severe ocular motility disturbances. However, if located in the anterior part and surrounded by more extensive connective tissue they frequently do. Rapidly growing tumours, benign (pseudolymphoma) or malign (non-Hodgkin lymphoma, adenocystic carcinoma, metastasis, melanoma) more generally cause diplopia whatever the location. The most severe motility disturbance may be often seen in metastasis of breastcarcinoma in which eye movement is limited in all directions. In these cases orthoptic examination is helpful for follow up and to determine whether treatment has been successful (chapter 24).

2. Graves, ophthalmopathy

Eye abnormalities due to thyroid disorders are called Graves' ophthalmopathy which may present in six different forms. 1. Signs with no symptoms (limited to upperlid retraction, stare and lidlag). 2. Soft tissue involvement (conjunctival and eyelid-oedema). 3. Proptosis. 4. Extra-ocular muscle involvement with diplopia. 5. Corneal involvement. 6. Visual loss due to optic nerve compression by muscle enlargement and/or intraorbital pressure rise.

Enlargement of eyemuscles in Graves' ophthalmopathy causes imbalance of eye movements. This enlargement is the result of a sterile, inflammatory process with reactive fibrosis resulting in impaired relaxation of eye muscles. Fibrosis in Graves' ophthalmology does not only affect eye muscles but also orbital connective tissue resulting in limit excursion of the eyeball. This is supported by high resolution CT scan examination showing increase of connective tissue in the orbit.

Beneficial results of strabismus surgery in patients with Graves' disease may be explained by the fact that the contraction power of the muscle is unaffected.

3. Orbital fractures

The assumption that eye-muscles are trapped in fractured bone should be abandoned as a basis for surgery. CT scan investigations and surgical exploration have demonstrated that eye muscles are hardly ever trapped in the fracture sutures. Extensive neuroradiological examination in orbital trauma has revealed other possible causes of eye motility disturbances which may be due to: 1. Posttraumatic oedema and bleeding. 2. Oculomotor nerve palsy. 3. Enophthalmos changing the contraction force of eye-muscles. Posterior displacement of the globe causes insufficient eyemuscle force causing double vision in extreme directions of gaze. 4. Scars formed in the connective tissue as seen on high resolution CT scan.

CT scan and clinical examination (cover test, forced duction test) and eye movement exercises are major factors in the decision between conservative or operative treatment.

4. Orbital myositis

Orbital myositis is a rare condition caused by a sterile inflammation of one or more eye-muscles. It may be to been distinguished from Graves' disease by pain during eye movement. Redness and vascular swelling around the insertion of the affected muscle in the conjuctiva supports the diagnosis. In contrast to Graves' ophthalmopathy, usually affecting the whole muscle, myositis only involves the posterior part leading to swelling as can be demonstrated on CT scan. Immediate treatment with steroids is of the utmost importance to avoid scar formation.

5. Intra orbital foreign bodies

Intra orbital foreign bodies, if located behind the globe, hardly ever cause limited eye movement. If however the intra-orbital foreign body is located in the anterior part at eyeball level or at the trochlea, motility disturbance may be severe. As already mentioned before, fibrosis around the foreign body is mainly responsible. It affects the normal function of the intraorbital connective tissue. Refined information can be gained by high resolution CT scan showing the exact location of the foreign body. Surgery can be performed together with resection of the scar tissue. To prevent adhesions 'Healon' is left behind.

Glass, caused by windscreen accidents is the most frequently observed foreign body. Incurable diplopia may result due to wood splinters. These should be removed immediately. They may give rise to even more scar tissue than glass.

References

Koornneef L, Melief CJM, Peterse HL, Wilmink JM (1983): Orbit II nr. 1 p. 1–10. Wegener's granulomatosis of the orbit, diagnostic and therapeutic problems.

vd Gaag R, Koornneef L, v Heerde P, Vroom ThM, Pegels JG, Feltkamp CA, Peeters HJF, Gillissen JPA, Bleeker GM, Feltkamp TEW (1984): Lymphoid proliferations on the Orbit: malignant or benign? Brit J Ophthal Vol. 68 p. 892–900.

Koornneef L (1984): Orbital bony and connective tissue anatomy. The eye and orbit in thyroid disease p. 5–23 Raven Press New York.

Mailette de Buy Wenniger-Prick LJJM, v Mourik-Noorderbos AM, Koornneef L (1986): Squint surgery in patients with Graves ophthalmopathy. Doc Ophthal 61 219–221.

Vascular causes of diplopia

R.J.W. DE KEIZER

The vascular system is an integral part of the anatomy and the functions of the muscles and nerve tissue. Abnormalities in this system can be a possible cause of neuro-ophthalmologic and orbital syndroms. Motility disturbances may be caused by excessive blood supply to the muscle with mechanical disturbances as well as by compression, dislocation or vascular disturbance of the nerve (e.g. geographical insufficiency for the large arterial vessel trunk or a local vasculopathy by diabetes mellitus).

In examining diplopia it is important to differentiate and determine on clinical grounds where the disorder is located in the chain formed by the unit: nucleus, nerve and muscle. The pattern of the motility disturbances, whether or not in conjunction with other symptoms, should lead to diagnosis. The role of the motility disturbances in the symptomatology can sometimes be a major one, at other times subordinate.

The next considerations start from that point of view where motility disturbances are regarded as most *important* expression of the symptomatology.

1. Aetiology

Disorders in the afferent and efferent system of the blood flow can cause an insufficiency of oxygen and nutrition at one side or a surplus of the same at the other. Origin of signs and symptoms depends on the quality of the blood, the vessel wall and the function of the collateral system. Disorders to be expected in the chain of nucleus, nerve and muscle are as follows.

1.1. Insufficiency of blood supply

1. Arterial deviations. a. Occlusion or stenosis of the arterial system in neck, skull base or orbit resulting in ischaemia or hypoxemia. b. Cardial or steal syndromes.

102

c. Spasm, under the influence of regulation or dysregulation of autonomic impulses such as migraine.

2. Malfunctions of the venous system. a. blockage, e.g. venous thrombosis, phlebitis, occlusion. b. stasis or reverse venous blood flow under higher pressure.

3. Combinations of 1 and 2. Such as arteriovenous fistulas or malformations. If a large shunt is present it is possible that the surroundings of the relevant artery lacks sufficient blood supply resulting in hypoxemia or ischaemia.

1.2. Oversupply of blood

Our body is built to cope with oversupply of blood under normal anatomic proportions. This coping however, depends on collateral circulation and a regulation mechanism. Secondary changes therefore can be the cause of signs and symptoms.

1. Arteriovenous fistulae. Local efferent disturbances and venous pressure increase with secondary hypoxemia can be the cause of neural and muscular disorders. An increase in volume of the muscle can also be a possible cause of motility problems.

2. Venous malformation, varix. The same disorders can be encountered as under 1.1., the local hypoxemia will be of lesser nature.

3. Blood vessel tumours, haemangiomas. These disorders can be the cause of bloodpooling with local disorders, as well as being the cause of steal phenomena. Capillary haemangiomas can induce mechanical astigmatism, or ptosis resulting in amblyopia.

1.3. Mechanical restrictions due to space-occupying processes

1. As 1.2.
2. Aneurysm in the orbit is a rare condition, however, more frequent is the giant aneurysm of the carotid artery near the ophthalmic branch, expressed in the orbital apex syndrome [1].
3. Haemorrhage in the orbit or conjunctiva.

The above mentioned disorders have in themselves again various causes which need to be detected. Some causes of the blocking or stenotic mechanism of the arterial and venous systems (groups 1.1.1a and 1.1.2a) are:
1. degeneration: atherosclerosis, fibromuscular dysplasia, Ehlers-Danlos syndrome, pseudoxanthoma elasticum.
2. inflammation of the vascular wall e.g. arteritis, syphilis.
3. vasculopathy: diabetes mellitus, hypertension, collagenousis, etc.
4. congenital: arteriovenous fistulae, haemangiomas, Sturge-Weber syndrome, and aneurysm.
5. traumatic: accidents, surgery.

2. Diagnostic procedures

A diagnostic procedure is proposed for examination of patients with oculomotor disturbances (Table 1). Previous history and the presence of other (ophthalmological) features are of main importance. Orthoptic investigation including Hess or Maddox procedure is necessary to localise abnormal eye movement.

Special attention has to be payed to the possibility of sympathic or parasympathic system involvement, which often interferes with third nerve palsies. Testing the pupils may distinguish the different causes. A third nerve palsy with abnormal delayed pupil or a sluggished pupillary reflex is strongly indicative for an aneurysm in the vicinity of the brainstem, while normal pupils point to diabetic autonomic neuropathy. A lesion of the third nerve nucleus is often bilateral, with asymmetrical signs. Detailed diagnostic procedures will be discussed further in the different types of vascular disorders. Lastly, vascular examination of the head and neck vessels by palpation, inspection and auscultation. The application of supporting examinations for localisation and possible therapy depends subsequently on the practical clinical diagnosis at the first instance.

2.1 Insufficient blood supply

In noninvasive examination of carotid stenosis the combination of Doppler ultrasound and oculoplethysmography (OPG) is able to detect vessel diameter reduction of 70% or more in at least 96% of the patients [2, 3, 4]. For exact location of the arterial lesions, Seldinger catheter angiography is most appropiate. For suspected venous abnormalities (orbital) venography is the method of choice. Intravenous subtraction angiography (iv-DSA) is a method which detects

Table 1. Order of clinical examination

- inspection of the face and eyelids (capillary or mixed haemangiomas, varix)
- external aspect of the eyeball (typical vascular loops, pulsating exophthalmus)
- visual acuity (apex syndrome)
- visual fields (chiasm, occipital lesion)
- fundus pathology (papilloedema, hydrocephalus, subdural haematoma)
  -diabetic retinopathy
  -ischaemia
  -venous congestion
  -arteriovenous malformation (Wyburn-Mason syndrome)
  -cilioretinal anastomosis (meningeoma)
- orbital inspection: exophthalmos, palpation, auscultation
- pupillary reactions
- trigeminal signs

both arterial and venous abnormalities [5, 6]. This method needs a low dose of contrast and small catheters and leads to less complications. A disadvantage is the possibility of less optimal visualisation. However, sometimes extensive radiological- and noninvasive examination is not necessary. An isolated sixth nerve palsy is usually due to self limiting nonspecific vasculopathies (hypertension, atherosclerosis, diabetic vasculopathy). This is valid as long as there is no progression caused by other underlying pathology [7].

2.2 Blood oversupply

In this case the noninvasive test as the Doppler velocity measurements, haematotachography, plays a prominent part [8, 9]. Special patterns are detected in the carotid- or the orbital vessels in case of dural- or direct carotid cavernous fistulas [8, 9, 10, 11]. A high 'venous flow' can be found in this Doppler method [8, 9] in the venous malformation with flow via the orbit. Doppler haematotachography, sometimes ultrasound and orbital venography can be useful, but to decide to surgical or invasive therapy (e.g. balloon embolisation) carotid angiography is necessary [9]. In space-occupying processes of the orbit ultrasonography is a first diagnostic examination and can produce quick results regarding localisation and type of tumour [12, 13].

2.3 Mechanical restriction due to space-occupying vascular lesions

In this group of disorders CT scan and ultrasonography are investigation methods of the first choice. Catheter angiography may be necessary to assure the diagnosis and sometimes to procede embolisation which then prevents surgery. Until recently the brainstem was rather unexplored, this because CT scan investigation often failed to detect lesions in such a small region. Nowadays, nuclear magnetic resonance imaging (MRI) [14] has become a diagnostic tool especially for the brainstem (i.e. vascular malformations resulting in oculomotor disturbance). But a final diagnosis cannot be made until during surgery or histological examination [15–17].

3. Signs and symptoms of ocular motility disturbances in relation to different vascular causes

3.1 Insufficient blood supply

3.1.1 Arterial system
Vertebrobasilar occlusion or stenosis. The major collateral system of the basilar

artery contains the Willis circle, the external carotid and the vertebral artery branches. Minor collateral circulation passes via the superior- and inferior cerebellar, the spino-radial and the arterio-cervical arteries. Gaze evoked nystagmus, horizontal gaze paralysis, internuclear ophthalmoplegia and cranial nerve abnormalities may occur in combination with ataxia and hemiplegia, uni- or bilateral. Eye symptoms (including motility disturbances) are found on about 50% with these disorders [18].

A transient motility disturbance or visual loss is often the presenting symptom of vertebro basilar stenosis caused by arteriosclerosis, embolia or arteritis [19].

Internal carotid stenosis. The features of internal carotid abnormalities vary largely and also depend on collateral circulation. Two-third of the cerebral hemispheres and both eyes, receive blood via the internal carotid arteries. The collateral circulation is made up by the contralateral internal carotid artery, both external carotid arteries, the circle of Willis and the basilar artery. Hemiplegia, amaurosis fugax and visual field defects form main events; ocular motility disturbances may occur but are not specific for the diagnosis (chapter 20).

Giant cell arteritis. Giant cell arteritis or temporal arteritis are well known causes of acute anterior ischaemic optic neuropathy (AION). Ophthalmoplegia in these conditions is less common. Arteritis involves either the supplying vessels of the nerves or the orbital branches supplying the ocular muscles [20].

An isolated six nerve palsy with normal erythrocyte sedimentation rate (ESR) excludes the possibility of arteritis and is more likely due to diabetes mellitus [7[.

Ophthalmoplegia due to diabetes mellitus. As already stated above, isolated third or six nerve palsy is often seen in the elderly and may be the first sign of diabetes mellitus (50%) [21]. This is a mononeuritis caused by a vasculopathy of supplying blood vessels. Histological findings are a pronounced enlargement and hyalinisation of the vessel wall in small arteries and capillary tissue with a stenotic microvascular ischaemic lesion. This is particularly seen in that part of the third nerve, which relates close to the cavernous sinus. The vasculopathy causes demyelinisation, which remyelinates spontaneously. It occurs often in the junction of two arterial supply systems [7].

From a diagnostic point of view one has to realise that oculomotor paresis in diabetes mellitus is seen in combination with normal pupil(-reaction). At present there is no good explanation for this phenomenon. However, suggestions have been made that it is probably due to the peripheral localisation of pupillary motor fibres [22]. If abnormal pupil reaction is found in a patient with already known diabetes mellitus it still points to an aneurysm, which should be investigated further. However, 'pupilsparing', third nerve palsy may occur in aneurysm. In patients with a normal pupillary reaction, aged 50 or more, and complete third nerve palsy angiography is not necessary. However, if incomplete third nerve palsy is present, particularly sparing the inferior oculomotor division, angiography has to be performed. In patients with a subnormal pupillary reaction and complete third nerve palsy an aneurysm has to be excluded by angiography, unless there are clear cut vasculopathic findings [40]. If third nerve palsy is found in a patient without known diabetes mellitus a glucose tolerance test has to be performed.

Ophthalmoplegic migraine. The clinical picture of migraine is: bilateral, central or paracentral scotomas suddenly occuring in the centre of visual field, enlarging and increasing in peripheral direction. This will last 20–40 minutes and may appear already in early youth together with pain around the eye. This occurrence is prevalent in children of approximately 10 years old, is accompanied with headache surrounding the eye. Headache is not always present [23]. In ophthalmoplegic migraine a third nerve palsy and pupil dilatation are often seen, which recover within one to four weeks. It is suggested that third nerve palsy results from enlargement and stretching of the carotid artery or spasm of the microvascular supply of the nerve itself. Ophthalmoplegic migraine in senility has to be distinguished from transient ischaemic attacks (TIA's), which often occur together with dizziness or more specific symptoms related to vertebrobasilar insufficiency [23].

3.1.2 Venous system

Cavernous sinus thrombosis. Septic or aseptic venous thrombosis may cause bizarre ocular motility disturbances, either or not in combination with frontal- and maxillary nerve or the fifth nerve abnormalities. A bilateral six nerve lesion is highly suspective for a cavernous sinus thrombosis or obstruction. Depending on the extent of the thrombosis one or more nerves may be affected unilaterally or bilaterally. This is certainly the case if primary infection is of facial origin. In the Parkinsonian concept [24] local venous thrombosis may occur after traumatic damage of the internal carotid artery in- or outside the cavernous sinus. Harris [25] histologically found an area with trabecular or cavernous aspects and a three part division: medial, antero-inferior and postero-superior part. Following the solid cramping of this area the bleeding will be blocked. These traumatic cavernous sinus events seemed to be of selflimiting origine.

The Tolosa-Hunt syndrome. This 'painful ophthalmoplegia' is caused by an unknown, nonspecific granulomatous inflammation of the superior ophthalmic vein or the cavernous sinus and is closely related to orbital pseudo-tumours. This inflammation spreads to the surrounding structures, such as adventitia of the carotid artery and the abducens nerve. No systemic reaction is found. Except for all three oculomotor nerves the ophthalmic trigeminal nerve root is involved, which results in pain or hypaesthesia in that region.

Mechanical movement disturbances may be also the results of myositis (and proptosis). The real Tolosa-Hunt syndrome often occurs acute and reacts well on treatment with steroids, which therefore can be used for diagnostic purposes. CT scan and blood analysis eliminate other conditions, i.e. collagen disorders, temporal arteritis, perinodal-arteritis, giant aneurysm, diabetic vasculopathy, lymphoma, carcinoma, meningioma and syphilis [26, 27]. The Tolosa-Hunt syndrome improves nearly always but may relaps thereafter.

The cavernous sinus inflammation reveals often parasympathic as well as sympathic pupillary signs. The pupil on the affected side is medium large and reacts poorly on light. Pharmacological pupil examination shows immediate reaction on pilocarpin 1/6% and adrenalin 1/1000 or one of both. Sometimes, both systems are either partially or totally affected.

The diagnosis is based on clinical features and radiological results, while surgical biopsy is not without risk and of small value [28]. A CT scan is necessary to exclude a tumour, which may give diagnostic difficulties while reacting on steroids. Orbital phlebography reveals (partly) occlusion of the superior ophthalmic vein or cavernous sinus, while arteriography demonstrates a minor restriction of the internal carotid artery in the cavernous sinus region.

Treatment with steroids results in immediate improvement but it is important to exclude a malignant tumour with CT because this tumour can react also for a period.

Stress may play an important role [41]. In theory a disturbance of adaptation on stress may induce an activation of the hypothalamic serotonin secretion and a spasm of the veins of hypothalamic region with decreasing of ACTH/steroid secretion. These reactions can be the impuls of inflammation and venous obstruction and a cause of the Tolosa-Hunt syndrome.

3.2 Surplus of blood supply

Carotid cavernous fistula (CCF). This is due to abnormal communication between either the internal or external carotid artery (or branches) and the cavernous sinus or the surrounding venous system. Fistulas strictly limited to the orbit may result in abnormal ocular motility [8].

Different types of CCF may be distinguished [9, 10].

1. The direct carotid-cavernous fistula. The internal carotid artery and the cavernous sinus fistel are either due to trauma or a ruptured aneurysm located in the cavernous sinus.

2. The dural CCF depends on: a) meningeal branches of the internal carotid artery = internal dural carotid cavernous fistulas; b) meningeal branches of the external carotid artery = external dural carotid cavernous fistulas.

Direct communications between internal carotid artery and cavernous sinus are prominent causes of pulsating proptosis, brisk ocular motility disturbances and glaucoma. A six nerve palsy results from marked increased pressure in the

108

cavernous sinus, which probably causes compression against the petroclinoidal ligament or the internal capsula, as well as poor arterial blood supply of the posterior meningeal artery. The abducens nerve is most vulnerable, because of running freely through the cavernous sinus and therefore susceptible for changes in intracranial pressure. Surprisingly, the sixth nerve sometimes has several roots all originating from the same nerve [25]. It is not clear, whether this variation contributes to or provides pathology. The abducens nerve is most vulnerable, which results in more longstanding abducens palsy than other oculomotor disturbance after trauma or successful embolectomy of a fistula.

The third and fourth nerve are embedded in connective tissue of two dura lamellae in the cavernous wall and therefore protected [24, 25]. Signs specific for dural fistula are exophthalmos, abnormal characteristic epibulbar vessel loops and glaucoma [8, 10, 12]. Abnormal ocular motility is frequent, however not specific (Fig. 1) [8, 12]. These features may have a mechanical origin, because the orbit is filled with venous congestive blood (Fig. 2) or by muscle expansion resulting from venous congestion and hypoxia [29]. Muscle thickening is clearly visible on CT scan examination and will disappear after successful treatment.

At present there is no eye movement abnormality specific for CCF (carotid

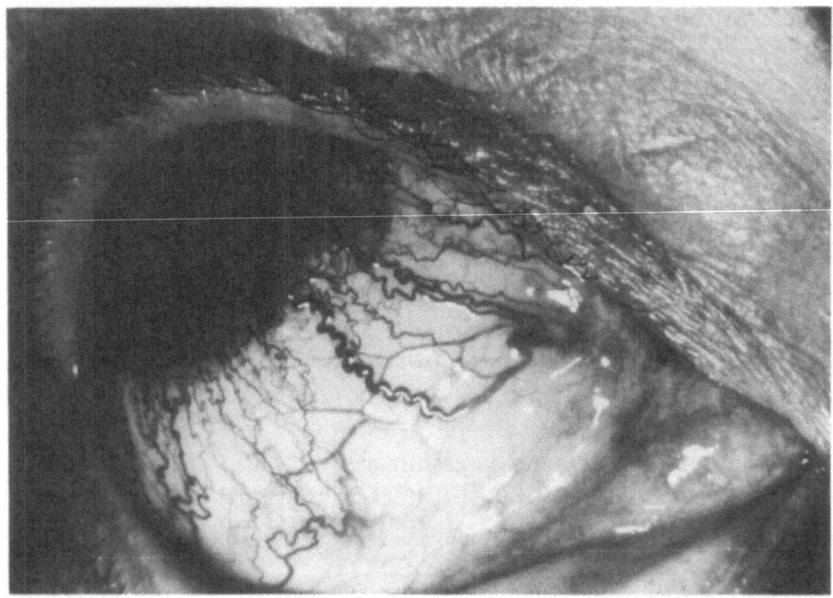

A

Figure 1. A) a 53-year-old woman with the special epibulbar loops of a spontaneous carotid cavernous fistula and a 7 mm proptosis of the right eye. B) motility is decreased downwards in the first period of signs and symptoms. C) motility disturbances are increased several months later. D) the angiography shows an internal carotid cavernous dural fistula on the right (+ left) side. Spontaneous recovery with conservative treatment.

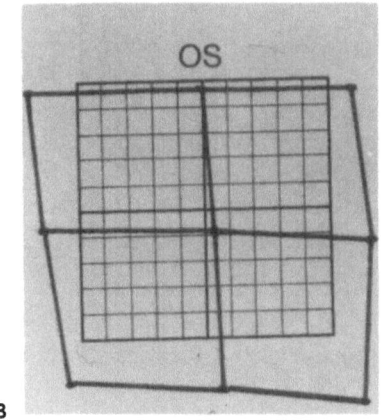 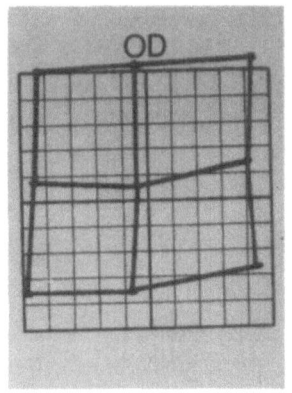

Figure 1.B) Hess chart.

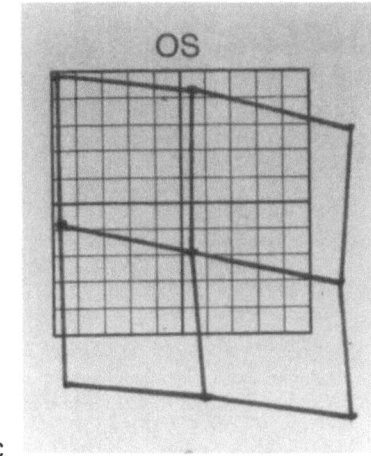 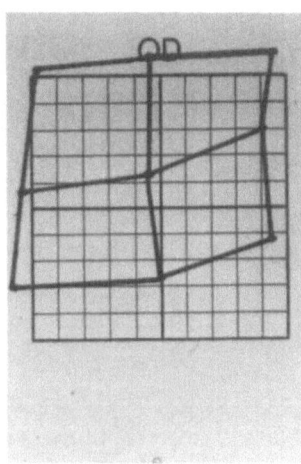

Figure 1.C) Hess chart 9 months later.

110

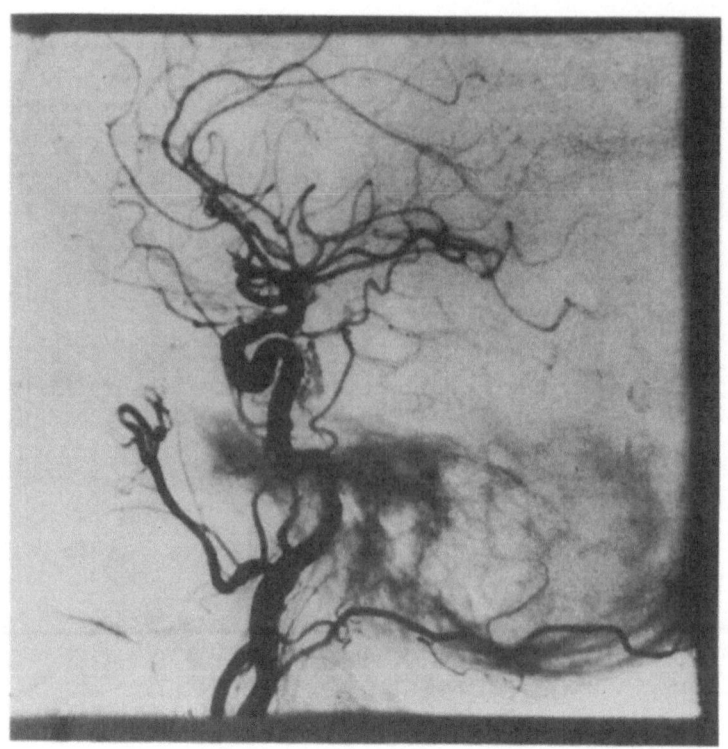

L.

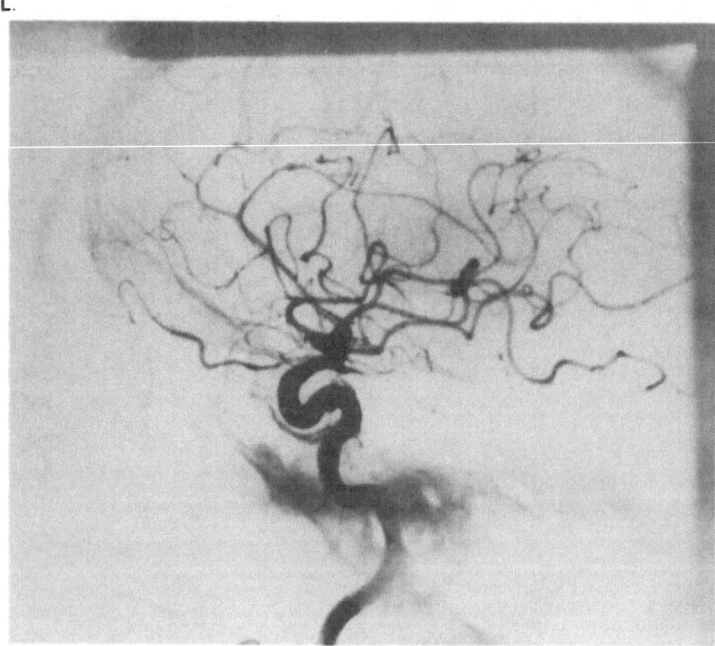

D   R.

Figure 1.D) Legend see page 108.

cavernous fistulas). However, Leonard [29] describes the six nerve as most frequently affected. He suggest that direct damage or pressure caused by the fistula is of main importance. Treatment of direct fistulas consists of balloon embolisation to eliminate the shunt and to remain intact flow of the internal carotid artery [9, 30]. If this is not successful muscle embolisation with proximal and distal closure of the carotid artery is applied (method Hamby [8]). Dural fistulae can demonstrate a spontaneous regression so invasive treatment is mostly not necessary. Observation and ophthalmological treatment (as therapy for the glaucoma) is the first choice and spontaneous thrombosis of the venous canal may occur [8, 10]. In progressive fistulas of the external carotid artery gelfoam embolisation may be considered [31].

Venous malformation varix haemangioma. Eye movement abnormalities in these conditions are due to impediments in the orbit or to local disorders in the muscle congestion (Fig. 3) [8, 12].

Capillary haemangioma. A capillary haemangioma is often visible at birth or shortly thereafter. The vascular tumour increases rapidly during the first year with a more gradual progression later (Fig. 4). Induction of astigmatism or ptosis may occur in this vessel tumour and therefore results in amblyopia. Intensive follow-up by an ophthalmologist and orthoptic treatment (training) are required [32]. Further therapy is preferably conservative. Only disfigurative swelling or growth over the pupil needs active treatment. Intra lesional steroids, surgery or radiotherapy can be performed [33]. Side effects of these treatments are meta-bolic disorders, serious loss of blood, traumatic injuries or decreased growth of facial bones. If progressive, capillary haemangioma have to be distinguished from arteriovenous malformations [8, 31]. Ocular motility disorders can be due to ptosis or occur if the orbit relates to the supply route. Displacement of the eyeball with disturbances of binocular vision may be seen in this stage. In serious facial disfiguration embolisation of the external carotid artery branches is considered and followed by local extirpation [31, 30].

The syndrome of Louis Barr. This is a seldom seen familiar phakomatosis with teleangiectasias of the conjunctival and small skin vessels, concurrent with neu-rological disturbances, i.e. progressive ataxia. The disorder starts with skin signs usually at 4 to 6 years ago (i.e. café au lait spots). The oculomotor disturbance is prominent as ocular motor apraxia.

3.3 Space-occupying vascular lesions

All under mentioned anomalies may space-occupying vascular lesions. Another

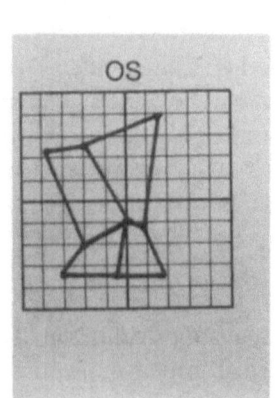

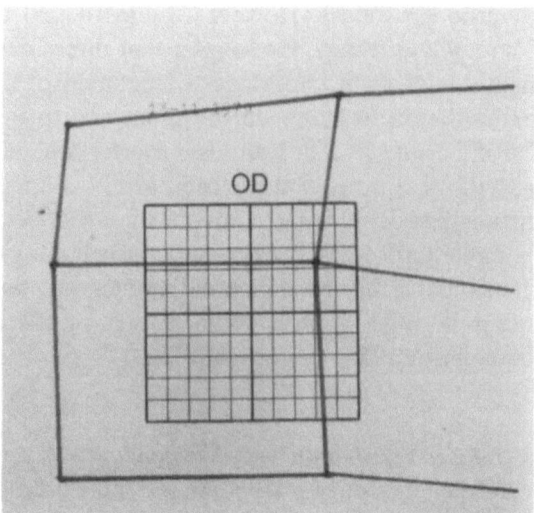

A

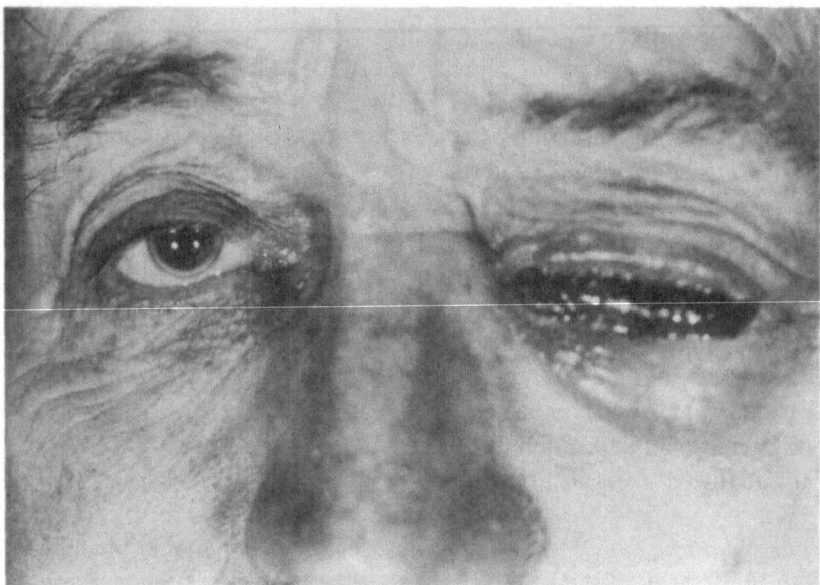

B

Figure 2. A) Hess scheme of a 65-year-old man with an internal carotid cavernous dural fistula of the left side with total ophthalmoplegia in the period of spontaneous thrombosis of the orbital veins and spontaneous recovery. B) clinical picture at that period. C) recovery with only an exotropia, later on an exophoria. D) clinical picture at that period.

113

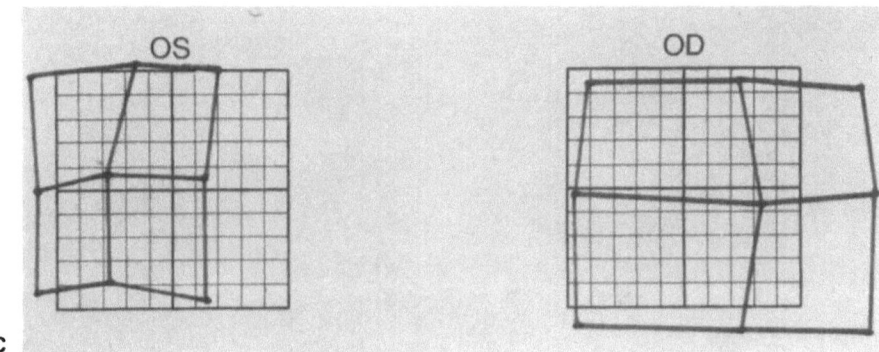

C

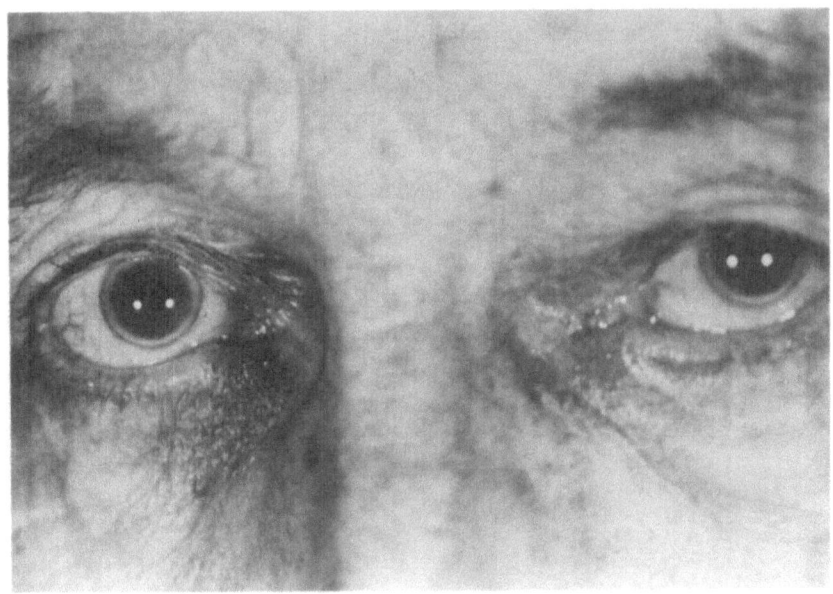

D

Figure 2.C) and D) Legend see page 112.

114

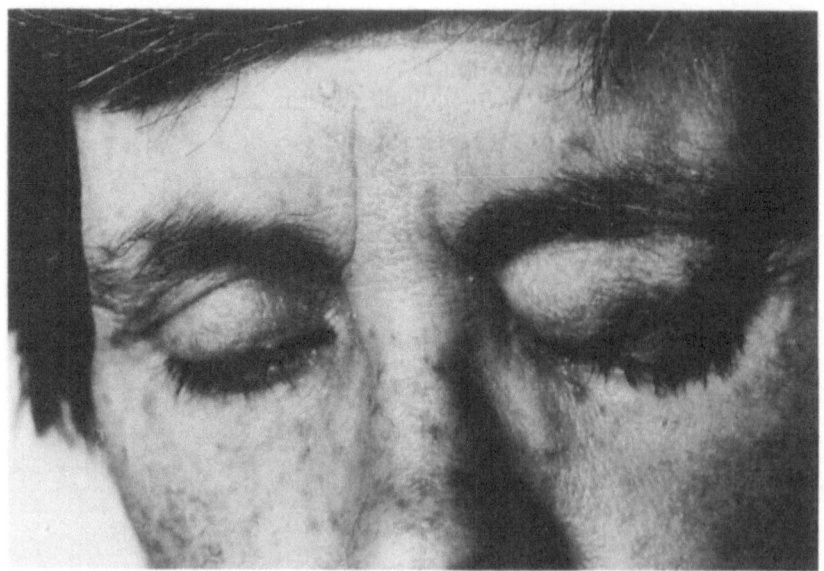

Figure 3. Clinical picture of a 60-year-old woman with an orbital varix before and after the Valsalva manoevre.

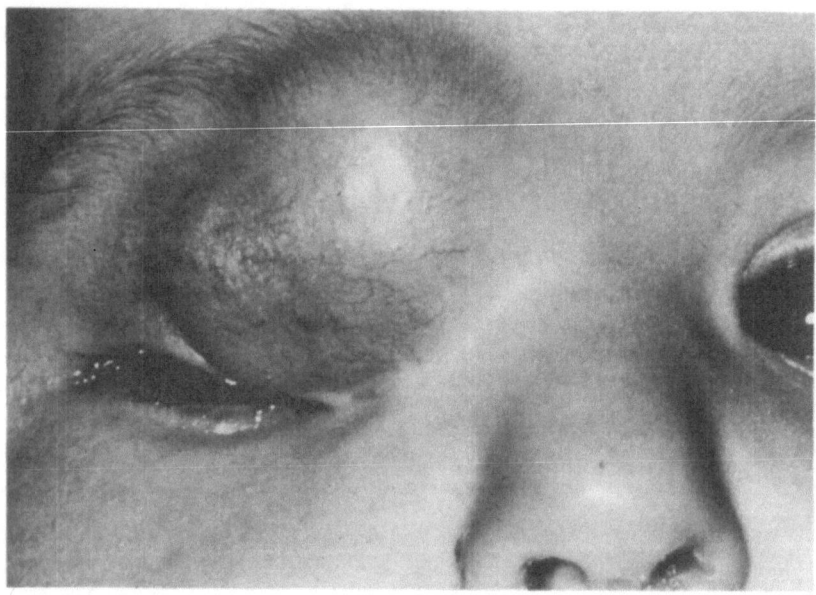

A

Figure 4. A) A 4-month-old patient with a capillary haemangioma. B) 4 months later, C) at 3 years of age.

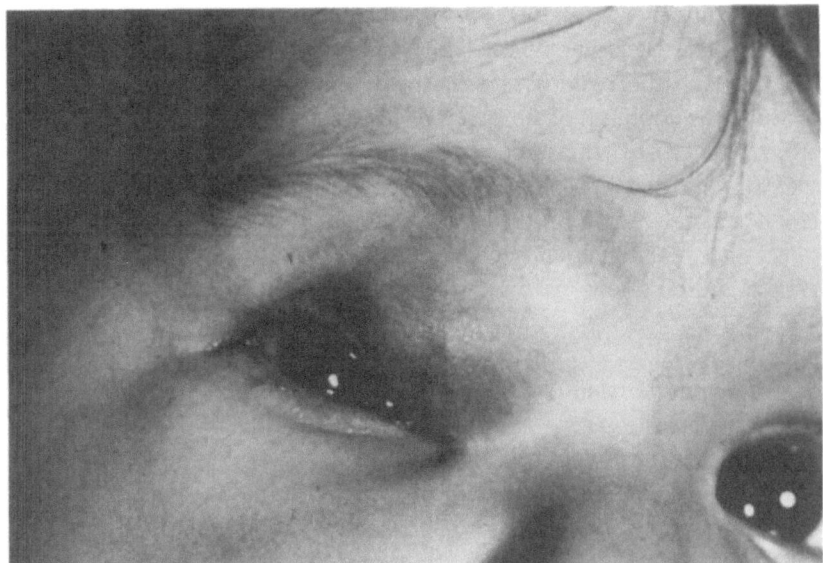

B

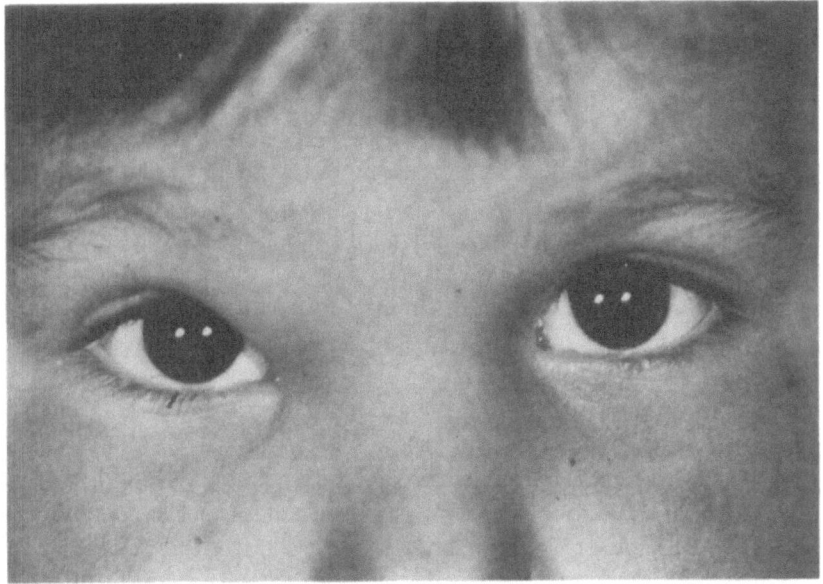

C

Figure 4.B) and C) Legend see page 114.

space-occupying vascular lesion is the aneurysm. Two types of aneurysms can be distinguished: a. saccular with a defect in elastic and muscular coat of the vessels (congenital, atherosclerosis, diseases of the collagen tissue), b. fusiform with gradual developing kinks over large trajects in the vertebral artery and basilar artery as result of atherosclerosis.

Symptoms depend on localisation, extension, eminent separation and also on blood leakage. Usually, paralytic (as result of extension) and apoplectic [34] (with recurrent subarachnoid haemorrhages) features occur. However, in most clinical presentations cases are difficult to dysentangle.

3.3.1 Localisation and clinical manifestation of the ocular motility disturbances

I. Vertebrobasilar aneurysm
Vertebrobasilar aneurysm may cause various brainstem signs, such as alternating quadriparese, visual field defects, horizontal and vertical gaze palsies or nystagmus. A bilateral six nerve palsy may be found in subarachnoid haemorrhage, which is due to its close relation to the enlarged and pulsating anterior inferior cerebellar artery. A paresis of the third and fourth nerve may develop under similar circumstances [35].

II. Internal carotid artery aneurysm
The communicans posterior. These aneurysms represent a large group (22–50%) of all intracranial aneurysms [21]. Because of the very close relation with the third cranial nerve, they often cause a complete oculomotor paralysis with pupil dilatation (mydriasis and cycloplegia). During spontaneous recovery or after clipping of the aneurysm improvement of adduction is most prominent but often incomplete [33]. This results in: a. retraction of the eyelid when trying to look down; b. adduction of the eye on attempt to look up; c. pupillary constriction in adduction (pseudo Argyl Robertson pupil); d. variation in the palpebral fissure at horizontal eye movement.

Aneurysms in the cavernous sinus occur in 1–2% of all intracranial aneurysms and are prevalent in women over the age of 40. The mass effect of these aneurysms may cause total unilateral or bilateral ophthalmoplegia [39]. The heralding symptom is pain followed by six and third nerve paralysis or total ophthalmoplegia. The pupil diameters are often fixed in midline due to simultaneous sympathic- and parasympathic fibre damage. There is no Horner syndrome, which can be proved pharmacologically. Pain is often more consistent than for example in trigeminal neuralgia. To differentiate from trigeminal neuralgia it has to be considered that concurrent areas of hypoaesthesia or anaesthesia are often found in one or more branches of the fifth nerve. For this reason the corneal reflex is of prominent importance because a loss of sensibility is often the only sign of the aneurysm [1]. The course of symptoms is rather specific, with after initial progression a more stationary course or improvement. The features of an intracavernous aneurysm depend on localisation in the sinus complex; particularly in the anterior part, symptoms indicating a suprasellar mass or enlarged fissure, exophthalmos, sensibility disturbance of the fifth nerve, visual loss and visual field defects may occur. In the posterior part it will be erosion of the petrosal bone, facial nerve lesion or deafness. An aneurysm in the middle causes erosion of the skull-base, bilateral ophthalmoplegia and decreased pituitary gland function, if present, inferiorly symptoms in the nasal-pharyngeal area are observed.

An X-ray of the skull may show a small curved line, suspect for a giant cavernous sinus aneurysm. The CT scan usually demonstrates a suprasellar process, which often angiographically appears to be a giant aneurysm. A carotid cavernous fistula may result in a ruptured carotid aneurysm [9].

Supraclinoid aneurysms. a. *The intracranial carotid aneurysms* at the origin of the ophthalmic artery from the internal carotid artery produce loss of vision and visual field defects in particular, and is not further discussed here [1, 34].

b. *Supraclinoid aneurysms* at the short initial segment of the proximal internal carotid artery before reaching the posterior communicans artery, are often of giant nature (larger than 2.5 cm) [36]. Prominent are the visual disturbances due to compression and the mass effect. The visual loss is slowly progressive and is concurrent with a variety of visual field defects. A third nerve paresis can sometimes occur: 1/3 in the series of Huber [34], 3/65 in the series of Vinuela [37] and identified as an orbital apex or fissure syndrome.

c. *The giant aneurysms* of the internal carotid bifurcation (proximate part of the anterior and medial cerebral artery) can also produce signs and symptoms of a third nerve disturbance with vision loss and visual field defects. The ones of the communicans anterior or anterior cerebral artery location sometimes produce visual loss and visual field defects, but both types are specially of apoplectic nature and are only recognisable after subarachnoid haemorrhage.

III. Aneurysms of the middle cerebral artery
These occur frequently and show a good prognosis, even after rupture. They seldom give neurological symptoms and, if they do, visual field defects are most frequent.

IV. Aneurysms of the posterior cerebral artery
In isolated cases, if large enough, they may produce hemi-anaesthesia, hemi-anopsia, isolated trochlear paralysis, progressive third nerve palsy or even a superior orbital syndrome with proptosis, trigeminal disturbances, oculomotor and trochlear paresis, as described by Coppeto [26].

The diagnostic procedure in aneurysms requires arteriography and CT scanning.

In 60% of the cases with giant aneurysms CT scan shows a thrombus mass, while the arteriography shows only a small part (or even a normal picture) as result of extensive thrombosis [36]. As therapy direct clipping of the aneurysm is preferred. If this does not belong to the possibilities, other technics, as internal carotid artery closing are available (chapter 25). Treatment is important because the haemorrhage percentage varies from 13–70%. An exception may be the more longstanding, not ruptured, giant aneurysm and the intracavernous located aneurysm.

3.3.2 Haematoma

Subdural haematoma
Ophthalmological signs and symptoms can prelude the more general features of subdural haematoma, papilloedema, optic disc atrophy, visual field defects, pupil abnormalities, gaze paralysis and oculomotor disturbances. The localisation of subdural haematoma varies from frontal to occipital region, with exclusion of the temporal part. A third nerve paralysis can occur in uncus herniation, which is seldom complete and most often affects pupillary motor fibres. A six nerve paresis, bilateral or unilateral, is often an accompanying symptom.

Orbital bleeding
Ocular motility disturbances resulting from orbital bleeding are often of acute nature, and cause a number of orbital signs, such as exophthalmos, blue swollen eyelids and blindness. The almost total ophthalmoplegia is of mechanical origine. The bleeding, fortunately rare, can be the result of a ruptured orbital aneurysm; rather a varix [38] and is frequent after trauma or surgical exploration. A high orbital pressure together with acute blindness requires immediate canthotomy or orbital exploration to prevent blindness.

Hyposphagma
In exceptional cases enormous conjunctival haematomas (hyposphagma) can be the cause of mechanical motility disturbances. For the differential diagnosis the patient has to look monocular and a slight improvement will be shown when trying out the direction of motility disturbances.

References

1. Huber A (1982): Eye signs and symptoms of intracranial aneurysm. Neuro-ophthalmol 2: 203–215.
2. Strik F (1981): Criteria for the evaluation of non-invasive testing for carotid artery stenosis. Neuro-ophthalmol 2: 17–22.

3. Strik F (1985): Carotid collateral circulation: relation between periorbital flow direction and ophthalmic artery pressure. Ultrasonoor Bulletin 2: 19–22.
4. Vrijghem JC, de Keizer RJW: Vascular and cardial disorders as cause of oculo-ischaemic disorders. (in preparation).
5. Hedges TR (1984): Intravenous digital subtraction angiography Proc. Neuro-Ophthalmology Antwerpen, 179.
6. de Schipper A, Stadnik T, Vereijcken H (1984): Intra-arterial digital subtraction angiography of the cerebral vessels. Proc. Neuro-Ophthalmology Antwerpen, 181.
7. Glaser JA (1982): Infranuclear Disorders of Eye Movements. In: Duane Th (ed.) Clinical Ophthalmology, vol. 2. Harper and Row, Philadelphia. Chapter 12.
8. de Keizer RJW (1981): Spontane carotico-caverneuze fistels. Thesis, Schipper Drukwerk Zaandijk.
9. de Keizer RJW, Peeters FLM, Veenhuyzen HB (1984): Diagnostic and therapeutic considerations in carotid cavernous fistulas as a cause of exophthalmos. Orbit 3: 153–169.
10. de Keizer RJW (1981): Spontaneous carotid cavernous fistulas. Neuro-ophthalmol. 2: 35–46.
11. de Keizer RJW (1982): A Doppler haematotachographic investigation in patients with ocular and orbital symptoms due to a carotid-cavernous fistula. Doc. Ophthalmol. 52: 297–307.
12. de Keizer RJW (1985): Vascular disorders in the orbit and in the orbital region. In: Ophthalmic tumours. Oosterhuis JA (ed.). Dr. W. Junk Publ. Dordrecht, 247–270.
13. Ossoinig KC (1981): Echographic differentiation of vascular tumors in the orbit. Doc. Ophthalmol. Proc. Ser. 29: 283–291.
14. de Keizer RJW, Vielvoye JG, de Wolff-Rouendaal D (in press): MRI in eye-and orbital tumours. Orbit.
15. Walsh FB, Hoyt WF (1969): Clinical Neuro-Ophthalmology. 3rd ed. vol. 3. Williams and Wilkins, Baltimore, 2414–2428.
16. Becker DH, Townsend JJ, Kramer R, Newton Th (1979): Occult cerebrovascular malformations. Brain 102: 249–287.
17. de Keizer RJW (1984): A diversity of ophthalmic signs and symptoms in superior sagittal sinus thrombosis. Proc. Neuro-Ophthalmol. Joint World Meeting. 5th Meeting Internat. Neuro-Ophthalmol. Soc. (INOS) and 7th Meeting Neurogenetics and Neuro-Ophthalmol. (WFN), May 1984, University of Antwerp, 187–191.
18. Minor RH, Kearns ThP, Millikan CH, Siekert RG, Sayre GP (1959): Ocular Manifestations of Occlusive Disease of the Vertebral Basilar Arterial System. Arch Ophthalmol. 62: 84–96.
19. Monteiro MLR, Coppeto JR, Greco P (1984): Giant cell arteritis of the posterior cerebral circulation presenting with ataxia and ophthalmoplegia. Arch. Ophthalmol. 102: 407–409.
20. Barricks ME, Traviesa DB, Glaser JS, Levy LS (1977): Ophthalmoplegia in cranial arteritis. Brain 100: 209–221.
21. Gittinger JW (1978): Disorders of the ocular motor nerves. Int. Ophthalmol. Clin. 18/1: 19–36.
22. Asbury AK, Aldedge H, Hershberg R, Miller Fisher C (1970): Oculomotorpalsy in diabetes mellitus. A clinico-pathological study. Brain 93: 555–566.
23. Hedges ThR (1972): Isolated ophthalmic migraine, its frequency, mechanisms and differential diagnosis. In: Smith JL (ed.) Neuro-Ophthalmology, vol. VI. Symposium of the University of Miami and the Bascom Palmer Eye Institute, Mosby and Co., St. Louis, Chapter 12: 140–149.
24. Parkinson D (1972): Venous Anatomy. In: Smith JL (ed.). Neuro-Ophthalmology, vol. VI. Symposium of the University of Miami and the Bascom Palmer Eye Institute, Mosby and Co., St. Louis, Chapter 12: 88–95.
25. Harris FS, Rhoton AL (1976): Anatomy of the cavernous sinus. J. Neurosurg. 45: 169–180.
26. Coppeto JR, Hoffman H (1981): Tolosa-Hunt syndrome with proptosis mimicked by giant aneurysm of posterior cerebral artery. Arch. Neurol. 38: 54–55.
27. Hunt WE (1976): Tolosa-Hunt syndrome, one cause of painful ophthalmoplegia. J. Neurosurg. 44: 544–549.

28. Schatz NJ, Farmer P (1972): Tolosa-Hunt syndrome; the pathology of painful ophthalmoplegia. In: Smith JL (ed.). Neuro-Ophthalmology, vol. VI. Symposium of the University of Miami and the Bascolm Palmer Eye Institute. Mosby and Co St. Louis, Chapter 9: 102–112.

29. Léonard TJ, Moseley IF, Sanders MD (1984): Ophthalmoplegia in carotid cavernous sinus fistula. Brit. J. Ophthalmol. 68: 128–134.

30. Vinuela FV, Brohm GM, Fox AJ, Kan S (1983): Detachable callibrated leak balloon for supraselective angiography and embolisation of dural arteriovenous malformation. J. Neurosurg. 58: 817–823.

31. de Keizer RJW, van Dalen JTW (1981): Wyburn Mason syndrome Subcutaenous angioma extirpation after preliminary embolisation. Doc. Ophthalmol. 50: 262–273.

32. Peeters HJF, Bleeker GM (1975): Orbital Haemangioma in Children. Proc. 2nd. Int. Symp. on Orbital Disorders, Amsterdam 1973. Mod. Probl. Ophthalmol. 14: 398–400.

33. Plessner-Rasmussen HJ, Marushak D, Goldschmidt E (1983): Capillary haemangiomas of the eyelids and orbit. Acta Ophthalmol. 61: 645–654.

34. Huber A, Yasargil MG (1983): Die Aneurysmen der Arteria ophthalmica. Klin. Mbl. Augenheilk. 182: 537–543.

35. Gittinger JW (1982): In: Lessell S and van Dalen JTW (eds.) Neuro-Ophthalmology, vol. II. Excerpta Medica, Amsterdam, Chapter 15: 215–220.

36. Pia HW, Zierski J (1982): Giant cerebral anrerysms. Neurosurg. Rev. 5: 117–148.

37. Vinuela FV, Fox A, Chang JK, Drake CG, Peerless SJ (1984): A clinical radiological spectrum of giant supraclinoid internal carotid artery aneurysm. Neuroradiol. 26: 93–99.

38. Szilvássy I, Gács Gy (1979): Akuter einseitiger Exophthalmus infolge Ruptur eines orbitalen venösen Aneurysmas. Klin. Mbl. Augenheilk. 175: 60–64.

39. Trobe JD, Glaser JS, Post JD (1978): Meningiomas and Auneurysms of the Cavernous Sinus. Neuro-ophthalmologic Features. Arch. Ophthalmol. 96: 457–467.

40. Trobe JD (1985): Isolated Pupil-Sparing Third Nerve Palsy. Ophthalmology 92: 58–61.

41. Hoes MJAJM, Bruyn GW, Vielvoye GJ (1984): The Tolosa-Hunt syndrome literature review: seven new cases and a hypothesis. Cephalgia 1: 181–194.

Section IV

Myogenic disorders

Histochemical fibre types in extraocular muscles

TJAARD U. HOOGENRAAD

The six extraocular muscles can be distinguished from other skeletal muscles by functional characteristics and by peculiarities in architecture, morphology, innervation and enzymehistochemistry. These differences are presented schematically in Fig. 1.

Functionally the extraocular muscles are unique since they generate not only extremely fast movements but also slow movements. Furthermore, the fatiguebility of these muscles is for various reasons very low.

Architecturally two areas can be discerned in extraocular muscles: a peripheral zone harbouring fibres with a small diameter and a very high mitochondrial content and a central (global) zone with fibres varying in diameter and mitochondrial content. The mean diameter of extraocular muscle fibres is less than in most other skeletal muscles [1].

By using light microscopy three muscle fibre types can be distinguished. 1) Fibres with a high content and a coarse distribution of the sarcoplasmatic intermyofibrillar material. These fibres are most frequently found in the periphery of the muscle. 2) Fibres with less intermyofibrillar material and a somewhat granular appearance with a regular sarcoplasmatic reticular network. These fibres predominate in the central parts of the muscle. 3) Fibres with only sparse intermyofibrillar material. These fibres often have a fine stippled appearance. They are found in the centre as well as in the periphery of the muscles [2].

Ultrastructurally it has been discovered that the extraocular muscles contain fibres with a more or less characteristic fibre type. These 'Felderstructur'-fibres have large myofibrils with indistinct margins. Much attention has been paid to the innervation of the extraocular muscles: it has been reported that in these muscles the number of muscle fibres innervated by one nerve fibre, the motor-unit, is much smaller than in other skeletal muscles. In most skeletal muscles one motor neuron innervates from several hundred to several thousand muscle fibres. In the ocular muscles only three to ten muscle fibres are innervated by a single neuron. Another peculiarity of extraocular muscles is that they contain some fibres that are multiply innervated. The endplates in these fibres have a grape-like ap-

124

DIFFERENCES IN ARCHITECTURE, MORPHOLOGY, INNERVATION AND
HISTOCHEMISTRY BETWEEN SKELETAL MUSCLES IN GENERAL AND
EXTRA-OCULAR MUSCLES

SKELETAL MUSCLES   **EXTRA-OCULAR MUSCLES**

ARCHITECTURE

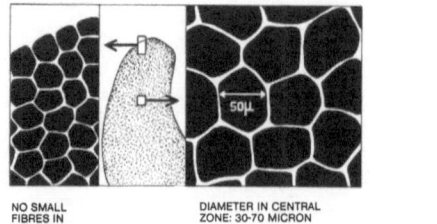 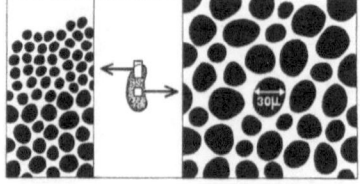

NO SMALL   DIAMETER IN CENTRAL   PERIPHERAL   DIAMETER IN CENTRAL
FIBRES IN   ZONE: 30-70 MICRON   FIBRES   AREA: 5-40 MICRON
PERIPHERY   SMALL
                                           DIAMETER

MORPHOLOGY

LIGHT-MICROSCOPY   ELECTRON-MICROSCOPY   LIGHT-MICROSCOPY   ELECTRON-MICROSCOPY

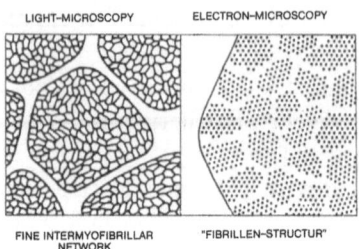 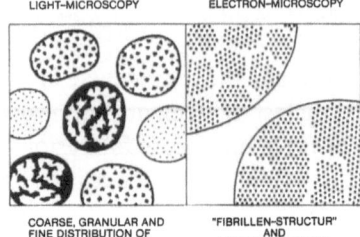

FINE INTERMYOFIBRILLAR   "FIBRILLEN–STRUKTUR"   COARSE, GRANULAR AND   "FIBRILLEN–STRUKTUR"
NETWORK   FINE DISTRIBUTION OF   AND
                                                INTERMYOFIBRILLAR   "FELDER-STRUKTUR"
                                                MATERIAL

INNERVATION

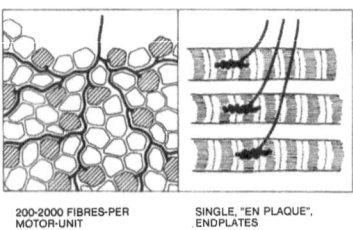 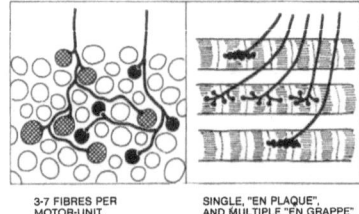

200-2000 FIBRES-PER   SINGLE, "EN PLAQUE",   3-7 FIBRES PER   SINGLE, "EN PLAQUE",
MOTOR-UNIT   ENDPLATES   MOTOR-UNIT   AND MULTIPLE "EN GRAPPE"
                                                               ENDPLATES

HISTOCHEMISTRY

ATP–ASE 9.4   NADH–TR   ATP–ASE 9.4   NADH–TR

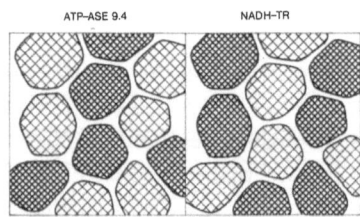 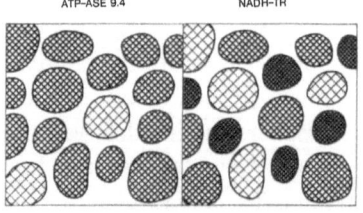

ALMOST COMPLETE RECIPROCITY   NO RECIPROCITY IN MAJORITY OF FIBRES

Figure 1.

pearance. However, most fibres in the extraocular muscles have single plate-like neuromuscular junctions like the endplates normally seen in skeletal muscles.

From the histochemical point of view the extraocular muscles can also be distinguished from most skeletal muscles [3]. In skeletal muscle type I and type II fibres have an almost exact reciprocity for the enzymes myosine ATP-ase and NADH-tetrazolium reductase (NADH-TR): high activity of myosine ATP-ase corresponds with low activity of the aerobic enzyme NADH-TR and vice versa. In the extraocular muscles reciprocity is present in the type I fibres but absent in most type II fibres that have high myosine ATP-ase activity at pH 9.4 and a high activity of NADH-TR.

1. The two fibre type system in skeletal muscles: the histochemical approach of classification and nomenclature

Myofibrillar ATP-ase activity (pH 9.4) is generally preferred for fibre typing of skeletal muscle fibres because it does not demonstrate intermediate fibre types: muscle fibres are either type I (weak reaction) or type II (strong reaction).

The type II fibres can be divided in sybtypes. In the skeletal muscles of many mammals these subtypes can be distinguished by differences in ATP-ase activity which are found after preincubation at pH 4.6 and pH 4.3. 'A' fibres have low activity after preincubation at pH 4.6 and at pH 4.3, 'B' fibres have high activity at pH 4.6 and low at pH 4.3 and 'C' fibres have high activity at pH 4.6 and also at pH 4.3. In this manner in most skeletal muscles type IIA and type IIB can be demonstrated. Theoretically type IIC fibres can be distinguished but these fibres are only seldom seen in human skeletal muscles. Dubowitz and Brooke [4] have shown that the activities of the aerobic enzyme NADH/TR and anaerobic enzyme alpha-glycerophosphate dehydrogenase (alpha-GPD) in the type II subtypes show a typical pattern: in the 'A' fibres aerobic and anaerobic enzyme activity is high, in the 'B' fibre the anaerobic activity is higher than the aerobic activity and in the 'C' fibre the aerobic activity is high and the anaerobic activity relatively low.

2. The two fibre system in extraocular muscles: the histochemical approach to classification and nomenclature

In 1979 we described a practical histochemical method by which the fibre types in the extraocular muscles can be classified [5]. It is based on the ATP-ase two fibre type system and resembles the method of classification and nomenclature of skeletal muscle fibre types. In our method, however, the subdivision of type II fibres is based on the relative activities of an aerobic and an anaerobic enzyme and not on the pH sensitivity of the ATP-ase reaction. The standard histochemical reaction for ATP-ase (pH 9.4) can be used to differentate type I from type II fibres but we found that the differences in darkness between type I fibres (dark) and type II fibres (light) were not pronounced and that after preincubation at pH 4.3 the distinction between the two fibre types is more marked: type I fibres stain extremely darkly and type II fibres extremely lightly (Fig. 2).

Type II fibres are divided into three subtypes based on the relative activities of the aerobic enzyme NADH-TR and the anaerobic enzyme alpha-GPD. IIA fibres have high aerobic and anaerobic activity, IIB fibres only high anaerobic activity and IIC fibres only have high aerobic activity.

Because the method is not completely identical with the method in common use for the classification of skeletal muscle fibres we have chosen for an nomenclature: type I-like and type II-like fibres.

2.1 Type IIC-like fibre, a typical ocular fibre: fast and unfatigueable

Type IIC fibres with type II ATP-ase activity, relative high aerobic activity and low anaerobic activity are seldom seen in skeletal muscles. In extraocular muscles, however, fibres with this histochemical profile are common. In the peripheral zone of the inferior oblique muscle we found that some 80% of the muscle fibres were characterised by this histochemical profile. In the central zone of this muscle approximately 30% of the fibres were type IIC-like.

If one tries to correlate the histochemical characteristics and the physiological properties of this fibre it seems justifiable to assume that it is able to make 'fast-twitch' that it is not easily fatigued because of its high content of aerobic enzymes.

2.2 Type I-like fibre: multiply innervated?

We have argued that the type I-like fibre in the human extraocular muscle is multiply innervated: Harker has shown that in sheep the multiply innervated fibre has a type I myosine ATP-ase activity [6]. Investigations on the ultrastructural level demonstrated that in human extraocular muscles the multiple inner-

Table 1. Histochemical reactions in human muscle

Muscle fibre type	I	IIA	IIB	IIC
Routine ATP-ase	+	+++	+++	+++
ATP-ase pH 4.6	+++	0	+++	+++
ATP-ase pH 4.3	+++	0	0	++
NADH-TR	+++	++	+	++
alpha-GPD	0	++	++	+

0 = very low, + = low, ++ = high, +++ = very high (after Dubowitz and Brooke, 1973)

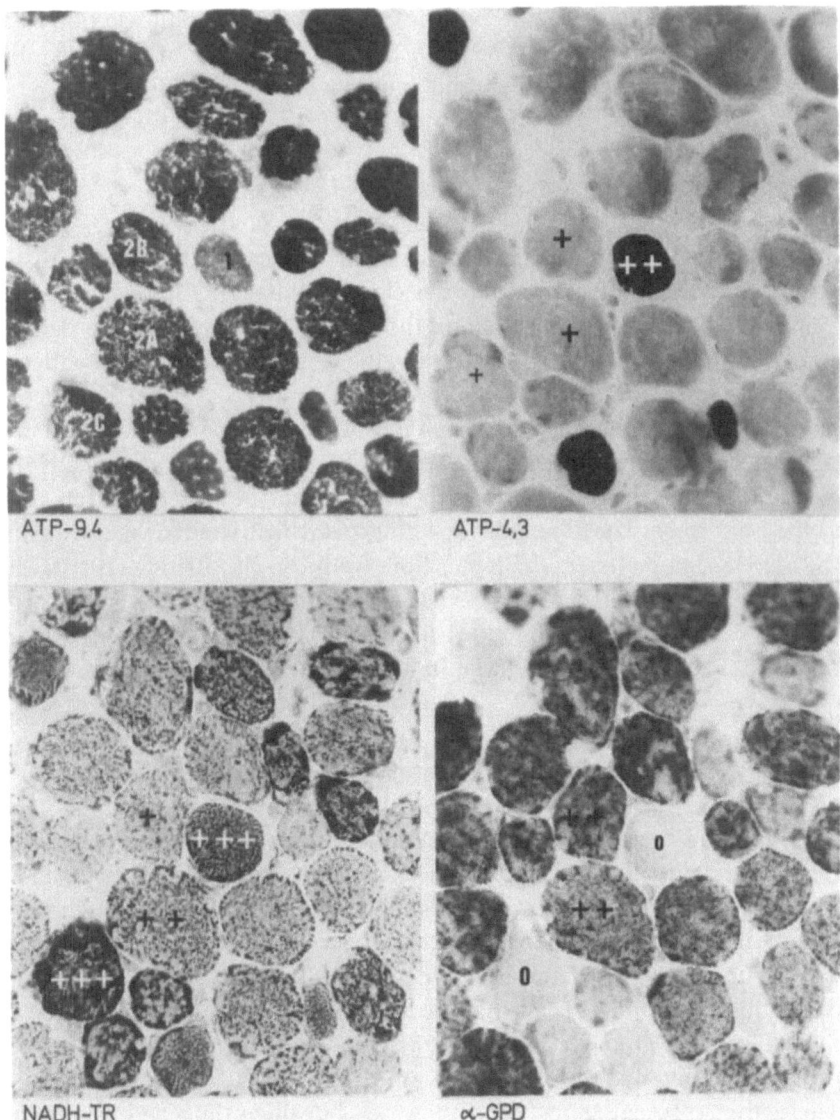

Figure 2. Male, 28 years old. Inferior oblique muscle. Central zone. Consecutive serial sections. The majority of the fibres has a type II-like myosine ATP-ase activity. In the section stained after preincubation at pH 4.3 type I-like fibres stain extremely darkly whereas the type II-like fibres stain lightly. The subtyping of three type II-like fibres has been indicated in the ATP-ase 9.4 section. The type IIA-like fibre has a relative high aerobic and anaerobic activity. The type IIB-like fibre has a relative low aerobic and a relative high anaerobic activity. The type IIC-like fibre combines a relative high aerobic activity with a low anaerobic activity.

vated fibre has a 'Felder-structur' pattern, whereas the other muscle fibres have the 'Fibrillen-structur' pattern. The histochemical profile of our type I-like fibre could well fit with those of a slow-tonic multiply innervated fibre.

3. Histochemical fibre types in the extraocular muscle of rabbits

Asmussen and Kiessling have described a histochemical method for the distinction of fibre types in the extraocular muscle of rabbits [7]. Although it uses the myosine ATP-ase reaction pH 9.4 and the aerobic enzyme succinate dehydrogenase without using an anaerobic enzyme, the results are comparable with ours. The nomenclature however is for human muscles.

These authors distinguished six fibre types: type 1 and type 2 are found in the peripheral parts of the muscle. The type 1 fibre has the histochemical profile comparable to our type IIC-like fibre, the type 2 would be classified in our system as a type I-like fibre. The fibre types 3, 4, 5 and 6 are restricted to the central parts of the muscle. In our system the type 3 fibre would be classified as type IIB-like, the type 4 as type IIA-like and type 5 as type IIC-like. The histochemical profile of the type 6 fibre resembles our type I-like fibre. Thus the results of these studies in rabbits are comparable with those in human extraocular muscle.

4. Classification based on other than pure histochemical characteristics

In 1974 Durston described a method by which fibres in the human extraocular muscles can be classified by morphological characteristics [2] and this method has been followed by others [8]. Durston distinguished three fibre types with various distributions of the intermyofibrillar material; a coarse, granular or fine pattern. He also defined the histochemical profile of these fibre types. If one compares this classification with ours it seems that the 'coarse' fibre corresponds with the type IIC-like fibre, the 'granular' fibre with the type IIB-like fibre and the 'fine' fibre with the type I-like fibre.

There are at present almost as many ways of distinguishing and naming fibre types as there are laboratories involved in the investigation of muscle. We think

Table 2. Histochemical reactions in human extraocular muscle

Ocular muscle fibre	I-like	IIA-like	IIB-like	IIC-like
ATP-ase pH 4.3	++	+	+	+
NADH/TR	++/+++	++/+++	+	++/+++
alpha-GPD	0/+	++	++	0/+

0 = -very low; + = low, ++ = high, +++ = very high

that Dubowitz and Brooke were right, who stated that whatever system is finely adopted it should fulfil the following criteria: 1) Nomenclature should be based on the parameter being studied: for the histochemist using myosine ATP-ase it is logical to distinguish type I and type II fibres but it would be illogical for him to distinguish fast and slow contracting fibres or 'coarse' and 'granular' fibres. 2) The various categories should be easily differentiated without a gradual transition from one fibre type to another or with many intermediate fibres. In the ocular muscles the ATP-ase pH 4.3 fulfills this criterion. 3) Any system of nomenclature must be useful when applied to experimental or pathological situations. A classification including too many fibre types is of theoretical interest but has little practical application in the evaluation of human diseases. A two fibre system is practical; a six fibre system is not. We feel that our system of classification and nomenclature fulfills these criteria and our experience suggests that the method is practicable when studying pathology in extraocular muscles [9, 10, 11].

5. Summary

In human extraocular muscles four types of fibres can be distinguished on the basis of histochemical stains; type I-like, type IIA-like, type IIB-like and type IIC-like fibres.

Using myosine ATP-ase, fibres in central and peripheral locations can be divided into two main fibre types: type I-like fibres and type II-like fibres. Using the aerobic enzyme NADH-TR and the anaerobic enzyme alpha-GPD, type II-like fibres can be subdivided into the three subtypes A, B and C. The A fibre has an intermediate activity of both aerobic and anaerobic enzymes, the B fibre has predominance of anaerobic activity and in the C fibre has predominance of aerobic activity.

In the extraocular muscles most fibres are type II-like. In the peripheral areas of the extraocular muscles most type II-like fibres belong to the type IIC-like subgroup. In the central areas the 3 subtypes of the type II-like fibres are more or less equally represented.

The histochemical profiles of these fibre types resemble those in other skeletal muscle. Extraocular muscles differ, however, from other skeletal muscles by the fact that the large majority of their fibres have a type II myosin ATP-ase activity and that most of these fibres have a predominance of aerobic activity. In most skeletal muscles type I and type II fibres are more or less equally represented and type IIC fibres do not occur.

References

1. Alvarado JA, van Horn C (1975): Muscle cell types of the cat inferior oblique. In: Basic mechanisms of ocular motility and clinical implications. Proceedings of the International Symposium, held in Wenner-Gren Center Stockholm, 1974. G. Lennerstrand and P. Bach-y-Rita, eds. Oxford, Pergamon Press. Wenner-Gren Center International Symposium Series nr. 24: 15–45.
2. Durston JHJ (1974): Histochemistry of primate extraocular muscles and the changes of denervation. British Journal of Ophthalmology 58: 193–216.
3. Harriman DGF (1975): Histochemical fibre types in human extraocular muscle. Bristol Medico-Chirurgical Journal 90: 27–29.
4. Dubowitz V, Brooke MH (1973): In: Muscle biopsy: a modern approach. Vol. 2 in the series: Major Problems in Neurology. London-Philadelphia-Toronto.
5. Hoogenraad TU, Jennekens FGI and Tan KEWP (1979): Histochemical fibre types in human extraocular muscles, an investigation of inferior oblique muscle. Acta Neuropathologica (Berlin) 45: 73–78.
6. Harker DW (1972): The structure and innervation of sheep superior rectus and levator extraocular muscles. Investigative Ophthalmology and Visual Sciences 11: 956–969.
7. Asmussen G, Kiessling A, Wholrab F (1971): Histochemische Characterisierung der verschiedenen Muskelfasertypen in der auszeren Augenmuskeln von Saugetieren. Acta Anatomica 79: 526–545.
8. Ringel SP, Wilson WB, Barden MT, Kaiser KK (1978): Histochemistry of human extraocular muscle. Archives of Ophthalmology 96: 1067–1072.
9. Hoogenraad TU (1982): Over uitwendige oogspieren. Microscopische en klinische studies, with a summary in English. Thesis. Elinkwijk Press. Utrecht.
10. Hoogenraad TU, Jennekens FGI, Tan KEWP (1977): Histochemistry of inferior oblique muscle in a case of congenital third nerve palsy. Documenta Ophthalmologica 44: 187–192.
11. Hoogenraad TU, Jennekens FGI, Tan KEWP (1978): Ophthalmoplegia due to myasthenia gravis. Histological and histochemical observations in the inferior oblique muscle. Docum Ophthal Proc Series, Vol 17: 27. Dr W Junk Publ, Dordrecht.

Ocular myopathies: syndromes with chronic progressive external ophthalmoplegia (CPEO)

L.A.K. BASTIAENSEN

An ocular myopathy is a degenerative disorder of extra-ocular muscles with the primary site of the lesion in the striated eye muscle cell itself. So ocular myasthenia and orbital thyroid disease are not discussed in this chapter. The clinical picture is dominated by blepharoptosis and restriction of eye movements. The course is usually chronic progressive, so the most important symptom of an ocular myopathy is chronic progressive external ophthalmoplegia (CPEO). This group of diseases is nearly always bilateral, with some asymmetry and asynchrony. Encephalomyopathies with CPEO form a quite distinct and important group. In these the ocular movement disorder can theoretically be ascribed to neuronal disorders as to myopathy of the extra-ocular muscles both. However, in the few autopsies in which data were obtained from the ocular motor nuclei and nerves no pertinent abnormalities were found. Myopathic changes on the contrary were common in the extraocular muscles and other, skeletal, muscles. The interpretation of extra-ocular muscular pathology is however very difficult: 'myopathic' changes have been shown to be concomitant with, or the result of chronic denervation [1].

In most general muscular diseases the extraocular muscles are not involved. The reason why is not clear but may probably be explained by the unique ultrastructure of the eye muscles (chapter 11).

1. Diagnosis

The diagnosis of an ocular myopathy is chiefly based on clinical signs and symptoms, but can be supported by: EMG of the extra-ocular muscles, determination in the blood of 'muscle enzymes', biopsy of extra-ocular or skeletal muscles.

The EMG of a normal extra-ocular muscle (by means of a concentric needle) is characterized by:

the limited number of eye muscle cells per motor unit (3 till 7): this is much less than in ordinary skeletal muscles, and results in a low voltage (300–1200 micron V) and short duration of the biphasic action potentials (1–3 msec).

Absence of action potentials during complete relaxation of the eye muscle: this occurs not in the rest-position of the eye but only in maximal contraction of the antagonist-muscle. Spontaneous activity in maximal relaxation (e.g. fibrillations) points to a neurogenic affection.

When contraction increases: the fast appearance (recruitment of motor units) of a high frequent pattern of discharges (interference pattern) with short-lasting (1–3 msec) biphasic action potentials (500–1200 micron V) in maximal con-traction.

A myopathic EMG derives its hallmarks form patchy loss of subunits (individ-ual muscle cells) of the motor units. This implies that the velocity and rate of recruitment of the motor units stay intact for a long time, just as the interference pattern. Even in a strongly paretic (myopathic) extra-ocular muscle, whereby scarcely any movement can be detected, the interference pattern can readily be found ('discrepancy' sign). The duration and amplitude of the action potentials shall decrease by the drop out of individual eye muscle cells per motor unit: this sign is difficult to spot because of the already existent short duration and highly interindividual variability of the amplitude of the action potentials. In the atro-phic endstage of an ocular myopathy whole motor-units shall eventually drop out: then the EMG can depict a lower frequency of discharges, but certainly much richer of action potentials than in a neurogenic paresis [2].

When the myopathic process spreads over more muscles than only the extra-ocular muscles, the activity of the disease can be estimated by determining the height of creatine-kinase and other 'muscular enzymes' in the blood. In such a case a high-normal to slightly elevated CK can be expected, buth other enzymes as aldolase, LDH and transaminases are only exceptionally elevated.

The technique and interpretation of extra-ocular muscle biopsy are difficult and only reliable in expert hands. So we rely mostly on a skeletal muscle biopsy if the skeletal muscles are also involved. Fortunately we can find specific histo-chemical and submicroscopical abnormalities even in clinically normal appearing skeletal muscles. For a general introduction in skeletal muscle biopsy see refer-ence [3].

2. Classification of ocular myopathies

There is considerable controversy regarding the nosological classification of ocular myopathies: of the ophthalmoplegia's several have been described [1]. The present classification of the ocular myopathies is based on clinical implications for the patient (Table 1).

2.1 Pure ocular myopathies (Myopathies restricted to the extra ocular muscles).

Congenital pure ocular myopathy
This is a very rare condition, when occurring without a wider myopathic context. An eventual heredity is not known. EMG and eye muscle biopsy show myopathic signs, and sometimes mitochondrial abnormalities [4]. Different forms of amino-aciduria can be seen in combination with congenital ocular myopathy. The extra-ocular muscles can be abnormally fragile [1]. Congenital ocular myopathy must be differentiated from other forms of congenital external ophthalmoplegia as: adhesion- and retraction syndromes, fibrosis of extra-ocular muscles, abnormal innervation, aplasia of extra-ocular muscles, -nerves or -nerve-nuclei. Of these the best known form of congenital external ophthalmoplegia is the 'autosomal dominant hereditary stationary external ophthalmoplegia' with varying expression, probably caused by hypoplasia of the nuclei and/or nerves to the extra-ocular muscles; it is certainly not an ocular myopathy.

Acquired pure ocular myopathies
When found at young age, we have probably to deal with a forme fruste of a late discovered congenital myopathy or a first manifestation of a general disease with ocular myopathy (see Ophthalmoplegia Plus).

A myopathy which remains restricted to the extra-ocular muscles manifests itself mostly on a mature age. The course is benign and the only signs are a progressive blepharoptosis and moderate to slight involvement of ocular movements. The three most important forms are discussed below.

Table 1. Classification of ocular myopathies

Pure ocular myopathies (restricted to the extraocular muscles)	Ocular myopathy as part of a more complex neurodegenerative disorder ('Ophthalmoplegia Plus')
– congenital	– congenital
– acquired	– encephalomyopathies
– Mitochondrial CPEO, restricted to the extraocular muscles	– Kearns' disease
– Chronic blepharoptosis in diabetes mellitus	– Leigh's syndrome
– Involutional blepharoptosis	– Canavan's disease
	– primary metabolic diseases with CPEO
	– primary cytochrome-c-oxydase deficiency
	– vitamin E deficiency
	– oculopharyngeal dystrophy
	– myotonic dystrophia
	– heredo-ataxia

134

Mitochondrial CPEO, restricted to the extra-ocular muscles
The patients are nearly always unaware of this condition; it is discovered acciden-
tally during a routine examination in the office of the ophthalmologist. There
exists hardly any clinical consequence, except that there is some need for ptosis
surgery in far progressed cases. Therefore the method of Blascovicz is prefered
(10 mm shortening of the m.levator palpebrae is nearly always sufficient) or the
Friedenwald-procedure (which has only a temporary result but the procedure can
be repeated 3 or more times and can be done as an out-patient). The affection is
autosomal dominant hereditary, but the heredity is difficult to study by the late
onset of the disease. In many instances a disturbed glucose-tolerance is found.
The condition may be considered as a form of mitochondrial CPEO with limited
expression [1].

Chronic blepharoptosis in longstanding diabetes mellitus
In a large consecutive population of patients with diabetes, who already had
micro-angiopathy, a considerable number of diminished height of interpalpebral
fissure was found, presumably caused by myopathy of the m.levator palpebrae
[5]. An insufficient oxygen uptake in this often used muscle with high energy- and
oxygen-need may contribute to this condition. No neurogenic condition nor
sympathetic denervation was detected sofar.

Involutional ptosis in senility
This is sometimes difficult to distinguish from desinsertion of the m.levator
palpebrae. In a levator biopsy myopathic signs are apparent in combination with
fatty degeneration [6, 7].

2.2 Ocular myopathies as a part of a more complex neuro-degenerative disorder.
(Ophthalmoplegia Plus).

Skeletal muscle affection is a common feature of the Ophthalmoplegia Plus
disorders. The affected muscles, in order of time of onset and severity are: facial
and other cranial muscles descending to: throat and neck muscles, proximal,
rump- and distal muscles of the extremities. Other organ systems may be affected,
such as heart, retina, nerve tissue, endocrine systems etc.

2.2.1 Congenital general myopathies with extra-ocular muscular involvement
Congenital myopathies are seldom accompanied by ophthalmoplegia. Sporadic
cases with extra-ocular muscle involvement have been described in: centronuclear, nemaline, reducing body, micro fibre and target fibre myopathy.
    Extra-ocular muscular abnormalities have also been described in congenital
familial myopathy with focal abnormalities of the cross-striation: central core
(minicore) disease [3]. A congenital ocular myopathy has been reported in

myopathy with fibretype disproportion. External ophthalmoplegia has been found in congenital type I [9], as well as in type II hypotrophy [10], sometimes in combination with other degenerative signs. The heredity of all these different syndromes is not clear: possibly sporadic or autosomal recessive.

2.2.2 Encephalomyopathies

Encephalomyopathies are commonly induced by mitochondrial defects. Completely different diseases belong to this group of affections, such as Menke's disease, Zellweger's syndrome (possibly a primary peroxisomal disorder), Leigh's syndrome, Alpers' disease and other progressive poliodystrophies, familial myoclonus epilepsy with ragged-red fibres, Canavan's disease, the newly described Melas syndrome [11] and the Kearns Sayre syndrome. With the exception of the latter these conditions occur mostly sporadically. The general signs of this heterogeneous group are: retarded growth, intellectual decline, fatiguability, epilepsy, ataxia, myoclonus, optic atrophy, pigmentary abnormalities of the ocular fundi, hypermetabolism with elevated serum lactate and pyruvate and occasionnally ophthalmoplegia.

The biochemical defects that have been found are heterogeneous. The following mitochondrial metabolic defects have been reported: disturbance of the pyruvate-dehydrogenase complex, decreased function of ATP-ase, NADH-oxidase, NADH-Coφ.reductase complex, cytochrome b, cytochrome-c-oxidase, succinate cytochrome-c-reductase, sometimes with loose coupling of oxidative phosphorylation and/or diminished ATP production [11, 12].

Generally spoken the biochemical dysfunction can be summarized as impaired substrate utilization, defective respiratory chain or impaired energy conservation and transduction, often each other overlapping in some way.

The mitochondrial dysfunction can easily be read out the morphological abnormalities of the mitochondria. On histochemical staining the muscle cells show subsarcolemnal mitochondrial aggregates with abnormal amounts of fat and glycogen between them. An usual method for screening these abnormal aggregates is the Gomoritrichrome staining method; the abnormal muscle cells show accumulations subsarcolemmaly where the abnormal functioning mitochondria are located: ragged-red fibres. With oxidative enzymatic staining methods the presence of excessive amounts of mitochondria can be confirmed. Electronmicroscopic investigation shows, besides an abnormal high number of mitochondria, marked changes in their external and internal structure.

It should be pointed out that none of these syndromes have specific mitochondrial defects. Not only there are large differences in clinical and biochemical abnormalities between the different syndromes, but there is also a large interindividual variability even in the same syndrome. It is even not known whether the biochemical dysfunction of the mitochondria is the cause or the result of these structural alterations. A proper nosological classification is hindered extra by the very probable occurrence of numerous phenocopies.

Mitochondrial CPEO, Kearns' disease. Mitochondrial abnormalities, as mentioned above, can be demonstrated in all organ systems involved. The disease may give rise to a variety of clinical signs and symptoms, in addition to CPEO; other signs may even dominate the clinical picture (Table 2).

Weakness, as in CPEO, or an increased fatiguability may be of neurogenous or myogenous origin, due to mitochondrial affection of both muscles and nerves. The rate of deterioration and the severity of signs and symptoms are mainly determined by the age of onset. Infantile onset gives a rapidly progressive, sometimes even fatal course (due to heartblock or CNS desease). The triad of 1. CPEO, 2. pigmentary retinopathy, 3. heartblock was previously named the Kearns-Sayre-syndrome. At present it is better to use this term for the whole infantile onset variant of mitochondrial CPEO.

On adult life (4–5th decade) this disease has a much more benign course, is slowly progressive, with less involvement of other organ systems. These clinical observations introduced the following classifications of mitochondrial CPEO or Kearns' disease [13]: infantile (first decade) or Kearns-Sayre-syndrome, juvenile (second decade), adult (third, fourth, fifth decade). All three forms present with a descending muscular weakness, although occasionally late-adult onset cases are restricted to the extra-ocular muscles only.

The pattern of inheritance of the disease is still disputed. In 25% of cases described until 1978 a familial occurrence had been reported [1]. However, in

Table 2. Clinical signs and symptoms of Kearns' disease

- Ptosis, CPEO, cranial and other skeletal muscle disease, fatigueability,
- retinal pigment degeneration (atypical, to even typical retinitis pigmentosa),
- cardiac abnormalities: progressive block, cardiomyopathy,
- central nervous system abnormalities: epilepsy, cerebellar, pyramidal, extra-pyramidal and dorsal tract signs, heat-intolerance, respiratory insufficiency, calcification of basal ganglia, alterations of the spinal fluid (increased protein content, abnormal proteins), spongiosis cerebri, progressive encephalopathy, especially the white matter, but also of the cerebral cortex,
- peripheral nervous system abnormalities: peripheral motor and sensory neuropathy,
- sensorineural degeneration: perceptive deafness, nystagmus, diminished excitability of labyrinths, optic atrophy,
- endocrine diseases: diabetes mellitus, adrenal medullary and cortical deficiency, retarded sexual maturation, disturbances of thyroid, parathyroid and aldosterone.renin system,
- retarded somatic growth, retarded bone-development,
- retarded or deteriorating mental development,
- skeletal anomalies: kyphoscoliosis, osteoporosis, dental anomalies,
- intestinal disturbances (especially of resorption), liver disease,
- further ocular abnormalities: corneal edema and clouding, exophthalmos, glaucoma simplex, pupillary anomalies,
- disturbed renal function: amino-aciduria,
- blood dyscrasias: anaemia, thrombocytopenia.

most cases the family history has not been adequately investigated and a familial case could have been missed easily.

Recently, a mitochondrial inheritance has been proposed for mitochondrial myopathies [14]. The mitochondrial DNA is nearly entirely derived from the mother, so maternal transmission is obligate in this form of heredity. In mitochondrial CPEO this is certainly not evident. In 83 families traced from the literature and our own files 89 maternal and 79 paternal transmissions were detected (paper in preparation). This makes a mitochondrial heredity of Kearns disease improbable. There still remains however the possibility of phenocopies with enzymatic defects encoded by mitochondrial genes, hitherto only documented in lower species. A more reasonable concept is that of an autosomal dominant transmission with varying expressivity and penetrance [15, 16, 17]. Consanguineous marriage in a former generation is suggestive of and autosomal recessive inheritance, but this is not sufficient proof.

The aetiology is completely unknown. In the past a mitochondrial enzymatic defect has been suggested. The finding of loose coupling of oxidative phosphorylation drew attention on this possibility [1]. In this situation mitochondrial respiration is not adequately regulated by the presence of ADP, but results nevertheless in a normal production of ATP. However, incomplete respiratory control occurs in various mitochondrial diseases and is accompanied by several different mitochondrial enzymatic defects (e.g. in other encephalomyopathies).

In other reports the pathogenesis was attributed to deficiency of cytochrome-c-oxidase, of carnitine, vitamine E and disturbance in folate metabolism of thiamin deficiency.

In 16 out of our own 20 patients with mitochondrial CPEO a biochemical mitochondrial investigation was performed. In only one a partial cytochrome-c-oxidase deficiency was found. Several publications have pointed to a partial shortage of cytochrome-c-oxydase in some muscle fibres in biopsy material, even in parts of healthy fibres [18, 19]. This finding has been proposed as a key to pathogenesis. More probable however is that any biochemical defect is secondary to structural defects of the mitochondrial and this aspecific. A slight (secondary) intramuscular carnitine defeciency was found in three of our patients.

In fact we only found a nonspecific disturbance of the mitochondrial functions [17], varying from decreased oxygenation of different substrates (malate, pyruvate) to slightly lowered oxydations and ATP production. In particular no clear enzymatic defect was discovered in the respiratory chain. These abnormalities, also described elsewhere [20], were considered secondary and other investigators have confirmed this [21]. Disturbance in folate metabolism, or shortage of vitamin E or thiamine were not detected in the 16 patients examined.

Histologically we found capillary proliferations with strongly thickened basal membranes just next to ragged-red fibres in the biopsies of skeletal muscles in mitochondrial CPEO [12, 22]. By measuring, these membranes turned out to be two or three times thickened compared to controles, even in the absence of a disturbed glucose tolerance in our patients. For this reason a concept of the microvascular pathogenesis of mitochondrial CPEO was introduced. Insufficient transport of oxygene and metabolites to the cell causes structural as well as functional alterations of mitochondria in an attempt to increase the metabolic rate: this is achieved by increase of number and volume of mitochondria, increase in the amount of cristae and swelling of the matrix. At a later stage decompensation occurs, speeded up by deposition of enzyme-negative crystals, which will diminish the metabolic rate further. Various secondary enzyme deficiences can be found at this stage, including partial cytochrome-c-oxydase deficiency and carnitine shortage. In the ultimate stages the mitochondria will atrophy or lyse. All these stages can be found in a skeletal muscle biopsy of patients with Kearns' disease.

This concept of a primary structural disorder is hardly to explain by autosomal recessive heredity, in which a primary enzymatic defect has to be expected. Our concept dealing with the postulated autosomal dominant heredity, points to a distinct nosological entity. For this entity the term Kearns' disease can be used, which however may be confused with Kearns Sayre syndrome, the presumed infantile variant of Kearn's disease. Very probably there are phenocopies with different or absent heredity, and possibly, with more or less causative enzymatic defects. It is also possible that the microvascular pathology, we found in Kearns' disease, is not specific, and that it will be found in other mitochondrial cytopathies, if specifically searched for. The pathogenesis of all these different diseases remains an enigma except in very few where specific enzyme defect has been found.

Occasionally an external ophthalmoplegia is found in other mitochondrial encephalomyopathies, as for example in juvenile spongiosis or Leigh's syndrome [23]. In some cases it seems from the case history, that these may in fact represent Kearns Sayre syndrome.

2.2.3 External ophthalmoplegia in metabolic disease

Primary carnitine deficiency can be classified in a muscular and a systemic form. The muscular form has a benign course and remains limited to the skeletal muscles only. In the systemic form liver, CNS and heart are also affected and the diagnosis is made by detecting carnitine deficiency in serum. The disease starts in early adolescense and is occasionally fatal. Extra-ocular muscles especially the m.levator palpebrae, may be involved. Skeletal muscle biopsy shows vacuoles of neutral fat and sometimes slight mitochondrial alterations with ragged-red fibres [24]. A secondary form of carnitine deficiency in the muscle fibre sometimes is found in combination of disturbance of the respiratory chain and in severe forms of Kearns' disease. Other secondary forms of carnitine deficiency occur in primary organic aciduries and due to proximal renal failure. In these last forms no ophthalmoplegia has been recorded.

A primary cytochrome-c-oxydase deficiency presents as a very severe, mostly

fatal, encephalomyopathy, which may occur in combination with external ophthalmoplegia [12, 25, 26]. In its complete form the disease is not compatible with
extra-uterine life. The heredity is probably autosomal recessive.

Vitamin E deficiency with successive external ophthalmoplegia has been described a few times [27, 28].

2.2.4 Oculopharyngeal dystrophy

This is characterized by progressive blepharoptosis and dysphagia, with onset in
late adult life (fifth decade). The underlying cause is of myopathic origin and
located in the extra-ocular muscles, especially the m.levator palpebrae and the
muscles involved in swallowing (pharynx and upper esophagus [1]). Ptosis can be
heralded by the dysphagia and vice versa. The disease was first reported in
French-Canadians [29]. The reports assumed an autosomal dominant heredity
with 100% penetrance and little variation in expression. Later associated signs
were detected: external ophthalmoplegia, dysphonia, involvement of other cranial and proximal muscles. In several cases the distal muscles of the limbs are
more affected than pharyngeal muscles: oculopharyngo-distal myopathy [30].

The disease has probably a pure myogenous origin, as proven at autopsy [1].
Infiltration of lymphocytes has been described occasionally in some skeletal
muscles at the onset of the disease [31]. Neurogenous features have been seen,
most probably due to accompanying conditions as cachexia (as a result of longstanding swallowing difficulties) and upper intestinal carcinoma, that concurs
remarkably often with oculopharyngeal dystrophy [32, 33, 34].

The diagnosis of these diseases mainly depends on the recognition of the
clinical picture, the heredity and finally a biopsy of a skeletal muscle. In the
biopsy of a proximal muscle we find small angular fibres which stain dark on
oxidative enzymatic stains, and 'rimmed vacuoles', subsarcolemmal vacuoles
with fine filaments radiating from the border. Hypertrophy of type II fibres is
often present [3, 35]. Nonspecific abnormalities are found on electron-microscopy. The disease has a slow progressive but otherwise benign course. Swallowing complaints, however may be so severe that death results from cachexia or
aspiration pneumonia. Cancer of the esophagus or stomach is found remarkably
often. The other possible diagnoses encompass all conditions where swallowing
complaints and external ophthalmoplegia ('oculopharyngeal syndrome') can occur: Kearns' disease, polymyositis, myasthenic syndromes, progressive bulbar
paralysis, lesions of the brainstem or cranial base, syphylis, cachexia.

2.2.5 CPEO in myotonic dystrophy

Blepharoptosis is seldom pronounced and involvement of ocular movement is
very rare. The disease is inherited in an autosomal dominant pattern with
extensive expression and penetrance. A clinical distinction with Kearns' disease
may be difficult, especially when general muscular weakness is accompanied by
pigmentary disturbances of the retina, cardiomyopathy, endocrine deficits, neu-

ronal deafness, dysphagia and dysarthria which may all occur in myotonic dystrophy. Muscular weakness however, may be more pronounced than in Kearns' disease.

Clinical and electrophysiological signs of myotonia and the typical lenticular abnormalities may provide a diagnosis at an early stage. In a skeletal muscle biopsy the most typical but not pathognomonic, abnormalities are nuclear chains and ring fibres. Atypical mitochondrial abnormalities are described in addition to nonspecific myogenic signs [1]. The extra-ocular muscular pathology has been described recently: the changes are typically myopathic [37].

2.2.6 CPEO in heredo-ataxias: myopathic?

Disturbed saccadic eye movements (e.g. slow saccades) frequently are reported in heredo-ataxias [1, 38]. A complete ophthalmoplegia is rare. Autopsy or biopsy findings of the extra-ocular muscles have seldom been reported. The oculomotor disorders are of a neurogenic (nuclear or supranuclear) nature and will not be discussed here, for it is beyond the issue of this chapter. In Friedreich's ataxia myopathic involvement of the extra-ocular muscles is occasionally described [39]. It is sometimes difficult to distinguish between a heredo-ataxia with partial CPEO, retinal pigmentary disturbances and cardiomyopathy and a form of Kearns' disease with abundant spino-cerebellar and cerebellar affection. A skeletal muscular biopsy and the type of heredity (autosomal recessive in Friedreichs ataxia) may be of help in these instances.

References

1. Bastiaensen LAK (1978): Chronic Progressive External Ophthalmoplegia. Stafleu Publ. Cy., Alphen a/d Rijn.
2. Bastiaensen LAK (1974): The diagnosis of myogenic ocular motor palsies. Short introduction to the electromyography of the external ocular muscles. Ophthalmologica 165: 513–516.
3. Dubowitz V, Brooke H (1973): Muscle biopsy. A modern approach. W.B. Sanders Cy, London.
4. Frazetto F, Streiff E, Forssmann W (1969): L'ophthalmyopathie congénitale. Ann Ocul. 202: 1228–1253.
5. Bastiaensen LAK (1985): Non-neurogenic blepharoptosis in diabetes mellitus. Neuro-Ophthalmology 5: 175–178.
6. Dortzbach RK, Sutula FC (1980): Involutional blepharoptosis, a histopathological study. Arch. Ophthalmol 98: 2045–2049.
7. Shore JW, McLord CD (1984): Anatomic changes in involutional blepharoptosis. Am.J.Ophthalmol. 98: 21–27.
8. Burck V, Brönneke J, Held KR (1983): Kongenitale Fehlbildungen im Bereich des Augen und deren Bedeutung für die Diagnostik über-geordneter Krankheitsbilder und die genetische Beratung. Klin.Mbl.Augenheilk. 183: 22–27.
9. Sugie SH, Hansen R, Rasmussen G, Verity MA (1982): Congenital neuromuscular disease with type I hypotrophy, ophthalmoplegia and myofibre degeneration. J.Neurol. Neurosurg. Psychiat. 54: 507–512.
10. Dubrovsky AL, Taratuto AL, Martino R (1978): Type 2 hypotrophy and ophthalmoplegia.

Another congenital neuromuscular disease? Abstr. 4th Congress Neuromusc. Dis. Montreal.

11. Pavlakis SG, Phillips PC, DiMauro SD, De Vivo DC, Rowland LP (1984): Mitochondrial myopathy, encephalopathy, lactic acidosis and strokalike episode: A distinctive clinical syndrome. Ann.Neurol. 16: 481–488.

12. Sengers RCA, Stadhouders AM, Trijbels JMF (1984): Mitochondrial myopathies. Clinical, morphological and biochemical aspects. Eur.J.Pediatr. 141: 192–207.

13. Bastiaensen LAK, Stadhouders AM, ter Laak HJ, Ruitenbeek W, Damen HAA, Frenken CWGM (1984): Kearns-Sayre Syndrome. Remarks on the pathogenesis with reference to a case with dwarfism and calcification of basal ganglia. Neuro-Ophthalmology 4: 55–63.

14. Egger J, Wilson J (1983): Mitochondrial inheritance in a mitochondrially mediated disease. New.Engl.J.Med. 309: 142–146.

15. Bastiaensen LAK, Joosten EMG, de Rooy JAM, Hommes OR, Stadhouders AM, Jaspar HHJ, Veerkamp JH, Bookelman H, van Hinsbergh UVM (1978): Ophthalmoplegia-Plus: a real nosological entity. Acta Neurol.Scandinav. 58: 9–34.

16. Bastiaensen LAK, Frenken CWGM, ter Laak HJ, Jaspar HHJ, Stadhouders AM. Ruitenbeek W, Veerkamp JH (1982): Kearns Syndrome: a heterogeneous group of disorders with CPEO, or a nosological entity? Doc.Ophthalmol. 52: 207–225.

17. Bastiaensen L, Stadhouders A, Trijbels J, Veerkamp J, Ruitenbeek W, Jaspar H, Ter Laak H (1981): Kearns Syndrome. Concept of a disease. In: Huber A, Klein D (eds) Neurogenetics and Neuro-ophthalmology, Elsevier North Holland Biomedical Press, Amsterdam. 205–211.

18. Müller-Höcker J, Pongratz D, Hübner G (1983): Focal deficiency of cytochrome-c-oxydase in skeletal muscle of patients with progressive external ophthalmoplegia. Virchows Arch. Pathol. Anat. 402: 61–71.

19. Johnson MA, Turnbull DM, Dick JJ, Sherratt HSA (1983): A partial deficiency of cytochrome-c-oxydase in chronic progressive external ophthalmoplegia. J. Neurol. Sci. 60: 31–53.

20. Allen PJ, DiMauro S, Coulter DC, Papadimitriou A, Rothenberg SP (1983): Kearns-Sayre Syndrome with reduced plasma and cerebro-spinal fluid folate. Ann. Neurol. 13: 679–681.

21. Mitsumoto H, Aprille JR, Wray SH, Nemni R, Bradly WG (1983): Chronic Progressive External Ophthalmoplegia (CPEO): clinical morphological and biochemical studies. Neurology 33: 452–461.

22. Stadhouders AM, Bastiaensen LAK, Jaspar HHJ, Ter Laak HJ (1981): Some new observations on ragged-red fibres in chronic progressive external ophthalmoplegia (CPEO). In: A Huber, D. Klein (eds). Neurogenics and Neuro-Ophthalmology, Elsevier North Holland Biomedical Press, Amsterdam. 223–227.

23. van Erven PMM, Gabreëls FJM, Ruitenbeek W, den Hartog MR, Fischer JC, Renier WO, Trijbels JMF, Hooft JL, Janssen AJM (1985): Subacute necrotizing encephalomyopathy (Leigh syndrome) associated with disturbed oxidation of pyruvate, malate and 2-oxoglutarate in muscle and liver. Acta Neurol. Scandinav. 72: 36–42.

24. Karpati G, Carpenter S, Engel AG, Watters G, Allen J, Rothman S, Klassen G, Mamer OA (1975): The syndrome of systemic carnitine-deficiency. Clinical, morphologic and patho-physiologic features. Neurology 25: 16–24.

25. Boustany RN, Aprille JR, Helperin J, Levy H, De Lory GR (1983): Mitochondrial cytochrome deficiency presenting as a myopathy with hypotonia, external ophthalmoplegia and lactic acidosis in an infant, and a fatal hepatopathy in a second cousin. Ann. Neurol. 14: 462–470.

26. DiMauro S, Mendell R, Schenk Z, Bachman D, Scarpa A (1978): Fatal infantile mitochondrial myopathy due to lack of cytochrome-c-oxydase. Abstract 4th Intern. Congress Neuromusc. Dis. Montreal.

27. Hoogenraad TU, Jennekens FGI, van Ketel BA, Staal GEJ, ten Thije OJ (1982): External eye muscle palsies and atypical retinitis pigmentosa in an adult with cystic fibrosis. Neuro-Ophthalmology 2: 267–274.

28. Tomasi LG (1979): Reversibility of human myopathy caused by vitamin E deficiency. Neurology 29: 1182–1186.

29. Barbeau A (1965): The syndrome of hereditary late onset ptosis and dysphagia in French Canada. In: E. Kuhn (ed). Symposium über progressive Muskeldystrophie-myotonie-myasthenie. Springer Verlag, Berlin.

30. Jaspar HHJ, Bastiaensen LAK, ter Laak HJ, Joosten EMG, Horstink MWI, Stadhouders AM (1977): Oculopharyngodistal myopathy with early onset and neurogenic features. Clin. Neurol. Neurosurg. 80: 272–282.

31. Bosch EP, Gowans JOC, Meursat T (1979): Inflammatory myopathy in oculopharyngeal dystrophy. Muscle Nerve 2: 73–77.

32. Kozachek JW, Wilson FJ (1982): Oculopharyngeal dystrophy: ultrastructure of muscles distant from the primary myopathy. Acta Neuropathol. 57: 7–12.

33. Krause KH, Schmitt HP, Houtman A (1981): Oculoparyngealy Muskel-dystrophie mit neurogener Muskelatrophie. Nervenarzt. 52: 79–84.

34. Probst A, Tackmann W, Stoechli HR, Junscau F, Ulrich J (1982): Evidence for a chronic axonal atrophy in oculopharyngeal 'muscular atrophy'. Acta Neuropathol. 57: 209–216.

35. Fukuhary N, Kumamoto T, Tsubeke T, Mayuzumi T, Nitta H (1981): Oculopharyngeal muscular dystrophy and distal myopathy. Intrafamilial difference in the onset and distribution of muscular involvement. Acta Neurol. Scandinav. 65: 458–467.

36. Couturier JC, Carrier H, Brunon AM, Davidas JL, Bady B (1981): La myopathie oculopharyngée: (à propos d'une observations familiale). Lyon Méd. 245: 109–113.

37. Kitano S, Yamashita H, Oohira A, Hori S, Ozawa T (1985): Findings in extraocular muscles in myotonic dystrophy. Ja. J. Neuro-Ophthal. 2: 159–165.

38. Cambier JM, Masson M, Prier S (1978): Etude électro-oculo-graphique d'un cas d'abolition des saccades horizontales avec viscosité du regard au cours d'une hérédo-dégénérescence cérébelleuse. Rev. Neurol. 134: 461–470.

39. Bastiaensen LAK, Jaspar HHJ, Stadhouders AM, Egberink GJM, Korten JJ (1977): Chronic progressive external ophthalmoplegia in a heredo-ataxia: neurogenic or myogenic? Acta Neurol. Scandinav. 56: 483–507.

Signs and symptoms of ocular myasthenia: a clinician's view

A.R. WINTZEN

In myasthenia gravis extra-ocular muscles are part of the motor system, which is, at least clinically, most consistently affected. The reason for this is not clear, but a possible explanation may be that extra-ocular muscles have little opportunity to recuperate, even during sleep. An other additional explanation may be found in the unique shape of their motor end-plates.

Although in myasthenia an extreme variability of muscular weakness during action may appear in any muscle, this variability is particularly marked in the oculomotor system [1]. Ptosis may change in time and the same occurs in the spectrum of images in patients with diplopia. Involvement of extra-ocular muscles is often asymmetric.

As regards treatment there is an important difference between skeletal and extra-ocular muscles; whereas any improvement in strength or indurance of skeletal muscles may result in substantial improvement, this is normally not the case in their extra-ocular counterparts; in the latter improvement less than complete recovery will not substantially change patients symptoms.

Therefore, ocular myasthenia poses grave and complex problems both for the patient and the physician. This paper is an attempt to arrange these problems in an orderly fashion.

Most neurological textbooks dealing with myasthenia gravis mention the various abnormalities of ocular movement that can be observed by the examiner. The functional consequences for the patients are mentioned only briefly, probably because it is considered self-evident that ptosis and ocular misalignment will impair visual function. However, this is only part of the story.

Objective signs of ocular myasthenia are:
- ptosis,
- limitation of movement (paresis) of individual ocular muscles,
- disconjugate movement of the eyes,
- 'jelly-like' movements, also referred to as 'quiver' or 'lightning' movements,
- pseudo-internuclear ophthalmoplegia.

1. Ptosis is obvious at first glance if it is unilateral or asymmetric and if it is gross.

If slight and symmetric, however, it can be easily overlooked, particularly in elderly people because of the redundant skin of their upper rim of the pupil being covered by the upper lid, but observation of raised eye brows or tilting of the head may be very helpful in detecting ptosis. As already mentioned, ptosis is rarely a constant phenomenon in myasthenia; close observation will reveal that in most cases it changes continuously, thus enabling to suspect a diagnosis of myasthenia immediately.

Discomfort resulting from ptosis varies. If gross and bilateral ptosis will obviously impair vision. On the other hand, if ptosis is unilateral in a patient with diplopia, it may be helpful from a functional point of view, except when the 'dominant' eye is covered. In the latter case the patient will do his utmost to look with the ptotic eye, despite severe and troublesome diplopia. But even if vision is not impaired because ptosis is slight and diplopia is unimportant or absent, the paretic levator palpebrae may still give trouble because of its important role in the facial expression of mood, interest and attention. Usually, this is not immediately perceived by the patient, but she/he may be confronted with unexpected questions, such as: 'Don't you enjoy the party?' or 'Are you tired?' or 'This doesn't seem to interest you very much, does it?'. In case of asymmetric ptosis an other mechanism becomes active. Whereas most can close one eye, i.e. innervate one orbicularis oculi muscle, nobody is able to raise one upper eyelid, i.e. innervate one levator palpebrae muscle, without raising the other at the same time. Because a myasthenic patient with unilateral or asymmetric ptosis tries to compensate ptosis, one eye will be closed too far (because of the paresis) and the other opened too wide (because of the bilateral effect of the attempted correction) for the intended facial expression [1]. The patients become aware of this discrepancy when facing a mirror and may comment that they are quite disfigured.

2. *Paresis of individual muscles* in eye movement may led to three specific subjective consequences: first, a sensation of movement of surrounding objects during eye- or head movement; secondly directional misprojection of fixated objects after such movement and thirdly, inability to quickly following moving objects [2]. The basis of this problem is the mismatch of intended and executed angle of eyeball rotation. There is no clinically detectable proprioceptive feedback of eye muscles; therefore, correct execution of their instructions seems to be self-evident to commanding oculomotor neurons. Minor inaccuracies are promptly corrected by retinal feedback. Major inaccuracies are perceived as object movement. This phenomenon is comparable to what one sees if an eyeball is rotated upward by one's own finger on the lower eyelid; as the backward rotation of the eyeball was not preceded by a corresponding oculomotor command, the result of no motor command and upward movement of the object over the retina is perceived as a downward movement of the object. This simple experiment shows that any movement of the image of an object over the retina, which is not accompanied by a corresponding oculomotor command, will be perceived as a movement of the object in a direction opposite to that as which of the eyeball was actually rotated.

It is very likely, that the discrepancy between the intended and actual ocular movement in myasthenic patients is responsible for their frequent complaints that a doorhandle or an outstretched hand was not found in the expected place, or that a doorstep did not have the expected height, thus explaining many of their stumbling. Many myasthenics state that they do not dare to cross roads, because they are not sure of exact direction and speed of motorcars. Likewise, they avoid driving a car, because they see apparently fixed objects, such as parked cars, appear to move up and down. Finally, the inability to quickly follow moving objects explains why myasthenics do not enjoy playing golf or tennis, because they loose sight of the ball they have just hit.

The recording of eye movement in myasthenic patients, especially of saccades, illustrates the complexity of the disturbance; both hypometric and hypermetric saccades can be observed in the same patient and even during the same movement [3–6]. This indicates, that extreme lability of neuromuscular transmission frustrates all efforts of the central nervous system to compensate for it. The efforts may even have an adverse effect. This inability of the central nervous system to cope with this problem may well be the neuronal basis of the patients' remarks about 'going mad' because of their eyes.

3. Disconjugate eye movement are caused by asymmetry of the neuro-muscular block; this results in diplopia and visual confusion. A characteristic feature of myasthenic diplopia, though not present in all patients, is continuous movement of two images with respect to each other, horizontally, vertically and torsion. Unlike other causes of diplopia, myasthenia frequently renders it very difficult for the patient to choose an angle of vision with minimal or no diplopia.

A myasthenic patient rarely benefits from having one eye covered, either because the unstable restriction of movement of the other eye obviates normal monocular function, or because the covered eye is the dominant one.

4. 'Jelly like' movements are quick nonconjugate oscillating movements [3, 7]. Similarly, 'twitch-movements' can be seen in the upper eyelids. They do not seem to bother the patient inordinately. Because they have not been reported in disorders other than myasthenia gravis, their presence may be useful for the diagnosis]7].

5. Distinction of pseudo-internuclear ophthalmoplegia from its brainstem-generated counterpart may be difficult, because myasthenia gravis and multiple sclerosis frequently occur in young women [6, 9]. Pseudo-internuclear ophthalmoplegia, however, is caused by impaired neuromuscular transmission and disappears with anti-cholinesterase drugs. Patients exhibiting this phenomenon usually have diplopia. The exact mechanism is not known.

References

1. Schmidt D (1975): Diagnostik myasthenischer Augensymptome, Klin. Mbl. Augenheilk. 167: 651–644.

146

2. Estânol B, Lopez-Rioz G (1984): Looking with a paralysed eye: adaptive plasticity of the vestibulo-ocular reflex. J. Neurol Neurosurg Psych. 47: 799–804.
3. Yee RD, Cogan DG, Zee DS, Bolok RW, Honrubia V (1976): Rapid eye movements in myasthenia gravis. Arch Ophthalmol. 94: 1465–1472.
4. Schmidt D, Dell'osso LF, Abel LA, Daroff RB (1980): Myasthenia gravis: Saccadic eye movement waveforms. Exp. Neurol. 68: 346–364.
5. Schmidt D, Dell'osso LF, Abel LA, Daroff RB (1980): Myasthenia gravis: dynamic changes in saccadic waveform, gain and velocity. J bid. 68: 365–377.
6. Spooner JW, Baloh RW (1979): Eye movement fatigue in myasthenia gravis. Neurol 29: 29–33.
7. Cogan D, Yee RD, Gittinger J (1976): Rapid eye movements in myasthenia gravis. Arch Ophthalmol. 94: 1083–1085.
8. Cogan D (1965): Myasthenia gravis. Arch Ophthalm. 74: 217–221.
9. Glaser JS (1966): Myasthenic pseudo-internuclear ophthalmoplegia. Arch. Ophthalmol., 75: 363–366.

Blepharoptosis

L.A.K. BASTIAENSEN, R.J.W. DE KEIZER

Blepharoptosis (ptosis) of the upper eyelid can be defined as a condition in which the margin of the upper eyelid is at a lower position than normal. In adults this is about 1.5 mm below the upper limbus of the cornea [1]. The interpalpebral fissure in a normal caucasion adult is 10 mm high [2]. The upper eyelid is elevated chiefly by action of the m.levator palpebrae, innervated by n-III, and partly by the m.tarsalis which has a sympathetic innervation.

The m.levator palpebrae has a common origin at the ligament of Zinn with the m.rectus superior. Embryologically they arise from the same origin and remain intimately connected in anatomical and functional respect during further life. This explaines elevation of the upper eyelid in upward gaze.

The m.orbicularis oculi closes the interpalpebral fissure; it is innervated by n-VII.

The opposite of ptosis, retraction of the upper eyelid, can be seen in conditions with overactivation of the sympathetic system (e.g. in Graves' disease), and of the ocular motor nerve (cyclic oculomotor spasms [3] or ocular motor synkinesis). Palsy of facial nerve results mainly in drooping of the lower eyelid and lagophthalmos.

The innervation of the m. levator palpebrae is derived from the central caudal nucleus in each ocular motor nuclear complex [4]. This subnucleus provides bilateral innervation of the levator muscles, so unilateral ptosis can hardly be explained by a nuclear lesion, except by extension outside the nuclear region.

Ptosis of the upper eyelid is a common and concomitant sign in many ocular motor disorders.

For introductory remarks on anatomy of the eyelids, clinical investigation of and therapeutic measures for ptosis, the reader is referred to ophthalmological, neurological and especially neuro-ophthalmological textbooks [5, 6, 7]. In general function of the upper eyelid depends on integrity of intrinsic muscles (m.levator palpebrae, m.tarsalis, m.orbicularis oculi) and their innervation; furthermore on other anatomic lid constituents (tarsus, ligaments, septum orbitale, conjunctiva and skin), surrounding structures of the eye and general, metabolic and neurological condition.

Investigation of a ptotic upper eyelid therefore encompasses:

– confirmation of the reality (cave pseudo-ptosis) and degree of ptosis (height of interpalpebral fissure).

– testing of function of the m.levator palpebrae. This is done by measuring differences in height of the interpalpebral fissure in extreme upward and downward gaze. The eyebrow position should be fixated to prevent contraction of the m.orbicularis oculi. The normal levator function is 10–14 mm.

– assessment of upper eyelid position in downward gaze with and without taking into account lower eyelid position. A retraction of the upper eyelid is better seen in this procedure. Furthermore, in some general muscular and neurogenous diseases, cachexia and senility, the lower eyelid moves down in the same proportion as the upper eyelid; sometimes there is in these conditions a lower lid lag in the primary position. In misdirection of n-III upper eyelid position can be oddly changed in looking down.

– establishment of presence or absence of lid fold. This is mostly absent in congenital ptosis and levator desinsertion. In this latter condition the upper eyelid is also thinner, sometimes even translucent. An intact lid fold points to a reasonably intact levator function.

– observation whether Bell's phenomenon is present; if positive in a condition with ptosis and restricted eye-elevation, points to a supranuclear origin. If negative, ptosis is associated with palsy of the superior rectus.

– assessment of any ocular or adnexal disease, and search for general, metabolic and neurological disturbances.

Establishment of site of the lesion in a case of ptosis may be supported by auxillary test methods. In case of a suspected general myopathy estimation of creatine-kinase and other muscular enzymes in blood can be helpful. Electromyography of the m.levator palpbrae is an infrequent used procedure which deserves more widespread application it can be done quickly and (nearly) painless, even in children; it is harmless and easily performed without local anaesthesia by instilling a coaxial facial needle under the upper orbital rim in a nearly horizontal direction through the m.orbicularis oculi and the orbital septum right into the belly of the levator, when patient looks down. A steady position of the needle in the muscle belly can easily be confirmed by asking the patient to look up: a massive recruitment of action potentials is immediately displayed on the EMG screen. This innocuous test (only 3 minor subcutaneous haemorrhages were seen in more than 300 procedures) can be of great help in making a distinction between myogenous, neurogenous and myasthenic causes [8].

A biopsy of the levator muscle is seldomly required, difficult to perform because of the long aponeurosis, and still more difficult to interpret. In cases of a suspected general muscular disease, a skeletal muscular biopsy deserves consideration.

1. Classification of blepharoptosis

1.1 Congenital [1, 6, 9–11]

Ptosis congenita occurs mostly sporadically but can be inherited as an autosomal dominant trait. Usually it occurs unilaterally. The syndrome of congenital ptosis with epicanthus inversus and blepharophimosis, is a bilateral condition and is mostly inherited in an autosomal dominant way. In about 10% of cases, congenital ptosis is associated with weakness of the m.rectus superior. The histo-pathological base for congenital ptosis is diverse. A neurogenous cause is common, but disturbances of anlage of levator muscle are also found (aplasia, hypoplasia, abnormal course of insertion, congenital fibrosis).

Congenital blepharoptosis is occasionally associated with disturbances of eye movement. Anomalous adhesions of the levator or anomalous innervation may result in ptosis in Duane's syndrome, Brown's syndrome and Marcus Gunn syndrome. Congenital external ophthalmoplegia, which can be inherited on an autosomal dominant way, is nearly invariably associated with severe ptosis. The cause can be nuclear, hypoplasia or myopathic.

Some general congenital conditions are associated with ptosis. These include:
chromosomal aberations: monosomy 4, trisomy 9-p, monosomy 18, trisomy 18, Turner syndrome;
first branchial arc syndromes: Hallermann-Streiff, Treacher Collins syndromes;
other congenital syndromes: syndromes of Ehlers-Danlos, Rubinstein-Taybi, Smith-Lemli-Opitz, Schwartz-Jampel, the Mail-Patella syndrome;
congenital general myopathies: nemaline myopathy, centronuclear myopathy, minicore myopathy, targetoid myopathy, microfibre myopathy;
orbital causes: neurofibromatosis, orbital or lid tumours (dermoid, hemangioma);
pseudo-ptosis: due to hypotropia of the fixing eye must not be overlooked.

1.2 Acquired [1, 7, 9]

Myogenous causes
1. *Myopathies.* See the chapter on Ocular Myopathies
2. *Ocular myositis.* The disease usually occurs as a pure ocular muscle disease with pain on ocular movement in the direction of the affected muscle, local eye redness and tendernes, exophthalmos, and occasionally blepharoptosis, when orbital involvement is more profuse. So it can be part of the spectrum of signs in the orbital pseudo-tumour syndrome.

Disturbances of neuromuscular transmission. Unilateral ptosis is a common sign in incipicient myasthenia gravis. Sometimes ptosis is compensated by superfluous innervation resulting in contralateral upper eyelid retraction and a normal palpebral height on the affected side: occlusion of the contralateral, retraction, side shall then reveal the ptosis on the affected side.

In oat-cell tumour of the lung a myasthenic syndrome with ptosis is not uncommon.

The diagnosis depends on the history (drooping of the eyelid more severe in the evenings) or clinical tests: drooping after sustained upward gaze, Cogan's lid twitch' sign, shivering of the lid. A tensilon test may demonstrate quite effectfully the blockage of the neuromuscular synapse by the immediate relief of ptosis some 15 seconds after i.v. injection. In old burnt-out cases of myasthenia however fibrosed levator muscle cells are not capable anymore for a visible effect on ptosis. In such case EMG control of the levator muscle during tensilon administration will reveal the myasthenic character of ptosis [12].

Oculomotor nerve paresis. The causes of n-III palsies are too numerous to name. The most common however, intra-cranial aneurysma and diabetes mellitus, deserve some comment.

Intracranial aneurysm is well known for its affection of n-III before rupture. The pupil is said to be almost invariably affected, often as the first sign. In longstanding diabetes mellitus ocular pareses by palsy of n-VI or III are nearly always self-limiting, spontaneously within 2 or 3 months. The pupil is known to be spared in diabetic n-III palsy. However, cases of intracranial aneurysma and n-III paresis without pupillary involvement, and cases of diabetes mellitus with n-III palsy including pupillary affection do occur!

Painful ophthalmoplegia is a syndrome of n-III and trigeminal involvement. Its eponyme, the syndrome of Tolosa Hunt, must be differentiated form intracranial aneurysma, tumours at the base of the skull (Chordoma!), and ophthalmoplegic migraine [18].

After longstanding n-III paresis, healing of the nerve can occur with aberrant regeneration: third cranial nerve misdirection syndrome. Typically is concomitant retraction of upper eye lid in downward gaze, or less frequently in adduction. Ptosis in abduction is also common.

Nuclear lesions of the n-III complex rarely cause ptosis except bilaterally, because of bilateral innervation of levator muscles; a crossed palsy of the superior rectus is typical for a nuclear lesion.

Cyclic oculomotor paralysis is a congenital or young acquired condition, with cycles of n-III palsy during every 2–3 minutes. It almost invariably concurs with severe disfiguring ptosis during the paralytic cycles.

Supranuclear palsies. Ptosis is rare in these conditions but is described in 'locked-in' syndrome and in mesencephalic lesions outside the oculomotor nuclear complex [14]. Cerebral palsy was recently described in which bilateral ptosis occurred after hemispheric infarction [15]. Apraxia of lidopening (e.g. in Huntington's Chorea) can mimic ptosis [1].

Sympathetic denervation. (Horner's syndrome is not commonly associated with a disturbance of eye movement. However in Wallenberg syndrome ocular lateropulsion, skew deviation, nystagmus and impaired smooth pursuit are accompanied by a homolateral Horner syndrome [16].

Tumours and vascular disorders of the upper eye lid or orbita, including haemangiomas, carotid-cavernous fistulas [17].

Desinsertion of the m.levator palpebrae. This occurs mostly in elderly and after trauma, including eye surgery. The upper eyelid is thinner and lacks the skin crease. Levator function, measured by methods described before, is remarkably intact.

Pseudoptosis is due to a variety of conditions. Anopthalmos, enophthalmos microphthalmos and phthisis bulbi concur with this form of ptosis because of insufficient support by the globe. In dermatochalasis and blepharochalasis drooping of the upper eyelid develops by excessive skin folds after loss of elasticity of the eye lidskin by degeneration respectively recurrent inflammation. Hysterical ptosis is caused by contraction of the orbicularis oculi muscles. In inflammatory conditions of the eye and its adnexae a thickened upper eyelid hangs down: the eyelid returns to its normal position inflammatory process is cured, except when levator desinsertion results form a longstanding inflammation. Ocular surgery can give the same transient aspect of ptosis.

References

1. Walsh TJ (1985): Ptosis. In: Neuro-Opthalmology. Clinical Signs and Symptoms. Walsh TJ (ed). 2e ed. Lee and Febiger, Philadelphia, 77–78.
2. Bastiaensen LAK (1985): Non-neurogenic blepharoptosis in diabetes mellitus. Neuro-Ophthalmology 5; 175–178.
3. Kommerell G, Mehdorn E, Ketelsen VP (1985): Okulomotorius Lähmung mit zyklischen Spasmen. Electromyographische und electronenmikroskopische Hinweise auf eine chronische Irritation des periphere nervs. Fortschr. Ophth. 82: 203–204.
4. Kobayaski S, Mukuno K, Tazaki Y, Ishikawa S, Okada K (1986): Oculomotor nerve nuclear complex syndrome. A case with clinicopathological correlation. Neuro-Ophthalmology 6: 55–60.
5. Walsh FB, Hoyt WF (1969): Clinical Neuro-Ophthalmology 3rd ed. Wiliams and Wilkins Cy. Baltimore.
6. Glaser JS (1978): Neuro-ophthalmologic examination: general considerations and special techniques, part 2. In: Glaser JS, ed. Neuro-Ophthalmology, Harper and Row Publish, Maryland, 37–46.
7. Burde RM, Savino PJ, Trobe JD (1985): Clinical decisions in Neuro-Ophthalmology. Mosby Cy. St. Louis. Chapter 8: 246–256.
8. Bastiaensen LAK (1972): The diagnosis of myogenic ocular motor palsies. Short introduction to the electromyography of the external ocular muscles. Ophthalmologica 165: 513–516.
9. Bastiaensen LAK (1978): Chronic Progressive External Ophthalmoplegia. Stafleu Publishing Cy. Alphen aan de Rijn.

10. François J (1969): Congenital Ophthalmoplegia. In: Brunette JR, Barbeau A eds. Progress in Neuro-Ophthalmology: Excerpta Medica, Amsterdam, 377–421.
11. Nema HV (1973): Ophthalmic syndromes. Butterworth & Cy, Publ., Edinburgh.
12. Bastiaensen LAK, van Gasteren JHM, Frenken CWGM, Leyten ACM (1979): Diagnostic problems in ocular myasthenia. Doc. Ophthalmol. 46: 381–390.
13. Bastiaensen LAK, Leyten ACM, Tjang TG, Misere JFMM (1983): Chondroid chordoma of the base of the skull: orbital and other neuro-ophthalmological symptoms. Doc. Ophthalmol 55: 5–15.
14. Leigh RJ, Zee DS (1983): Diagnosis of central disorders of ocular motility. In: Leigh RJ, Zee DS (eds). The neurology of eye movement. Davis Cy FA. Philadelphia. 191–262.
15. Caplan LR (1974): Ptosis. J. Neurol. Neurosurg. Psychiat. 37: 1–7.
16. Leigh RJ, Zee DS (1983): Wallenberg Syndrome. In: Leigh RJ, Zee DS (eds) The Neurology of eye movement. Davis Cy FA. Philadelphia: 214.
17. de Keizer RJW (1985): Vascular disorders in the orbit and in the orbital region. In: Oosterhuis JA (ed), Ophthalmic Tumours. Dr. W Junk Publish. Dordrecht 247–271.

Section V

Neurology

The interpretation of nystagmus

A.G.M. VAN VLIET

Most classifications and pathophysiological explanations of nystagmus are still rather arbitrary and inadequate. Thus, the best way is to hold on to a pure-descriptive definition like the one used by Leigh and Zee [1]: 'Nystagmus is a repetitive, to-and-fro movement of the eyes that includes smooth sinusoidal oscillations (pendular nystagmus) and alternation of slow drift and corrective quick phase (jerk nystagmus)'.

Nystagmus was traditionally subdivided into two types: pendular nystagmus and jerk nystagmus. The direction of the fast component defines the nystagmus direction. Improvement of the equipment in the recording of eye movements have allowed better definitions of nystagmus forms and gave new insight into their pathophysiology. According to Leigh and Zee [1] nystagmus may perhaps be best conceptualized as being due to disorders of the mechanisms that hold fixation steady: the vestibular, optokinetic and pursuit systems that act to hold images steady on the retina in primary position, and a network (the neural integrator) that enables to hold eccentric positions of gaze. Based on the slow-phase wave form of nystagmus, now four common types of nystagmus have been differentiated (Fig. 1).

1. Nystagmus. Mechanisms

1. The first type of disturbance causes the eyes to deviate at an ever increasing speed. This increasing speed of slow phase results in a jerk nystagmus, which is almost always congenital, or a pendular nystagmus, which can be either congenital or acquired.

2. Nystagmus resulting from vestibular tone imbalance. This causes a constant velocity drift of the eyes. The added quick phases give a 'saw-tooth' appearance. The amplitude becomes smaller on fixation and larger in the dark, behind Frenzel spectacles or record when the eyes are closed.

3. Nystagmus resulting from a leaking integrator. The integrator is a neural

156

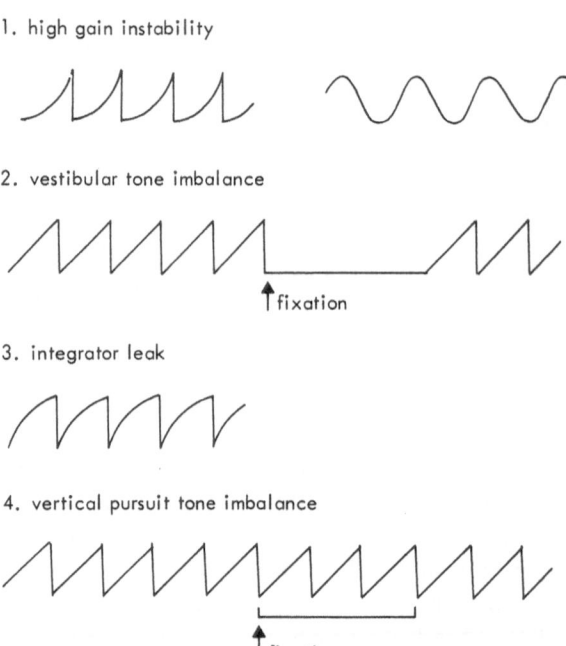

1. high gain instability

2. vestibular tone imbalance

↑fixation

3. integrator leak

4. vertical pursuit tone imbalance

↑fixation

Figure 1. Defects in SEM subsystem which produce nystagmus.

network that produces a signal proportional to eye position to hold horizontal eccentric gaze. If the integrator is 'leaky' the eyes drift towards the primary position with an exponentially decreasing speed of slow phase. This nystagmus is known clinically as gaze-evoked nystagmus and gaze paretic nystagmus.

4. Finally, nystagmus resulting from pursuit tone imbalance, which is only found in vertical eye movements, gives rise to upbeat or downbeat nystagmus. The linear slow phase of this true saw-tooth nystagmus is not inhibited by fixation.

Although these new insights provide a more scientifically based classification of nystagmus this is still far from ideal, however, practical diagnostic differentiation of nystagmus on clinical grounds is still the easiest approach. Differentiation of nystagmus on clinical grounds is based on criteria concerning form, direction, intensity, fixation and association with other signs.

2. Classification of nystagmus

If nystagmus is found on examination, on the basis of the above criteria, the following questions may be asked: 1. Is it physiological or pathological? If physiological nystagmus is ruled out, the following question is: 2. Is it congenital or acquired? If we conclude that the nystagmus is not congenital, the next question is: 3. Is it labyrinthine or central? If we are certain that a nystagmus is not labyrinthine but central: 4. What is then the localization of this central lesion?

2.1. Physiological nystagmus

One has to consider whether nystagmus is physiological or not. Nystagmus is physiological if: a. it is an saw-tooth nystagmus resulting from physiological stimuli, such as vestibular and optokinetic stimuli; b. it is an end-point nystagmus, which is not pathological; c. it is a jerk nystagmus that occurs on extremes of lateral gaze and diminishes as eccentric gaze is maintained. In poor vision however, this does not extinguish on prolonged gaze-holding. The most important feature is that the nystagmus disappears when the eyes return even a few degrees from extreme position, although this nystagmus may begin on lateral gaze of only 20°. End-point nystagmus often has a latent period of several seconds before it starts, has a small amplitude, is irregular, sometimes dissociated and is also present in the dark. The shape of the slow phase shows a more linear than exponential fall. This makes differentiation from the pathological gaze paretic nystagmus possible.

Rule of thumb: an end-point nystagmus is rarely pathological.

2.2. Congenital or acquired

If nystagmus is pathological, is it congenital or acquired? Congenital nystagmus is usually characterized by a form deviating from the saw-tooth form, which is the primary position clinically often resembles pendular horizontal nystagmus of large amplitude, but on recording is seen not to be a true sinusoidal movement (Fig. 2). In the horizontal direction of gaze this nystagmus changes to a rapid jerk nystagmus with the fast component. A useful differential diagnostic aid between congenital and acquired nystagmus is examination of nystagmus during vertical eye movements. Congenital nystagmus tends to remain horizontal while pendular in acquired (pendular) nystagmus, such as uni-ocular pendular nystagmus rarely seen in multiple sclerosis, and spasmus nutans, which will be discussed later. Congenital nystagmus becomes more obvious by attempts fixate; the intention to look is the main driving force [2]. But labyrinthine nystagmus, which is suppressed by optical fixation, may only become manifest in darkness or if fixation is removed (e.g. behind Frenzel lenses). Convergence appears to reduce congenital nystagmus. Congenital nystagmus is not accompanied by vertigo or oscillopsia. Inversion of the optokinetic nystagmus is typical for many cases of congenital nystagmus.

Rule of thumb: a coarse irregular horizontal nystagmus, when the patient is

158

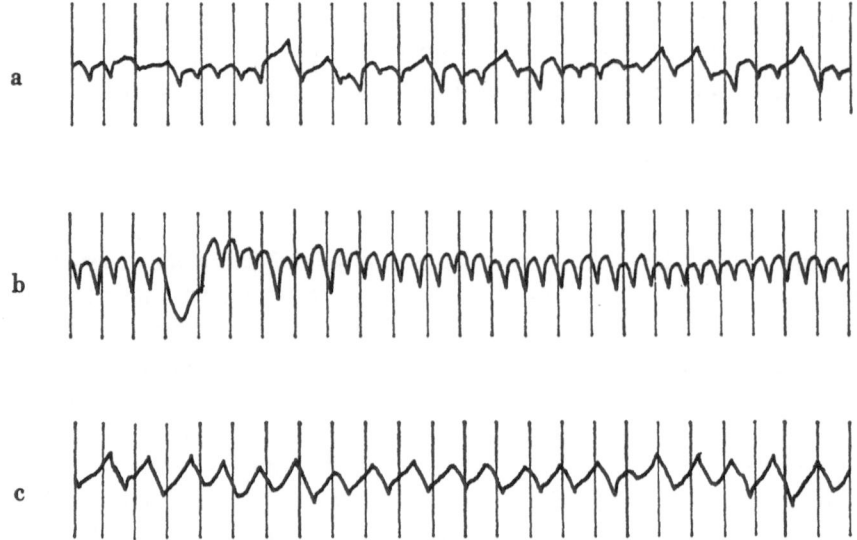

Figure 2. Different wave forms of congenital nystagmus (3).

looking straight forward and is not dizzy, is nearly always congenital.

Latent nystagmus and manifest latent nystagmus are types of congenital nystagmus that are elicited by looking with one eye [3]. This is a conjugate jerk nystagmus with the fast phase towards the fixing eye. Although latent nystagmus is congenital, the slow phase has an exponentially decreasing angular velocity, in contrast to congenital jerk nystagmus which usually has an exponentially increasing angular velocity. Manifest latent nystagmus occurs in amblyopia or strabismus on monocular fixation even with both eyes open. The direction of the manifest latent nystagmus in patients with alternating fixation is always in the direction of the fixating eye. In these patients the diagnosis of congenital nystagmus is usually made because nystagmus is present when both eyes are open. The change in direction of nystagmus when viewing with the other eye opposite to the fast phase of the manifest nystagmus and the recording of an exponentially decreasing angular velocity of the slow phase confirms the diagnosis of manifest latent nystagmus.

As already mentioned above, a *pendular nystagmus* may also be acquired, although it is more commonly congenital. This nystagmus is usually horizontal but sometimes vertical and is associated with oscillopsia and sometimes with a head tremor. It can have a fast jerk component in the direction of gaze when the eyes are moved horizontally. If the eyes move vertically, the nystagmus may become vertical pendular, as distinct from congenital nystagmus in which the movements in most cases remain horizontal. Acquired pendular nystagmus indicates a dysfunction of brain-stem and/or the cerebellum. According to Ell et al. [4] over 50% have multiple sclerosis, 30% brain-stem vascular disease (stroke or

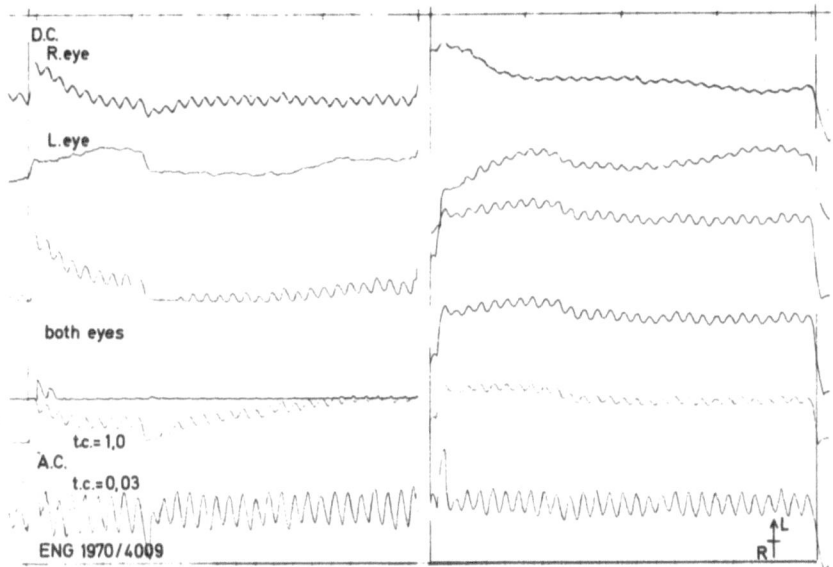

Figure 3. Spasmus nutans. Dissociated pendular nystagmus, at first monocular in the right eye (a), then with the larger amplitude in the left eye (b).

angioma). Differentiation between acquired pendular nystasmus in multiple sclerosis and congenital pendular nystagmus is possible by using next criteria. Congenital pendular nystagmus is seldom pure sinusoidal, has no vertical component and is never disssociated. Acquired pendular nystagmus in multiple sclerosis, on the other hand, often has vertical components and is usually dissociated. In addition, acquired pendular nystagmus often shows postsaccadic inhibition: after a saccade the pendular nystagmus is inhibited for 1–2 seconds. Finally, oscillopsia and neurological signs (in 92% cerebellar signs), except for head tremor, are never found in patients wit congenital nystagmus.

Spasmus nutans consists of nystagmus associated with head nodding and an abnormal position of the head. The disease affects children and usually begins between the ages of 3 and 18 months, but never later than the third year. Nodding of the head is usually the first and most obvious sign. Nystagmus however is essential. It has a number of typical characteristics which by themselves are sufficient to make the diagnosis of spasmus nutans almost certain. The direction can be either horizontal or vertical. Spasmus nutans is the primary cause of monocular vertical nystagmus in young children. Most cases of spasmus nutans with vertical nystagmus are bilateral, asymmetrical in a way that it appears to be unilateral. The horizontal nystagmus is pendular, remarkably fine and fast, viz. between 6 and 8 Hertz, and dissociated in a characteristic manner, i.e. more marked in one eye, or even strictly unilateral, and in the same patient sometimes in the right and sometimes in the left eye (Fig. 3). In some cases this asymmetry depends on the direction of gaze. The cause of spasmus nutans is not known. Recently, there have been a number of reports on the association of a tumour affecting the optic nerve and the chiasma resulting in spasmus nutans.

Decreased vision can also be the cause of nystagmus. This so-called *ocular nystagmus* is characterized by a combination of a pendular or jelly-like eye movements and an irregular jerk nystagmus with a slow drift of the eye out of the primary position and a corrective jerk towards the primary position.

2.3. Labyrinthine or central

If it is decided that a nystagmus is not congenital, one has to determine whether the nystagmus is labyrinthine (inclusive of neuronal vestibular) or central. The following criteria can help us with the differential diagnosis between labyrinthine and central:

a. The principal direction of labyrinthine nystagmus is horizontal or horizontal-torsional, sometimes associated with a slight vertical component. A pure torsion or pure vertical nystagmus is never labyrinthine but always central.

b. A second criterion is the intensity decline, which is the difference in the intensity of the nystagmus in the different horizontal directions of gaze. In Alexander's classification of first-degree nystagmus (weak nystagmus) nystagmus is present only if the patient looks in the direction of the fast phase. In second-degree nystagmus (moderate nystagmus) nystagmus also occurs if the patient looks straight ahead. In third-degree nystagmus (intense nystagmus) the nystagmus persists if patient looks in the direction of the slow phase. Thus, it is beating opposite to the gaze direction as contrasted with a symmetrical gaze evoked nystagmus, i.e. the fast phase of nystagmus is in the direction of gaze and there is no nystagmus in primary position. In labyrinthine nystagmus the intensity decline is small; a large decline in intensity suggests central nystagmus. As differences of intensity in various positions of third-degree nystagmus cannot be large, this is usually labyrinthine.

c. For another reason, third-degree nystagmus is usually labyrinthine. Labyrinthine nystagmus only occurs if there is a relative imbalance in the activity between the left and right vestibular nuclei, and is directed towards one side, in the direction of the labyrinth which initiates the most stimuli. A labyrinthine nystagmus is thus per definition directed only to one side (i.e. asymmetric). In a third-degree nystagmus this asymmetry is very strong. On the contrary, a symmetric gaze-evoked nystagmus is always central.

d. We already mentioned that labyrinthine nystagmus increases in darkness or when fixation is removed (e.g. behind Frenzel lenses), while fixation causes labyrinthine nystagmus to decrease. This is a specific influence of the cortex on the vestibular nystagmus. There are other non-specific influences. The intensity of the labyrinthine nystagmus increases by alertness and stress, and decreases through tiredness. This explains why a slight labyrinthine nystagmus is not necessarily present each occasion of examination.

e. In labyrinthine nystagmus, various signs harmonize: falling tendency, past pointing, deviation in Unterberger's stepping test (the blindfolded subject steps without moving from the spot where he is standing) are all in the direction of the slow phase of the nystagmus, i.e. in the direction of the affected labyrinth.

f. Finally, it is obvious that injury to the labyrinth can easily lead to involvement of the adjacent cochlea, so that auditory symptoms or signs may support the diagnosis of labyrinthine nystagmus.

On the basis of these criteria one never can say with certainty that a nystagmus is labyrinthine, because the central nervous system is able to imitate labyrinthine nystagmus, we only definitely can say whether nystagmus is not labyrinthine. In that case we are dealing with a central nystagmus.

Rule of thumb: a symmetric gaze-evoked nystagmus is always central.

Rule of thumb: a pure torsion or vertical nystagmus is always central.

2.4. Anatomical location

Direction of this nystagmus often indicates a more precise localization. *Horizontal nystagmus* of central origin often has characteristics of a gaze nystagmus. This is the form of nystagmus most commonly met with in clinical practice. It is a jerk nystagmus induced by an attempt to keep the eye in an eccentric position; in the primary position there is no nystagmus. The slow phase of gaze nystagmus can be linear or show exponentially decreasing speed like gaze paretic nystagmus. In absence of sedatives and anti-epileptic drugs a horizontal gaze nystagmus indicates a lesion of the brain-stem and/or the cerebellum; a more exact localization is not possible without analysis of the accompanying neurological symptoms and signs. Bilateral gaze nystagmus is often associated with a vertical gaze nystagmus in upward direction; this is seldom seen other than with bilateral horizontal gaze nystagmus. Gaze nystagmus in downward direction is usually absent. The most common cause of bilateral gaze nystagmus is the use of sedative and anti-epileptic drugs. If there is an obvious asymmetry in the amplitude of the nystagmus between the eyes, this is called 'dissociated nystagmus'. The most common form of dissociated nystagmus is that of the abducting eye in internuclear ophthalmoplegia. Precise recording shown that the speed of the slow phase of this nystagmus decreases exponentially and that the fast phase of the abducting eye is always associated with hypometric saccades in the adducting eye. If the angle of gaze is chosen so that it is within the range of poorly functioning adducting eye, abduction nystagmus will stop as soon as the adducting eye has attained its object (Fig. 4). A myasthenic, paretic nystagmus of the abducting eye, associated with an adduction paresis, can often imitate abduction nystagmus of internuclear ophthalmoplegia. Anti-cholinesterase medication resolves this reveals the diagnosis.

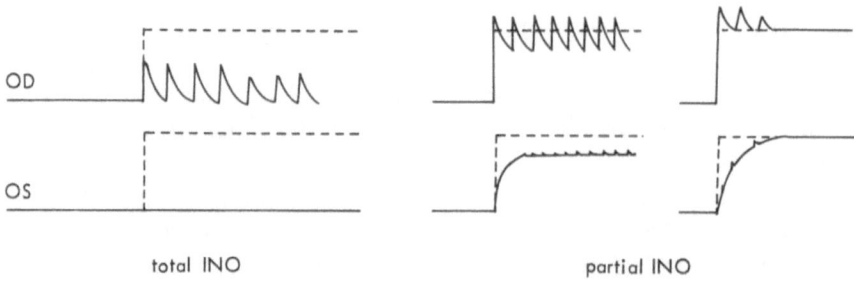

OD

OS

total INO   partial INO

Figure 4. Dissociated nystagmus of the abducting eye in internuclear ophthalmoplegia.

Internuclear ophthalmoplegia implies a lesion of the medial longitudinal fasciculus, if peripheral causes such as myasthenia gravis are excluded. The most frequent cause of internuclear ophthalmoplegia in young adults, especially bilateral, is multiple sclerosis. In the elderly a vascular stenosis is the most common cause. The combination of a gross ipsilateral gaze nystagmus, due to compression of the brain-stem, and a fine vestibular nystagmus towards the healthy side, caused by loss of the ipsilateral vestibular nerve, is called Bruns' nystagmus and is the typical nystagmic picture of an acoustic neurinoma in an advanced stage. In addition, on upward gaze the contralateral vestibular nystagmus increases and on downward gaze it changes into an ipsilateral nystagmus, the so-called diagonal division. If the eyes are closed, nystagmus towards the normal side predominates. Other nystagmus patterns, however, may also be seen in tumours of this cerebellopontine angle.

In connection with *vertical nystagmus,* between *upbeat* and *downbeat nystagmus* are distinguished. Two types of upbeat nystagmus exist. Type I has a large amplitude, which increases on upward gaze according to Alexander's law, i.e gaze in the direction of the fast component increases the frequency and amplitude, while gaze in the opposite direction has the reverse effect. Static tilt to prone and supine positions usually alters the characterstics of the type I upbeat nystagmus, e.g. modification of the amplitude of upbeat nystagmus or reversal of the direction of the nystagmus to downbeating. Primary position upbeat nystagmus occurs predominantly with intra-axial lesions of the tegmental grey matter at the pontomesencephalic and pontomedullary junctions, but from the literature there is also evidence of intrinsic cerebellar lesions, probably involving the brachium conjuctivum [5]. The variation in amplitude of upbeat nystagmus in response to static tilt implies an otolith-related component in the genesis of this nystagmus.

Type II has a small amplitude and decreases on upward gaze, contrary to Alexander's law, and indicates an intrinsic lesion of the medulla oblongata. There is also an intermediate form which behaves like type II, but in the primary position it has an amplitude of more than 5°. This intermediate form is usually seen in untreated cases of Wernicke's disease.

Downbeat nystagmus, contrary to Alexander's law, is not maximal on extreme downward gaze, but usually has its maximal intensity on lateral gaze, just beneath the horizontal axis. Downbeat nystagmus strongly suggests a lesion of the craniocervical junction, such as in Arnold-Chiari malformation. Downbeat nystagmus has also been described in patients with a presumably parenchymal cerebellar condition, especially in patients with a heredodegenerative disease.

Pure torsional nystagmus is almost only seen in syringobulbia.

An extraordinary combination of torsional and vertical oscillations has been found in the see-saw nystagmus. This is a conjugate, pendular, torsional oscillation (in all fields of gaze) with a superimposed disjunctive vertical vector (only in the primary position or on downward gaze). The eye with intorsion rises while the opposite eye with extorsion falls. See-saw nystagmus is an entity which is generally associated with chiasmal lesions of various etiology with bitemporal hemianopia. It is occasionally congenital.

3. Paroxysmal nystagmus

Up to now the permanently present nystagmus has been discussed. We can add a new dimension to our diagnostic approach if the duration or the behaviour of the nystagmus in the course of time is taken into consideration. Then, we could make a difference between: 1. permanent nystagmus, that is as long as the affection is present, 2. gradually decreasing nystagmus, and 3. paroxysmal nystagmus.

A lasting nystagmus usually indicates a lesion in the brain-stem, i.e. a central nystagmus. A peculiar behaviour in the course of time is that of the periodic alternating nystagmus (nystagmus alternans), in which a persisting horizontal jerk nystagmus periodically changes direction. There may be a fixed sequence every ninety seconds with a pause of ten seconds, but in many patients the timing is very asymmetric. Periodic alternating nystagmus can be either congenital or acquired. Differentiation is possible with help of the wave form of slow phase.

A nystagmus which after an acute onset gradually decreases in intensity and disappears in one or two weeks, is typically for labyrinthine nystagmus in case of an acute loss of the function of one labyrinth.

The paroxysmal nystagmus practically only occurs in the form of a benign paroxysmal positional nystagmus. This leads to discussion of positional nystagmus.

A *positional nystagmus* depends on a certain postural change or a certain position of the head in space. Therefore, we distinguish between a positional nystagmus of the benign paroxysmal type and a positional nystagmus of the central type. Fig. 5 shows the technique of eliciting the positional nystagmus of the benign paroxysmal type. Patient is seated on a couch with his gaze fixed on the examiner's forehead. The head turned to one side is than grasped firmly between examiner's hands and carried back briskly into the position shown. After a latent

164

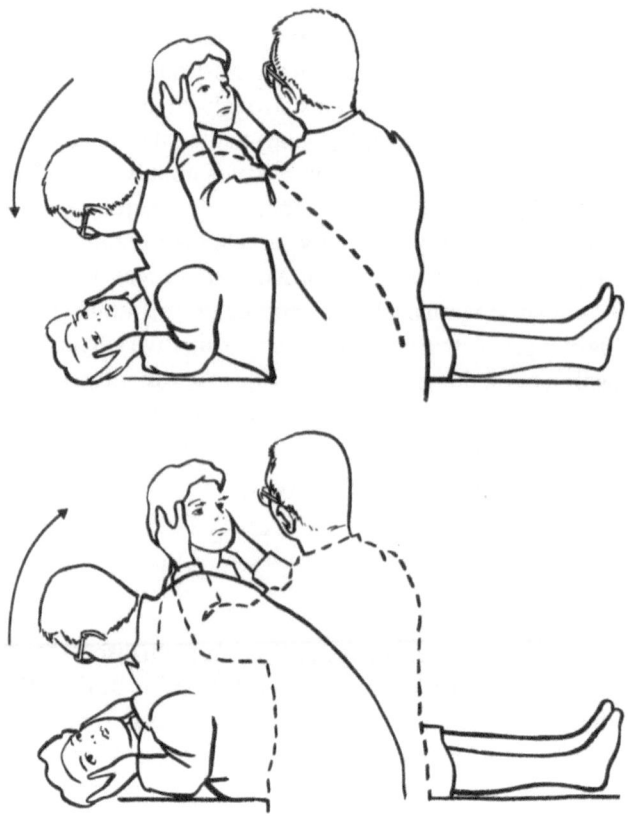

Figure 5. Technique for inducing paroxysmal positional nystagmus (From Leigh & Zee [1]).

period of a few seconds an episode of vertigo occurs accompanied by a mixed vertical torsional nystagmus in the direction shown, that is to say, it exhibits both vertical and rotatory components which are directed towards the ear placed undermost in test position. The onset of nystagmus is nearly always preceded by distress; patient's colour may change and he may close his eyes and cry out. The nystagmus increases to a rapid crescendo in a period which may be as short as 2 to 3 seconds, or as long as 10 seconds; it then rapidly declines together with the vertigo and distress. If the patient is then set up, a recurrence of vertigo in a milder form is generally noted and nystagmus may be observed, the direction of which is reversed. If vertical position is again resumed, nystagmus may reappear in a diminished form and be of shorter duration or it may not be possible to elicit it again until after a period of rest. A positive response if it occurs, typically does so with the head turned to one side but not to the other. Hence, if the test gives a negative response with the head turned to the right, it has to be repeated with the head turned to the left. The positional nystagmus of the benign paroxysmal type is the commonest cause of vertigo following head injury and also occurs after a rigid rest cure.

It was further demonstrated that it was this manoeuvre and not any neck twisting that provided the essential stimulus for eliciting an attack.

Rule of thumb: dizziness on upward gaze or on lying backwards nearly always points to a paroxysmal positional nystagmus and is hardly ever caused by torsion of the neck.

Unlike the positional nystagmus of the benign central type there is the positional nystagmus which lasts as long as the defined position is maintained, namely the positional nystagmus of central type. It is mostly horizontal, often towards the ear placed uppermost in the test position and mostly not accompanied by vertigo. This nystagmus can be the first sign of a tumour of the posterior fossa, but we do need to exclude a toxical positional nystagmus. A positional nystagmus with the rapid phase towards the ear placed undermost is specific for an alcohol intoxication, and appears within 30 minutes after the intake of alcohol, the so-called positional alcohol nystagmus I.

This first phase lasts approximately $3^1/_2$ hours. The second phase begins several hours after the end of the first phase. The direction of positional nystagmus is then away from the pillow to uppermost ear and lasts up to ten hours after intake of alcohol, this is the so-called positional alcohol nystagmus II.

Rule of thumb: a symmetric positional nystagmus without alcohol: always immediately refer to a neurologist.

References

1. Leigh RJ, Zee DS (1983): The neurology of eye movement. FA Davis Company, Philadelphia, p. 194.
2. van Vliet AGM (1963): Zur Diagnostik des kongenitalen Nystagmus. Ophthalmologica 145: 453–459.
3. van Vliet AGM (1973): On the central mechanism of latent nystagmus. Acta Ophthal 51: 772–781.
4. Ell JJ, Gresty MA, Findley LJ (1983): Acquired pendular nystagmus. J Neurol Neurosurg Psychiatry 46: 189.
5. Fisher A, Gresty M, Chambers B, Rudge P (1983): Primary position upbeating nystagmus. Brain 106: 949–964.

General information

Baloh RW, Honrubia V (1979): Clinical neurophysiology of the vestibular system. FH Davis Company, Philadelphia, pp. 101–124.

Vestibular eye movement disorders

W. BLES

The vestibular system comprises the semi-circular canals and the otoliths to sense angular and linear accelerations. Detection of these accelerations results in compensatory eye movements (vestibulo-ocular reflex) subserving gaze stabilization in space. Eye movements due to semi-circular canal stimulation are well documented, especially the horizontal following stimulation of the horizontal semi-circular canals.

The effect of otolith stimulation on eye movements is less clear. This may be due to the complicating factor that with linear movements of the head the magnitude of the compensatory eye movements depends on the eye-object distance (which is not the case with rotations). Changing the orientation with respect to the gravitational vector induces only minor counter rotation of the eyes. This is the reason why otolith induced eye movements are only occasionally used for clinical diagnosis. A further complicating factor is that it is impossible to stimulate the otoliths separately. Moreover, because of the multidirectional orientation of the hair cells on the macula, a sudden loss of function of an otolith should not result in typical eye movements or change in gaze. Since this book is clinically orientated, otolith induced eye movements will not be discussed. Of interest however, is that patients complain about oscillopsia of the horizon whilst walking or driving. This (transient) complaint is due to the absence of vertical eye movements, caused by otolithic malfunction. Patients with unilateral loss of vestibular function seldom complain of this phenomenon. This complaint may help to diagnose a bilateral loss of vestibular function since the absence of nystagmus and vertigo would normally not suggest vestibular involvement.

For a better understanding of the (pathological) eye movements due to canal stimulation the physiology of the semi-circular canals will be briefly summarized; more details are provided by e.g. 1. The hair cells that cover the crista ampullaris are arranged very regularly with all kinocilia located proximally to the utriculus. To understand the meaning of this one should be aware of the resting discharge activity of the cells on the vestibular nerve. Bending of the stereocilia in the direction of the kinocilium results in an increase of the discharge frequency (hyperpolarization). Bending in to the opposite was in a decrease (hypopolarisation). This implies a cooperation of the semi-circular canals on both sides because of their anatomical symmetry. Rotation of the head e.g. to the left results therefore in an increase of the discharge frequency in the left labyrinth and a decrease in the right labyrinth. The neural pathway via Scarpa's ganglion and the vestibular nuclei to the eye muscle nuclei evokes a compensatory eye movement to the right, subserving gaze stabilization. Together with the fast 'reset' into the opposite direction, these eye movements comprise the slow and fast phase of the vestibular nystagmus. Because of the mechanics of the cupula-endolymph system it reacts to accelerations. Further integration within the central nervous system leads to fully adequate compensatory eye movements in the frequency range of normal head movements. In a systems analysis of vestibular nystagmus the velocity of the slow phase can be modelled by postulating that behind the cupula-endolymphe integrator (short time constant) both a direct and an indirect pathway to the eye muscle nuclei exist. The indirect pathway does so via the socalled 'central velocity storage mechanism' (long time constant) which subserves also the optokinetic after nystagmus [2].

Vestibular eye movement disorders may be encountered in different ways: a. an acute unilateral lesion, causing imbalance between both labyrinths results in a spontaneous nystagmus, b. the system reacts on a certain stimulus in an unexpected way, or not at all, c. a certain movement produces an unexpected (abnormal) vestibular stimulus.

The eye movement disorders which are diagnostically most relevant will be discussed shortly. It should be clear, however, that any final diagnosis depends not only on the eye movement disorder but on other findings like e.g. vestibulospinal reflexes and the clinical history as well. These topics will not be covered here.

a. Spontaneous nystagmus is defined as the nystagmus which is present when the patient's head is in the normal upright position in the absence of recent vestibular or visual stimulation. Spontaneous nystagmus of peripheral vestibular origin is almost always strictly horizontal. When the patient is in a normally illuminated room, looking at a point at a distance of about 1 meter, a classification according to Alexander can be made. A nystagmus is classified as first degree if it can be observed only when the patient is looking in the direction of the fast phase component. It is second degree if it is also seen when looking straight ahead, and third degree when observed in addition, in the direction of the slow phase. Except in the acute phase, spontaneous nystagmus will be suppressed by visual fixation. This means that the patient's eyes must be kept closed and that ENG methods should be used to record the spontaneous nystagmus.

The observation that spontaneous nystagmus is suppressed by visual fixation strongly suggests a peripheral vestibular disturbance. A sudden loss of function of one of the labyrinths may be the cause of a nystagmus in the contralateral direction. However, one must be careful in defining the site of the lesion, because of the possibility that the primary nystagmus has developed into a secondary nystagmus of contralateral direction. The decay time of the primary spontaneous nystagmus varies from days to weeks or even months which implies that only in the acute phase some definite identification of the site of the lesion is possible.

Recording of the spontaneous nystagmus during the attack and in the next few hours, in patients suffering from Ménière's disease, [3] has revealed that the nystagmus beats towards the healthy side during the attack, but changes its direction within a few hours. This finding is at odds with the former notion of hyperfunction during the attack. McClure [3] advocates his recording method because the site of the lesion can be indicated by correlation with the attacks which may be of special importance when the other labyrinth gets involved as well. In Ménière's disease the labyrinth that gives the poorest response to caloric irrigation is not always causing the attacks.

b. Two important vestibular stimuli can be produced in the clinic by means of a rotation chair and by caloric irrigation. Although it has recently been re-evaluated [4] the caloric irrigation technique is uniquely equiped to differentiate between the left and the right labyrinth. Usually there will be no problems interpreting caloric nystagmograms. If the nystagmus slow phase velocity is taken as parameter, a difference of 22% or more between both labyrinths in reaction to caloric irrigation is considered as pathological [5]. The assumption is that the anatomy of both ears is identical and that the same irrigation media (water, air) are used. A unilateral low response may be seen e.g. in case of neuritis vestibularis, acoustic neurinoma or Ménière's disease.

The conclusion that a labyrinth is functioning may be drawn only if it is possible to induce a nystagmus in both directions by means of caloric irrigation. Especially irrigation with cold water (or air) may result in an aspecific response mimicking a normal response. By changing the head pitch angle over 180° the nystagmus will be inverted in case of real labyrinthine functioning. Another problem may be encountered in hot air caloric irrigation which is the appropriate irrigation technique in case of middle car pathology.

Due to evaporative cooling of the mucous layer the nystagmus may mimic the response on cold air stimulation. Here too, a change of head position is the appropriate manoeuvre to determine labyrinthine functioning. Vuyk [6] advocates in case of abnormal middle ear anatomy to use only cold air but with head pitching after appearance of the nystagmus. This procedure is justified since only a qualitative assessment of labyrinth function is allowed in these patients.

The diagnosis of bilateral dysfunction due to caloric insensitivity of both labyrinths has to be verified using a rotation chair, preferably with the aid of Coriolis techniques.

The advantage of modern rotation chair tests is that well-defined reproducible stimuli are applied. Because of this, variation of the respective parameters in the mathematical model of the VOR can be achieved. It also provides a systematic way to study the interactions with optokinetic and cervical stimuli [7]. Although unilateral labyrinth lesions as a group are statistically different from controls in that they show a lower gain and shorter time constants during rotation chair examinations, asymmetric gain and time constants for nystagmus to the left or right in case of labyrinthine left/right differences is not an obligatory observation.

Difficulties in the interpretation of nystagmus arise especially if there is only a poor nystagmic reponse on rotatory chair stimulation. Interpretation in terms of 'some minor vestibular activity' is very common but most probably not correct. Baloh et al. [8] suggest the presence of a very short time constant, which might explain the absence of nystagmus with caloric irrigation in these patients. However, if head tilt during full speed rotation does not evoke Coriolis effects, absence of any vestibular function should be considered as a possible cause. The nystagmus found might be interpreted as due to somatosensory stimulation, the varying contact between the chair and the patient's back in view of the finding that gain of somatosensory nystagmus in patients with labyrinthine loss of function is twice as high as in controls [9]. The optokinetic nystagmus is of less intensity in these patients and the optokinetic after nystagmus is absent, because the already mentioned 'central velocity storage mechanism' does not function anymore in these patients.

c. Vestibular eye movement disorders are encountered in patients suffering from the socalled benign paroxysmal positional vertigo. This vertigo is induced mostly by rolling over from one to the other side or by rising quickly from a lying position. The associated nystagmus is tested by moving the patient rapidly from the sitting to the lying position, flexing the neck and with the head turned to the left or to the right. Normally such a quick manoeuvre results in vestibular stimulation only during the movement with compensatory eye movements of very short duration. The patients, however, produce a nystagmus after a latency of several seconds, lasting about 20–30 seconds. If the manoevre is repeated afterwards, there may not be a further response. The nystagmus is mainly a geotropic rotatory nystagmus.

Because of the rotatory character recording with EOG techniques is impossible. This type of nystagmus can be observed easily with Frenzel glasses or even without glasses (rotatory nystagmus is not suppressed by visual fixations) and is a strong indication that there is a peripheral vestibular lesion. The difference with a positional nystagmus of central origin is the immediate onset of the nystagmus and the non-adaptation of this type of nystagmus. In case of a labyrinth fistula this manoeuvre is said to induce nystagmus but seldom a rotatory nystagmus.

An explanation for this benign positional nystagmus and vertigo has been suggested by Schuknecht [10] and has been called 'cupulolithiasis'. The hypothesis is that inorganic material from the utriculus otolith gravitates and gets attached to the cupula of the posterior canal which is situated inferior to the utriculus when the head is upright. When the provocative manoeuvre is executed the inorganic material is thrown of the cupula which results in a repositioning of the cupula and therefore in vertigo and nystagmus. Although this mechanism is not generally accepted, Brandt and Büchele [11] claim a remarkably high percentage of clinical remission by treating these patients with provocative head positions on a repeated and consecutive basis. The other routine vestibular examinations are mostly negative in these patients which is in accordance with this hypothesis.

References

1. Kandel ER, Schwartz JH (1981): Principles of neural science. Arnold Publishers, London.
2. Raphan T, Matsuo V, Cohen B (1979): Velocity storage in the vestibulo ocular reflex arc (VOR). Exp Brain Res 35: 229–248.
3. McClure JA (1983): Electronystagmographic monitoring in vestibular disorders. Adv ORL (Karger, Basel) 30: 193–200.
4. Von Baumgarten et al (1984): Effects of rectilinear acceleration and optokinetic and caloric stimulations in space. Science 225: 208–212.
5. Baloh RW, Honrubia V (1979): Clinical neurophysiology of the vestibular system. FA Davis Company, Philadelphia.
6. Vuyk HD, Bles W, Feenstra L (1983): Inverted nystagmus with caloric stimulation. Clin Otolaryngol 8: 290.
7. Bles W, de Jong JMBV (1982): Cervico-vestibular and visuo-vestibular interaction. Self-motion perception, nystagmus and gaze shift. Acta Otolaryngol 94: 61–72.
8. Baloh RW, Hess K, Honrubia V, Yee RD (1984): Low and high frequency sinusoidal rotational testing in patients with peripheral vestibular lesions. Acta Otolaryngol (Stockholm), Suppl 406: 189–193.
9. Bles W, de Jong JMBV, de Wit G (1983b): Somatosensory compensation for loss of labyrinthine function. Acta Otolaryngol (Stockholm) 97: 213–221.
10. Schuknecht HF (1974): Pathology of the ear. Harv Univ Press, Cambridge.
11. Brandt Th, Büchele W (1983): Augenbewegungsstörungen. Gustav Fischer Verlag. Stuttgart-New York.

Disorders of horizontal and vertical gaze

DAVID S. ZEE

1. Neural control signals

To interpret ocular motor pathology, it is helpful to understand the nature of the neural signals that drive the ocular motor neurons and the eye muscles during the various types of eye movements. Recordings from ocular motor neurons in alert monkeys as well as ocular electromyographic studies in human beings have shown that the innervational change during all types of eye movements consists of a phasic (proportional to eye velocity) and tonic (proportional to eye position) component [1].

For saccadic eye movements, this neural signal has been called the pulse-step change in innervation. The *pulse* is an eye velocity command that generates the high-frequency burst of innervation seen during the saccade. It moves the eye rapidly from one position to another against orbital viscous forces. The *step* is an eye-position command that generates the appropriate level of tonic innervation at the end of the saccade to hold the eye in its new position against orbital elastic-restoring forces. Normally the saccadic pulse and step must be appropriately matched to prevent post-saccadic drift. It is thought that the immediate premotor command for the pulse change in innervation is created by cells located in the pontine and mesencephalic paramedian reticular formation called burst neurons. These neurons are normally silent but burst at a high frequency immediately preceding and time-locked to the high-frequency burst of neural activity that occurs in ocular motor neurons during a saccade. The step of innervation is thought to be created by a central neural network or neural integrator that integrates (in the mathematical sense) the saccadic eye-velocity command (pulse) to produce the appropriate position-coded information (step) for the oculomotor neurons. The cerebellar flocculus, the medial vestibular nucleus and the rostral portion of the nucleus prepositus (one of the perihypoglossal nuclei located just behind and medial to the medial vestibular nucleus) have been shown to be necessary for normal function of the brain stem neural integrator [2, 3].

Similar considerations apply to eye velocity commands from the pursuit and vestibular (including optokinetic) systems. They are passed directly to the ocular motor neurons to create the phasic change in innervation and also indirectly through the neural integrator to produce the appropriate tonic change in innervation. Both theoretical considerations and neurophysiological evidence point to a single common integrator that integrates all types of conjugate eye-velocity commands.

2. Horizontal gaze mechanisms

2.1 Abducens nucleus

Commands for adduction during all types of conjugate movements project to the medial rectus subset of oculomotor neurons via the medial longitudinal fasciculus (MLF). They arise from cells within the contralateral abducens nucleus that are called internuclear neurons. These cells are intermingled among abducens motor neurons; the latter innervate the ipsilateral lateral rectus for abduction. Thus, one can explain the observation that a lesion of the abducens nucleus causes a conjugate ipsilateral gaze palsy for all types of versional eye movements. Such lesions usually occur in conjunction with a facial palsy because the VII nerve courses over the abducens nucleus. Likewise, as patients with a conjugate gaze palsy recover, they often show a residual VI nerve palsy probably due to fascicle involvement.

2.2 Pontine paramedian reticular formation

Supranuclear inputs to abducens interneurons include a projection from neurons within the adjacent rostral medullary and pontine paramedian reticular formation (PPRF). A lesion within the PPRF causes an ipsilateral conjugate gaze palsy for versional eye movements although there is a suggestion that vestibular (and perhaps optokinetic) eye movements can be occasionally spared with more rostral PPRF lesions. Likewise VII nerve paralysis is often absent with PPRF lesions. Injection of kainic (or ibotenic) acid, which destroys cell bodies but leaves fibers intact, into the PPRF leads to a selective disorder of saccadic eye movements [4]. Pursuit, gaze-holding and vestibular responses are left intact. Horizontal saccades are affected, probably because the burst neurons that generate horizontal saccades are destroyed. Bilateral kainate lesions in the caudal but not rostral PPRF also lead to disorders of vertical saccades. Presumably this occurs because caudal kainate lesions also destroy pause cells (see below) and thereby interfere with the mechanisms of control over the mesencephalic burst neurons that produce vertical saccades.

Physiological recordings of single-unit activity of neurons in the caudal pons

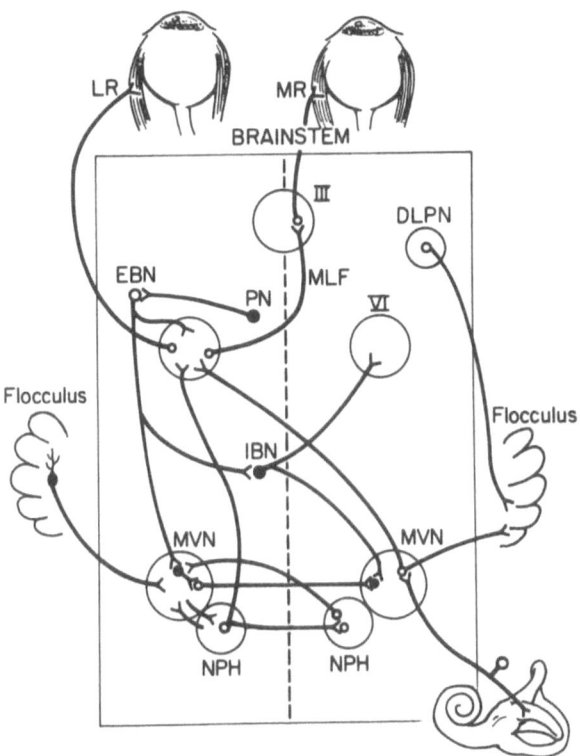

Figure 1. Pathways important for horizontal gaze. The abducens nucleus (VI) contains motor neurons that innervate the ipsilateral lateral rectus muscle (LR) and internuclear neurons with axons that ascend in the contralateral medial longitudinal fasciculus (MLF) to contact medial rectus (MR) motor neurons in the contralateral third nerve nucleus (III). From the lateral semicircular canal, primary vestibular afferents project mainly to the medial vestibular nucleus (MVN). Vestibular commands are then carried to the contralateral abducens nucleus. Saccadic inputs reach the abducens nucleus from ipsilateral excitatory burst neurons (EBN) and contralateral inhibitory burst neurons (IBN). Eye position information (the output of the neural integrator) probably reaches the abducens nucleus from neurons within the MVN and nucleus prepositus hypoglossi (NPH). Pursuit commands reach the flocculus from the dorsolateral pontine nuclei (DLPN). This projection is drawn here as being ipsilateral although the size of the contralateral projection is larger.

reveal a number of cells that discharge in relation to horizontal eye movements. In the PPRF there are the *burst neurons* that create saccadic eye velocity commands. *Pause neurons*, which are located in a midline caudal pontine nucleus called the nucleus raphe interpositus, discharge tonically except just prior to and during saccades. These neurons presumably exert a tonic inhibitory influence upon saccadic burst neurons and so prevent extraneous saccades when fixation is desired. It has been proposed that malfunction of specific cell types within the PPRF may give rise to specific ocular motor disorders. For example, slow saccades may arise from burst cell dysfunction and saccadic oscillations (ocular flutter and possibly opsoclonus) may arise from pause cell dysfunction [5]. Recent pathological study of a patient who had slow horizontal saccades with olivopontocerebellar atrophy revealed a loss of large neurons in the nucleus gigantocellularis in the PPRF [6]. These cells were presumably burst neurons and their degeneration was responsible for the slow saccades.

2.3 Vestibular and perihypoglossal nuclei

In addition to the PPRF, the vestibular nuclei and perihypoglossal complex (especially the nucleus prepositus hypoglossi) also project directly to the abducens nucleus. Since the cerebellum has both strong afferent and efferent connections to both the vestibular nuclei and perihypoglossal complex, one mechanism by which the cerebellum influences horizontal gaze (and especially smooth pursuit eye movements and gaze-holding) may be through connections from these caudal brain stem structures to the VI nerve nuclei. Ibotenic acid lesions within the rostral portion of the medial vestibular nucleus and the adjacent nucleus prepositus hypoglossi interfere with vestibular and optokinetic eye movements as well as the neural gaze-holding network or neural integrator that creates the saccadic step of innervation [3]. Such animals are unable to hold eccentric positions of gaze and have gaze-evoked nystagmus.

2.4 Topical diagnosis of horizontal conjugate gaze palsies

It follows from the above considerations that a pontine lesion can cause a conjugate gaze palsy by virtue of an isolated abducens nucleus lesion, an isolated PPRF lesion, or a combined abducens nerve (fascicle) lesion and contralateral MLF lesion [7]. The last is suggested if the gaze palsy is not perfectly conjugate. A PPRF lesion is suggested when vestibular movements are spared and the ipsilaterally directed saccades made in the contralateral part of the orbit are extremely slow. An abducens nucleus lesion is suggested when vestibular induced movements are also impaired and when ipsilaterally directed saccades made in the contralateral part of the orbit are rapid (since inhibitory projections from the PPRF to the intact abducens nucleus are spared). Midbrain lesions can also produce horizontal conjugate gaze palsies – usually for contralaterally directed saccades and ipsilaterally-directed pursuit. Vestibular eye movements are intact [8].

3. Vertical gaze mechanisms

3.1 Mesencephalic control of vertical eye movements

Vertical gaze ultimately is elaborated through mesencephalic structures although ascending influences from the pons are also important [9, 10]. Vertical vestibular (and in part, pursuit) commands are carried up to MLF; presumably their cells of origin are within the vestibular nuclei including the so called Y-group. Hence, patients with bilateral internuclear ophthalmoplegia have disorders of vertical pursuit, vertical vestibular eye movements and vertical gaze-holding as well as impaired horizontal ocular motility. There is also an ascending MLF projection from the perihypoglossal complex. Commands from the caudal PPRF are also carried rostrally in a juxta-MLF pathway that impinges upon a group of cells comprising the rostral interstitial nucleus of the MLF (riMLF). This nucleus is located at the ventral mesencephalic-diencephalic junction and contains neurons that discharge in relationship to both up and down vertical saccadic eye movements. The existence of vertical saccadic disorders after bilateral caudal PPRF lesions may reflect involvement of this pontine projection to the riMLF. The riMLF projects through the posterior commissure to its analog on the other side of the mesencephalon as well as directly to the oculomotor nucleus. Vertical eye movements are affected by lesions within the posterior commissure; upgaze is primarily disturbed. More ventral lesions, closer to the riMLF may affect both up and downward gaze or affect downward gaze alone. The interstitial nucleus of Cajal (INC) also appears to be important for vertical gaze, probably in the generation of slow eye movements and for vertical gaze-holding. The INC projects both contralaterally through the posterior commissure to the oculomotor subnuclei for upward movements and ipsilaterally directly to the oculomotor subnuclei for downward movements.

3.2 Topical diagnosis of vertical conjugate gaze palsies

Upgaze palsies are characteristic of lesions in the posterior commissure. The palsies may be limited to saccades with pursuit and vestibular movements intact. Some patients, while not able to make saccades above the midline, can make perfectly normal upward (and downward) saccades in the lower field of gaze [11]. This finding implies that, in these patients, the vertical saccadic burst neurons in the riMLF must be intact. The paralysis of upgaze appears to reflect an inability to program a command to move the eyes above a certain point. This is a higher level type of saccadic disorder related to defects in internal processing of signals related to target or eye position. There is evidence that caudal thalamic lesions may also lead to this type of disorder [12].

If the riMLF itself is involved, saccades become slow or absent. Isolated

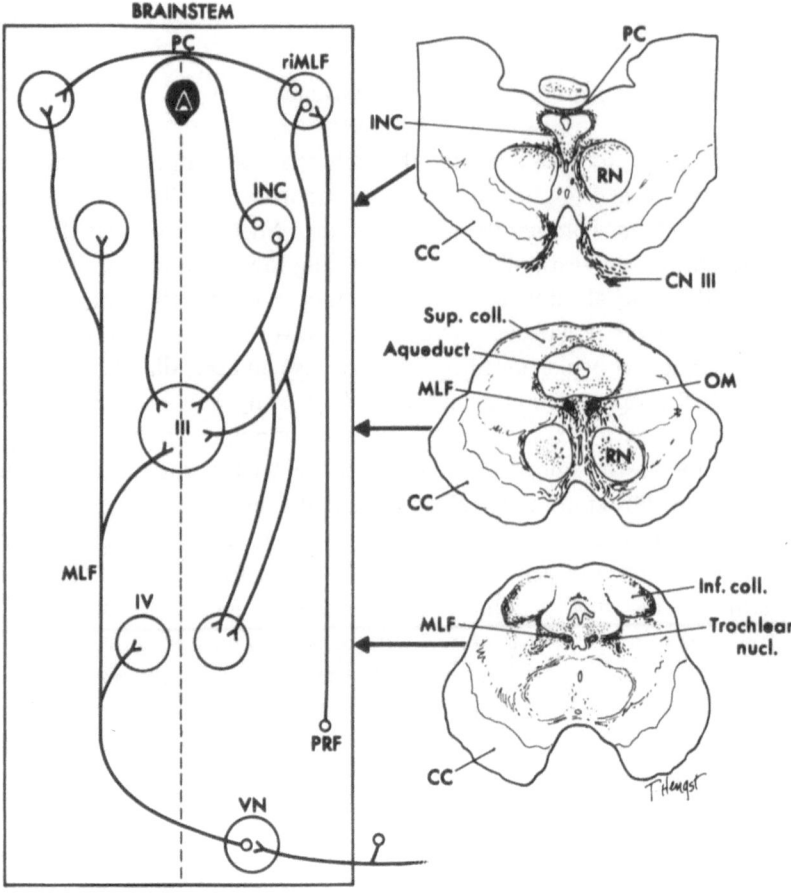

Figure 2. Anatomical pathways important in the synthesis of vertical versional eye movements. Vestibular inputs from the vertical semicircular canals synapse in the vestibular nuclei (VN) and ascend in the medial longitudinal fasciculus (MLF) and brachium conjunctivum (not shown) to contact neurons in the trochlear nucleus (IV), oculomotor nucleus (III), interstitial nucleus of Cajal (INC), and rostral interstitial nucleus of the medial longitudinal fasciculus (riMLF). The riMLF, which lies in the prerubral fields, also receives an input from neurons in the pontine reticular formation (PRF). The riMLF contains burst cells that pass saccadic commands to the neurons of III and IV as well through the posterior commissure (PC) to the contralateral riMLF. The INC also projects to III and IV: projections to the elevator subnuclei (innervating the superior rectus and inferior oblique muscles) pass above the aquaduct of Sylvius (A) in the posterior commissure, projections to the depressor subnuclei (innervating the inferior rectus and superior oblique) pass ventrally.

downgaze palsies probably reflect partial involvement of the riMLF or of its efferent pathways to the oculomotor nuclei. Other signs of lesions in this region include convergence-retractory nystagmus, skew deviation, head tilt, lid retraction and pupils that respond better to light than to accommodative stimuli.

4. Cerebral control of saccadic and pursuit eye movements

4.1 Saccades

Recent neurophysiological studies have demonstrated neurons within the frontal eye fields (FEF) and the superior colliculi (SC) that discharge before and are specifically related to contralaterally-directed visually-guided saccadic eye movements [13]. The PPRF itself receives direct inputs both from the contralateral FEF and from the contralateral SC. Disruption of either the FEF or SC alone causes subtle and transient deficits. Paired lesions, however, of both the SC and FEF create a marked deficit in production of saccades [14]. Thus, there are two parallel pathways – one via the FEF, the other via SC – that can trigger saccadic eye movements. The FEF, though, also project to the SC via both direct and indirect (through the basal ganglia) pathways. There is also evidence for a division of labour between FEF and SC pathways in the generation of saccades; the former being more concerned with internally-generated, voluntary saccades, and the latter with externally-triggered, reflexive saccades. Furthermore, saccades to remembered targets seem to depend upon a FEF-caudate-substantia nigra, pars reticulata-SC pathway [15, 16].

In normal circumstances, the FEF may trigger saccades through the superior colliculus, both directly and via the FEF-caudate-substantia nigra, pars reticulata-SC pathway. The latter appears to act as an inhibitory gate upon the SC so that when fixation is desired the SC is prevented from responding to novel visual stimuli. When a voluntary change of fixation is desired, the SC is disinhibited so that a saccade can be generated.

Experimentally, FEF lesions alone lead to deficits in generation of voluntary saccades to the remembered locations of targets [17]. Likewise, in human patients with frontal lobe lesions saccades can not be made away from a target stimulus [18]. Patients compulsively look toward the peripheral target even when instructed to look in the opposite direction. Patients with Huntington's disease show a similar deficit in this task [16]. In experimental animals SC lesions alone lead to an increase in saccade latencies for visually-guided saccades and to a decrease in distractability; the brief glances that are made to a suddenly appearing peripheral visual stimulus even during attempted straight ahead fixation [19]. Combined FEF and SC lesions lead to a global deficit in the generation of saccades of all types.

4.2 Pursuit

The smooth pursuit pathway is less well known. While unilateral parietal and unilateral cerebellar lesions create predominantly ipsilateral pursuit deficits, the precise pathways by which these structures influence the brain stem conjugate gaze centers are not known. The occipital-mesencephalic projections of the internal sagittal stratum do not appear to be crucial for pursuit since their unilateral disruption causes no pursuit deficit. Recent evidence suggests that structures located at the temporal-parietal-occipital junction (area MT, MST, FST) and their projection to the dorsolateral pontine nuclei (DLPN) are important for pursuit eye movement [17, 21]. DLPN in turn projects to the flocculus from which pursuit commands are carried to the medial vestibular nuclei for horizontal pursuit and to the Y-group of the vestibular nuclei for vertical pursuit. Finally recent evidence and physiological studies also implicate the FEF in generation of pursuit eye movements [22] and bilateral FEF lesions disrupts smooth pursuit [23, 24].

4.3 Cerebellum

The cerebellum appears to play a major role in the control of all types of eye movements although the exact anatomical pathways by which such control is exerted are not well understood. Presumably cerebellar effects are mediated by connections with the vestibular nuclei, perihypoglossal complex and reticular formation via the deep nuclei. Thus far at least four types of ocular motor functions can be attributed to the cerebellum: 1) control of saccade amplitude, 2) stabiliation of images upon the fovea during both fixation and smooth tracking, 3) adjustments of the duration of vestibulo-ocular responses (as reflected in the time constant of the vestibulo-ocular reflex) and 4) repair of ocular motor dysmetria. The dorsal cerebellar vermis and underlying fastigial nuclei appear to be most important in the control of saccade amplitude; saccadic dysmetria is an important sign of lesions in this region [25]. The cerebellar flocculus appears to be important for a variety of retinal image-stabilizing reflexes [2]. Lesions here produce abnormalities in smooth pursuit, fixation suppression of vestibular nystagmus, and the ability to hold eccentric positions of gaze (resulting in gaze-evoked nystagmus). The latter abnormality reflects a poor ('leaky') neural integrator. Precise matching of the saccadic step to the saccadic pulse, so that post-saccadic drift does not occur, also appears to be a function of the flocculus. The cerebellar nodulus is important for decreasing the duration of vestibular responses if there is a visual-vestibular or otolith-semicircular canal conflict [26]. Finally, the cerebellum appears to play a role in repair of ocular motor dysmetria [27]. For example, if saccade size is inappropriate (such as caused by a peripheral nerve or muscle paralysis), an intact dorsal cerebellar vermis and the underlying fastigial nuclei are necessary for the proper readjustment of saccade amplitude and for the elimination of dysmetria. Similarly, if the amplitude (gain) or direction of the vestibulo-ocular reflex is inappropriate, or if the saccadic step and pulse are not appropriately matched, an intact vestibulo-cerebellum is necessary for the proper readjustment of the VOR and for the elimination of post-saccadic drift. The vestibulo-cerebellum receives mossy fiber inputs about movement of the head, movement of the eyes and movement of images on the retina as well as a climbing fiber input about movement of images on the retina. The perihypoglossal nucleus also projects to the vestibulo-cerebellum. The Purkinje cells of the vestibulo-cerebellum project back to the vestibular nuclei directly. Thus, a rich anatomical substrate exists for cerebellar-vestibular interaction.

References

1. Leigh RJ, Zee DS (1983): The Neurology of Eye Movement, FA Davis, Philadelphia.
2. Zee DS, Yamazaki A, Butler PH, Gucer G (1981): Effects of ablation of flocculus and paraflocculus on eye movements in primates. J Neurophysiol 46: 878–899.
3. Cannon SC, Robinson DA: The final common integrator is in the prepositus and vestibular nuclei. In: Adaptive Processes in Visual and Oculomotor Systems, Keller EL and Zee DS (eds), Pergamon Press, Oxford, in press.
4. Henn V, Lang W, Hepp K, Reisine H (1984): Experimental gaze palsies in monkeys and their relation to human pathology. Brain 107: 619–636.
5. Zee DS, Robinson DA (1979): A hypothetical explanation of saccadic oscillations. Ann Neurol 5: 405–414.
6. Buttner-Ennever JA, Wadia NH, Sakai H, Schwendemann G (1985): Neuroanatomy of oculomotor structures in olivopontocerebellar atrophy (OPCA) patients with slow saccades. J Neurol, in press.
7. Pierrot-Deseilligny Ch, Chain F, Serdaru M, Gray F, Lhermitte F (1981): The 'one-and-a-half' syndrome. Electro-oculographic analyses of five cases with deductions about the physiological mechanisms of lateral gaze. Brain 104: 665–699.
8. Zackon DH, Sharpe JA (1984): Midbrain paresis of horizontal gaze. Ann Neurol 16: 495–504.
9. Buttner-Ennever JA, Buttner U, Cohen B, Baumgartner G (1982): Vertical gaze paralysis and the rostral interstitial nucleus of the medial longitudinal fasciculus. Brain 105: 125–149.
10. Pierrot-Deseilligny Ch, Chain F, Gray F, Serdaru M, Escourolle R, Lhermitte F (1982): Parinaud's syndrome. Electro-oculographic and anatomical analyses of six vascular cases with deductions about vertical gaze organization in the premotor structures. Brain 105: 667–696.
11. Baloh RW, Furman JM, Yee RD (1985): Dorsal midbrain syndrome: clinical and oculographic findings. Neurology 35: 54–60.
12. Albano JE, Wurtz RH (1982): Deficits in eye position following ablation of monkey superior colliculus, pretectum, and posterior-medial thalamus. J Neurophysiol 48: 318.
13. Bruce CJ, Goldberg ME (1985): Primate frontal eye fields. I. Single neurons discharging before saccades. J Neurophysiol 53: 603–635.
14. Schiller PH, True SD, Conway JL (1980): Deficits in eye movements following frontal eye-field and superior colliculus. J Neurophysiol 44: 1175.
15. Hikosaka O, Wurtz RH (1983): Visual and oculomotor functions of monkey substantia nigra pars reticulata. IV. Relation of substantia nigra to superior colliculus. J Neurophysiol 49: 1285–1301.
16. Zee DS, Lasker AG, Hain TC, Folstein SJ, Singer HS: Eye movement disorders in basal ganglia disease. In: Movement Disorders II: Neurology of the Extra-pyramidal Systems, Findley LJ and Gresty M (eds), Macmillan Press, in press.
17. Deng S-Y, Goldberg ME, Segraves MA, Ungerleider LG, Mishkin M: The effect of unilateral ablation of the frontal eye fields of saccadic performance in the monkey. In: Adaptive Processes in Visual and Oculomotor Systems, Keller EL and Zee DS (eds), Pergamon Press, Oxford, in press.

18. Guitton D, Buchtel HA, Douglas RM (1985): Frontal lobe lesions in man cause difficulties in suppressing reflexive glances and in generating goal-directed saccades. Exp Brain Res 58: 455–472.

19. Wurtz RA, Albano E (1980): Visual-motor function of the primate superior colliculus. Ann Rev Neurosci 3: 189.

20. Newsome WT, Dursteler MR, Wurtz RH: The middle temporal visual area and the control of smooth pursuit eye movements. In: Adaptive Processes in Visual and Oculomotor Systems, Keller EL and Zee DS (eds), Pergamon Press, Oxford, in press.

21. Suzuki DA, Keller EL (1984): Visual signals in the dorso-lateral pontine nucleus of the alert monkey: Their relationship to smooth-pursuit eye movements. Exp Brain Res 53: 473–478.

22. Bruce CJ, Goldberg ME, Bushnell MC, Stanton GB (1985): Primate frontal eye fields. II. Physiological and anatomical correlates of electrically evoked eye movements. J Neurophysiol 54: 714–734.

23. Keating EG, Gooley SG, Kenney DV (1985): Impaired tracking and loss of predictive eye movements after removal of the frontal eye fields. Soc Neurosci Abstr 11: 472.

24. Lynch JC, Allison JC (1985): A quantitative study of visual pursuit deficits following lesions of the frontal eye fields in rhesus monkeys. Soc Neurosci Abstr 11: 473.

25. Optican LM, Robinson DA (1980): A cerebellar dependent adaptive control of the primate saccadic system. J Neuro-physiol 44: 1058–1976.

26. Waespe W, Cohen B, Raphan T (1985): Dynamic modification of the vestibulo-ocular reflex by the nodulus and uvula. Science 228: 199–202.

27. Berthoz A, Melvill Jones G: Adaptive Mechanisms in Gaze Control, Elsevier, Amsterdam, 1985.

Syndromes of the medial longitudinal fasciculus

E.A.C.M. SANDERS

The medial longitudinal fasciculus (MLF) is the main pathway subserving horizontal and vertical gaze movements. The MLF extends from the superior and medial vestibular nuclei at the level of the pons to Perlia's nucleus in the rostral mesenchephalon. Its exitatory fibres cross the midline at the level of the abducens (sixth) nucleus to terminate in the oculomotor (third) nucleus [1].

The MLF is surrounded by other structures thought to be associated with pre-motor control of vertical and horizontal eye movement. They include Cajal's interstitial nucleus, the nucleus of the posterior commissure in the pretectum and the posterior commissure itself (Chapters 1, 2 and 3).

The centre for horizontal gaze is located within the pontine tegmentum near the sixth nerve nucleus. The latter contains two populations of neurons: abducens motor neurons, which supply the lateral rectus muscle and abducens internuclear neurons which project via the MLF in order to contact motor neurons of the lateral oculomotor nucleus.

The rostral mesenchephalon region that is crucial for the generation of vertical saccades, has been called the rostral interstitial nucleus of the MLF (ri MLF). The neural signals necessary for vertical vestibular, saccadic and smooth pursuit eye movement and for the maintenance of vertical eye position are carried, in part, via fibres of the MLF [2].

Deficits caused by lesions of the MLF depend mainly on the exact site of the lesion. Rostral lesions, involving also the oculomotor nucleus may impair convergence, but more caudal lesions do not. Bilateral experimental lesions of the ri-MLF in monkey cause a vertical saccadic deficit more pronounced for downward eye movement. Bilateral lesions of the MLF impair vertical saccades and pursuit eye movement but often spare vertical up and downward saccades.

1. Vertical gaze disorders

It has been emphazised that vertical gaze paralysis is produced by a bilateral lesion of the brainstem. While this principle appears to be generally correct it is evident that unilateral lesions can give rise to upward or upward plus downward gaze paralysis [3]. Both experimental and clinico-pathological evidence suggest an important role for the ri-MLF in the initiation of vertical eye movement (Chapter 3). At present a similar role is assumed for Cajal's interstitial nucleus, also called the interstitial nucleus of the MLF [4]. In man, the ri-MLF lies dorsomedial to the anterior pole of the red nucleus rostral to the interstitial nucleus of Cajal and lateral to the Darkschewitsch' nucleus.

2. Internuclear ophthalmoplegia

2.1 Adduction

The syndrome of internuclear ophthalmoplegia (INO) is a well recognized disorder of horizontal eye movement often seen in multiple sclerosis patients [5]. It is manifested by impairment of adduction of the eye on the side of the MLF lesion and abduction overshoot eventually followed by a nystagmus of the abducting eye [6]. In the classical case the medial rectus can still be driven by the convergence mechanism (Fig. 1).

Unilateral impairment of adduction was probably first described by Sauvineau [7] in 1895, a sign for which Lhermitte [8] introduced the term 'Paralysie Internucleaire'. Spiller [9] was the first to describe a clinico-pathological observation. He reported paralysis of ocular adduction with preservation of convergence. The lesion actually was a large softening located in the tegmentum of the upper third of the pons. Cogan [10] and Christoff [11] presented four histo-pathologically confirmed cases with small vascular lesions of the MLF, who all showed a homolateral impairment of adducting gaze in combination with preserved convergence. From these and other studies it is assumed that an INO can be attributed to a lesion of the MLF between the levels of the third and sixth nucleus. It has been assumed that the lesion affects axons arising from cells in the paramedian pontine reticular formation (PPRF) but this idea was later refuted [12]. The impairment of adduction is variable, the most severe lesions causing complete loss of adduction beyond the midline during contralateral gaze. In early reports the clinical diagnosis of INO depended on the recognition of a limited range of adduction. Wilson [13] drew attention to the nystagmus which may be seen in the abducting eye. The origin of this nystagmus is still controversal [14, 15].

A less severe lesion may cause no apparent limitation in the excursion of the adducting eye; the and only manifestation of the lesion may be reduced adduction velocity during a horizontal saccade. It has been shown that a saccade is the result of a pulse-step change in innervation in which there is activation of the agonist and disinhibition of the antagonist. In patients with INO the peak angular saccadic velocities were significantly lower than in normal subjects and were also

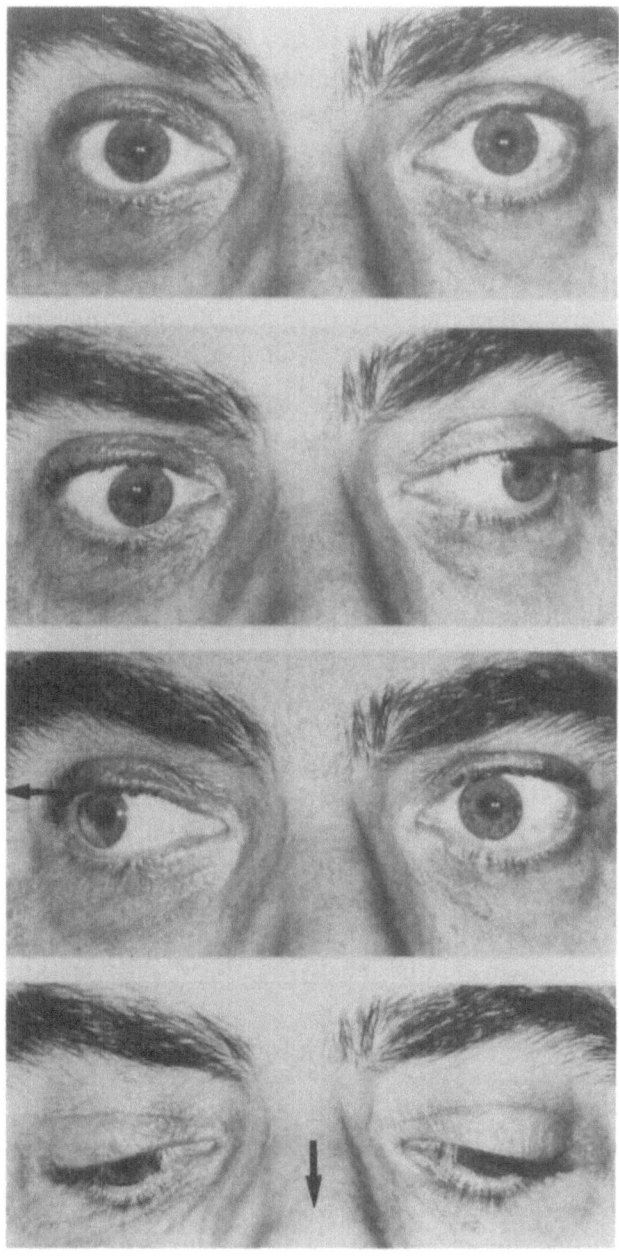

Figure 1. Eye movements of a 50 years old multiple sclerosis patient with bilateral slowing of adduction indicating a bilateral internuclear ophthalmoplegia.

significantly lower than abduction velocities. However, the INO abduction velocities were lower than those of the healthy control persons. Accordingly one may infer that measurement of the peak angular velocities during saccadic eye movement may be useful in detecting INO at an early stage [16]. Loss of adduction of the ipsilateral eye is easy to understand since excitatory fibres ascend in the MLF to innervate the medial rectus muscle. Other aspects of the eye movement disorder have been less satisfactory explained. The reduction of saccadic velocity as one of the characteristic and first symptoms could be explained by the idea that the pulse- is more affected than the step- mechanism. In demyelination the burst fibres cannot carry a high frequency discharge, this may contribute to reduced peak angular velocity. However the finding of saccadic intrusions* in INO suggests disordered supranuclear control of pause cells by releasing burst neurons [17].

2.2 Abduction

Lutz [18] divided INO into anterior and posterior types according to whether the medial or the lateral rectus muscle was paralysed on attemped conjugate gaze. The latter will cause an INO affecting abduction. It seemed to be difficult to distinguish INO of abduction from abducens paralysis if convergence is still possible. Only few cases have been reported in the literature [19]. The centre for lateral gaze is supposed to lie in the paramedian pontine reticular formation (PPRF). This structure is situated close to the abducens nucleus so that a discrete lesion of connections between the centre for lateral gaze and the ipsilateral abducens nucleus becomes improbable. Any infarction, tumour or multiple sclerosis plaque will most likely damage not only the connections between but, in addition, the centre for lateral gaze or the abducens nucleus itself. In these mixed lesions, which may occur quite frequently, an INO would be masked by conjugate gaze paresis or abducens palsy.

3. The one-and-a-half syndrome

Combined lesions of the PPRF and adjacent MLF on one side of the brainstem may cause an ipsilateral horizontal gaze palsy and contralateral INO [20]. This combination of eye movement disorders is called the 'one-and-a-half syndrome'. This is a clinical disorder characterized by a lateral gaze palsy in one direction and a INO in the other direction. In the complete form one eye lies fixed at the midline for all horizontal lateral movements. The other eye can only abduct and exhibits horizontal jerk nystagmus (Fig. 2).

*saccadic oscillations that transiently interrupt fixation.

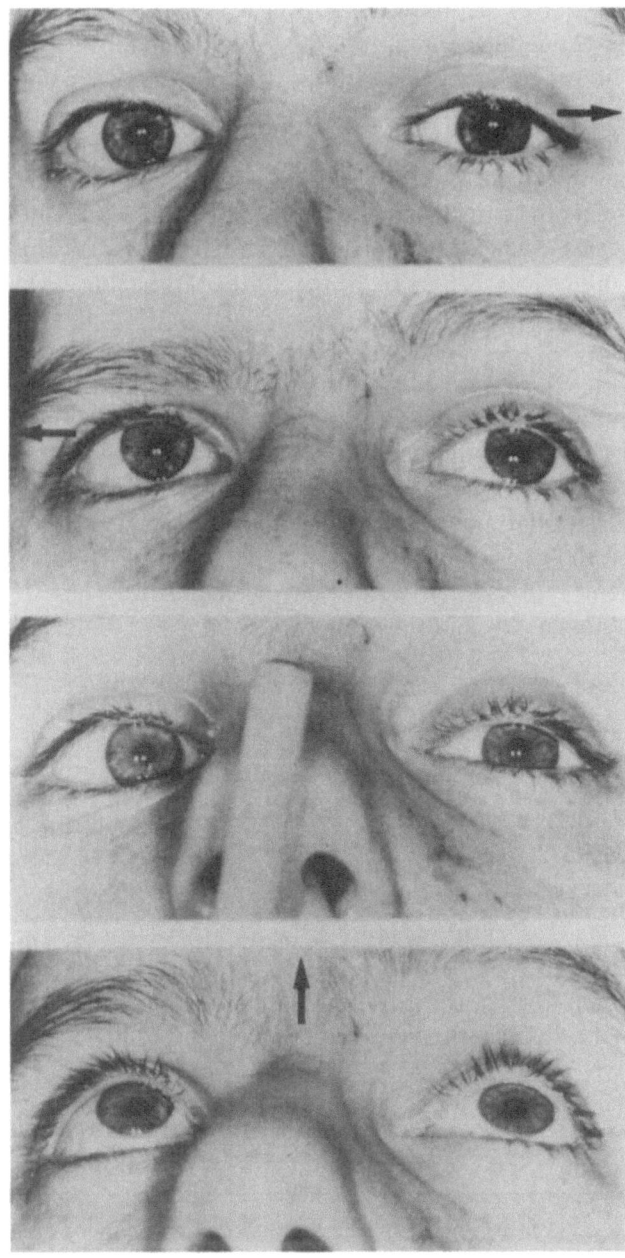

Figure 2. One-and-a-half syndrome in a 19 years old patient with a brainstem glioma.

Usually the syndrome is produced by a single unilateral lesion of the dorsal part of the lower pontine tegmentum, affecting the ipsilateral PPRF, the abducens nucleus and internuclear fibres of the ipsilateral MLF. A comparison of the clinical features of INO and 'one-and-a-half syndrome' is presented in Table 1.

It was Miller Fisher [21] who presented the first clinico-pathological report of this syndrome. Pierrot-Deseilligny [22] described four main theoretical variations. They relate to distinctive features of the deficient lateral gaze. The lateral gaze palsy may be produced by damage to 1. both PPRF and abducens nucleus; 2. to the abducens nucleus; 3. to both the root fibres of the abducens nucleus and the contralateral MLF when two lesions are involved and 4. to the pontine reticular formation only.

Patients with a 'one-and-a-half syndrome' may show exotropia when attempting to look straight ahead. The eye opposite the side of the lesion is deviated outward [23]. This strabismus has been attributed to the unopposed drives of the contralateral intact pontine gaze centre and had been called paralytic pontine exotropia. This ocular motor disturbance can be explained by a single paramedian lesion in the pons probably more rostral in the PPRF than the 'one-and-a-half syndrome'. In case of bilateral involvement of the pons a total loss of horizontal conjugate eye movement may be seen.

4. Skew deviation and incyclorotory nystagmus

Horizontal oculomotor disturbances in MLF lesions are well known. Little attention has been payed to the vertical abnormalities in for example INO. Meienberg [24] reported a case of an oculomotor syndrome with paresis of the homolateral oblique muscles. This patient showed a dissociated 'gaze paretic' unilateral nystagmus, synchronously, the right eye showed a cyclorotatory nystagmus. It was suggested that the lesion responsible for the motility disturbance interrupted fibres ascending from the left vestibular nucleus to the nuclei that innervate the left inferior rectus and right superior oblique muscles. Because

Table 1. Comparison between the features of an internuclear ophthalmoplegia and the one-and-a-half syndrome.

Internuclear ophthalmoplegia	One-and-a-half syndrome
– Ipsilateral impairment of adduction	– Ipsilateral gaze palsy
– Contralateral nystagmus	– Contralateral INO
– Normal convergence	– Either no convergence or an exotropia contralateral to the lesion
– Unilateral lesion in the FLM between the IIIth and VIth nucleus	– Unilateral MLF VIth and PPRF lesion

no INO was seen a lesion of the MLF seemed unlikely and it was presumed that the fibres ascending from the vestibular nucleus were interrupted before entering the MLF. In a more recent paper a similar case was described which however was accompanied by an INO [25]. This strongly suggests that the MLF carries horizontal as well as vertical tonic fibres including those related to vestibulo-ocular function.

5. Summary

Lesions of the MLF produce a variability of eye movement disorders varying from subclinical to a complete horizontal gaze palsy. Depending on the brainstem level location, the lesions led to vertical, horizontal or a combination of gaze disorders. The uni- or bilateral internuclear ophthalmoplegia is most striking related to the MLF and causes an uni- or bilateral INO. Bilateral INO is often accompanied by a vertical gaze disorder or vertical nystagmus. The other described syndromes are caused by involvement of the MLF and surrounding structures (ri-MLF, PPRF, abducens or vestibular nucleus).

References

1. Nieuwenhuys R, Voogd J, van Huyzen (1979): The human nervous system. Springer Verlag Berlin, Heidelberg, New York, first edition.
2. Buttner-Ennever JA, Buttner U (1978): A cell group associated with vertical eye movements in the rostral mesencephalic reticular formation of the monkey. Brain research Amsterdam, 151: 31–47.
3. Buttner-Ennever JA, Buttner U, Cohen B, Baumgartner G (1982): Vertical gaze paralysis and the rostral interstitial nucleus of the medial longitudinal fasciculus. Brain 105: 125–149.
4. Pisak P, Pisak T, Bender M (1976): The pretectal syndrome in the monkeys. I Disturbances of gaze and body posture. Brain 92: 521–534.
5. Reulen JPH, Sanders EACM, Hogenhuis LAH (1983): Eye movement disorders in multiple sclerosis and optic neuritis. Brain 106: 121–140.
6. Cogan DG, Kubik CS, Smith WL (1950): Unilateral internuclear ophthalmoplegia; Report of eight clinical cases with one postmortem study. Arch Ophthalm 44: 783.
7. Savineau 1895): Une nouveau type de paralysie associee des mouvements horizonteaux des yeux. Bull Soc Franc Ophthal 13: 524–534.
8. Lhermitte J (1922): L'encephalite, l'ethargique. Questions neurologiques d'actualite. Masson (ed) Paris 163–203.
9. Spiller WC (1924): Ophthalmoplegia internuclearis anterior; a case with necropsy. Brain 47: 345.
10. Cogan DG (1970): Internuclear ophthalmoplegia typical and atypical. Arch Ophthalmol 40: 583–589.
11. Christoff N, Anderson PJ, Nathanson M, Bender MB (1960): Problems in anatomic analysis of lesions of the medial longitudinal fasciculus. Arch Neurol 2: 293–304.
12. Bird AC, Leech J (1976): Internuclear ophthalmoplegia: An electrooculographic study of peak angular saccadic velocities. Br J Ophthalmology 60: 645–651.
13. Wilson SA (1906): Case of disseminated sclerosis with weakness of each internal rectus and

nystagmus on lateral deviation to the other eye. Brain 29: 298.

14. Pola J, Robinson DA (1978): Oculomotor signals in medial longitudinal fasciculus of the monkey. J Neurophysiol 41: 245–259.

15. Leigh RJ, Zee DS (1983): The neurology of eye movement. Contempory neurology series. FA Davies Phyladelphia.

16. Crane TB, Yee RD, Baloh RW, Hepler R (1983): Analysis of characteristic eye movement abnormalities in internuclear ophthalmoplegia. Arch Ophthalmol 101: 206–210.

17. Herishanu YO, Sharpe JA (1983): Saccadic intrusions in internuclear ophthalmoplegia. Ann Neurol 14: 67–72.

18. Lutz A (1923): Ueber die Bahnen der Blickwendung und deren Dissocierung. Klin Monatsbl Augenh 70: 213–235.

19. Kommerell G (1975): Internuclear ophthalmoplegia of abduction. Arch Ophthalmol 93: 531–534.

20. Wall M, Wray SH (1983): The one-and-a-half-syndrome. A unilateral disorder of the pontine tegmentum. A study of 20 cases and a review of the literature. Neurology 33: 971–980.

21. Fisher CM (1967): Some neuroophthalmological observations. J Neurol Neuros Psychiatry 30: 383–392.

22. Pierrot Deseilligny Ch, Chain F, Serdaru M, Gray F, Lhermitte F (1981): The one-and-a-half-syndrome. Brain 104: 665–699.

23. Sharpe JA, Rosenberg MA, Hoyt WF, Daroff RB (1974): Paralytic pontine exotropia. Neurology 24: 1076–1081.

24. Meienberg O, Rover J, Kommerell G (1978): Prenuclear paresis of homolateral inferior rectus and contralateral superior oblique eye muscles. Arch Neurol 35: 231–233.

25. Nozki S, Mukuno K, Ishikawa S (1983): Internuclear ophthalmoplegia associated with downbeat nystagmus and contralateral incyclotory nystagmus. Ophthalmologica 187: 210–216.

Oculomotor disturbances in extra-pyramidal disorders. A review of the literature

E.L.E.M. BOLLEN, W. VAN DER KAMP, J.C. DEN HEYER,
J.G. VAN DIJK, R.A.C. ROOS, O.J.S. BURUMA

Oculomotor disturbances have been described in Parkinson's disease, in progressive supranuclear palsy (Steele-Richardson-Olszewski's disease), in Wilson's disease and in Huntington's chorea.

1. Parkinson's disease

Parkinson's disease is a disturbance of motor function of unknown aetiology. The major neurological abnormalities are hypokinesia, slowing of movement, muscular rigidity and tremor. These are usually attributed to cell loss in the substantia nigra and its efferent projection sites. A parkinsonian syndrome may be introduced by neuroleptics and it has been described after encephalitis lethargica. Several oculomotor disturbances have been found in Parkinson's disease.

1.1. Saccadic eye movements (SEM)

a. *The latency of saccadic eye movements (SEM) is moderately increased* in Parkinson's disease (Table 1) [1]. The cause of this latency increase is unknown. The increase in the latency of SEM is larger if the fixation time before the target jump is smaller (Table 2) [1, 2].

SEM latency increase has also been described in Alzheimer's disease [3, 4]. Parkinson's disease may be associated with dementia and show an Alzheimer's type of pathology. The latency increase, however, is also found in Parkinson patients with normal intellectual function [1].

b. *Peak velocity of SEM is lowered* in Parkinson's disease (Table 1) [1]. Damage to the pontine paramedian reticular formation has been shown to cause SEM slowing [6]. However, structural damage to the pons has never been observed in Parkinson's disease [7]. Inappropriate co-activation of agonist and antagonist ocular muscles has been described in Parkinson's disease [8, 9] and has been invoked to explain the decrease in the peak velocity of SEM [1]. Such cocontraction may be caused by impaired activation of agonist on direction burst cells, antagonist off direcon burst cells and inhibitory burst cells [8, 9]. Dysfunction of higher oculomotor centers however (frontal eye fields, substantia nigra or superior colliculi) may also be responsible for the decrease in the peak velocity of SEM [1].

c. *SEM are hypometric* in Parkinson's disease. Multiple step saccades are required to obtain a desired eye position. The hypometria of SEM is striking in patients who are instructed to refixate between two stationary targets as rapidly as possible [35] and in patients who voluntarily refixate back and forth between far left and far right without any specific target present [27].

d. *Square wave jerks are saccades of small amplitude* that interrupt fixation by taking the eyes away from, then after several hundred msec back to the target. They occur frequently in Parkinson's disease. They are also seen in progressive supranuclear palsy, cerebellar disease and in focal cortical disease [10]. Their origin in Parkinson's disease is not known.

Table 1. Latency and peak velocity of saccadic eye movement.

	Normals	Patients	
		Mild	Advanced
Latency(ms)	220 ± 40	270 ± 80	360 ± 90
	Mean peak velocity (deg/s)		
Saccade amplitude			
4 deg	176 ± 15	157 ± 36 *	130 ± 34 ***
10 deg	314 ± 43	288 ± 49 ***	246 ± 56 **
18 deg	396 ± 54	387 ± 66	296 ± 55 ***

* $P < 0.05$ ** $P < 0.01$ *** $P < 0.001$

Table 2. Fixation time in saccadic eye movement.

Subjects		Fixation time (ms)					
		<200	<300	<400	<500	<800	>800
Normals	L A T E N C Y	390	370	320	270	240	210
Mild patients		440	340	350	250	220	210
Advanced patients		670*	630*	400*	380	330**	260*

* $P < 0.05$ ** $P < 0.01$. Latencies are the mean of the mean values for each subject

After White OB et al., Brain (1983) 106: 571–587.

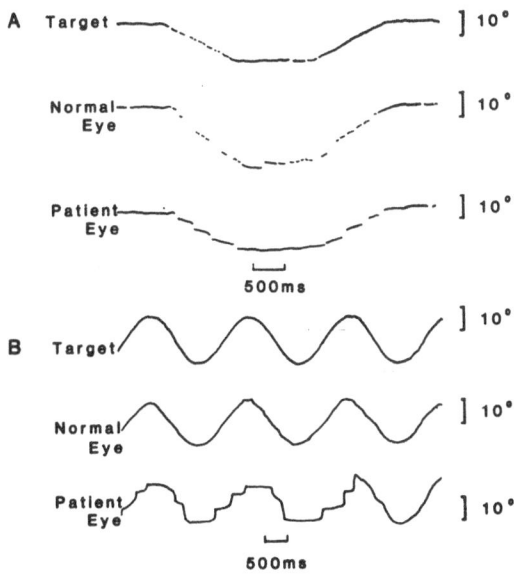

Figure 1. Examples of digitized smooth pursuit movements made by patients with advanced disease and normal subjects. A, single repeated ramps. B, sinusoidal target. Right is upward, left downward. After White OB et al., Brain (1983) 106: 571–587.

2. Smooth pursuit

Smooth pursuit is also abnormal in Parkinson's disease. The gain (ratio of smooth eye velocity to target velocity) is low and catch up saccades may occur with target velocities as low as 10 degrees per second (Fig. 1) [1]. The diminished pursuit gain in Parkinson patients is constant for target velocities up to 407 per second, but further decreases with higher target velocities to values lower than that found in normals (Fig. 2–3) [1]. Abnormalities in SEM and smooth pursuit are more obvious in advanced disease [1]. Both are ameliorated after treatment with L-dopa [1].

3. The vestibulo-ocular reflex (VOR)

The VOR assures good vision during head movements by stabilizing the eyes relative to the visual environment. The VOR gain (ratio of smooth velocity to head velocity) is about 1.0 when a stationary target is fixated during head rotation. In the dark, the VOR gain is less than 1. However, normal subjects can enhance their VOR gain in the dark by imagining a stationary target. Conversely, the VOR must be suppressed for clear perception of moving targets, while tracking them with the head. In the dark normal subjects can, to a certain extent

194

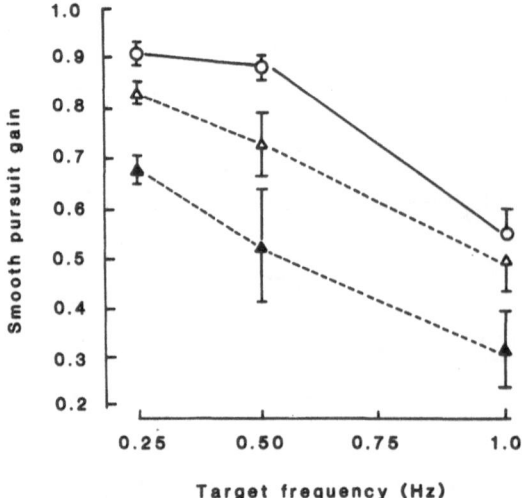

Figure 2. Graph of smooth pursuit gain VS target frequency for sinusoidal targets. Patients with advanced disease (▲). Normal subjects (o). Error bars indicate ± 1 SD. After White OB et al., Brain (1983) 106: 571–587.

[11], voluntarily suppress the VOR by imagining a target moving with the head. Parkinson patients have a lower VOR gain than controls, with a visible stationary target as well as in the dark. In advanced stages of the disease they are unable to raise the VOR gain to normal levels by imagining a stationary target in the dark. Parkinson patients also less effectively suppress their VOR and paradoxically increase their VOR gain when attempting suppression (Fig. 4–7, Table 3) [11].

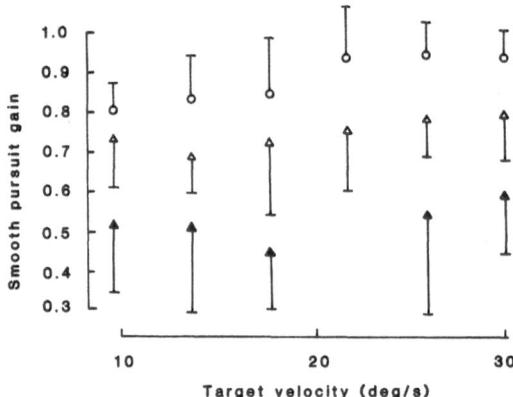

Figure 3. Graph of smooth pursuit gain VS target velocity for a sinusoidal target at 0.5 Hz. Patients with advanced disease (▲). Patients with mild disease (△). Normal subjects (o). After White OB et al., Brain (1983) 106: 571–587.

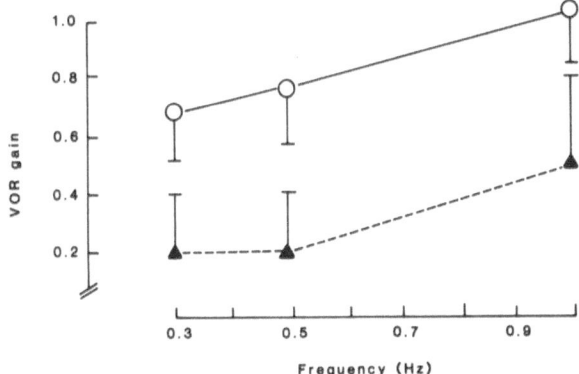

Figure 4. Graphs of mean VOR gain in darkness at 3 rotational frequencies. Patients with advanced disease (▲). Normal subjects (o). Error bars represent 1 SD. After White OB et al., Brain (1983) 106: 555–570.

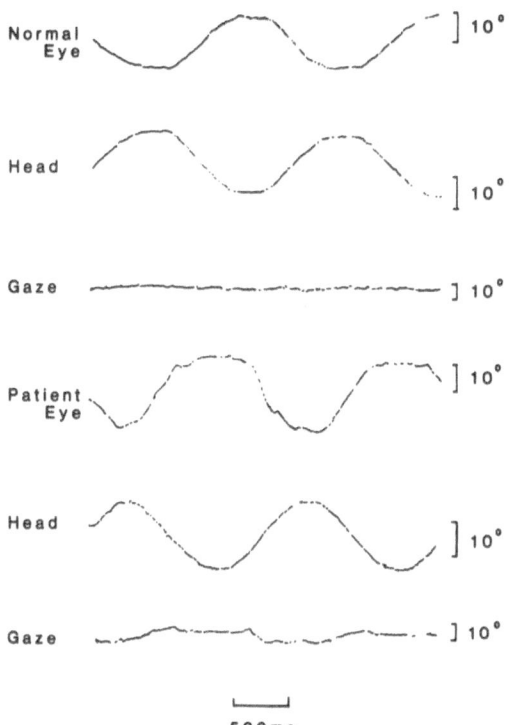

Figure 5. Recordings of horizontal eye, head and gaze (eye plus head) positions obtained while subjects fixated a stationary target. Gaze channels show retinal image motion in patients compared with normal subject. Right is upward, left downward. After White OB et al., Brain (1983) 106: 555–570.

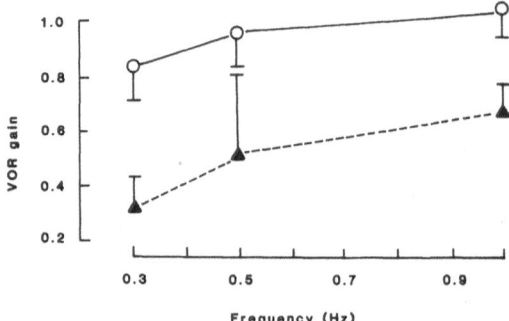

Figure 6. Graph of mean VOR gain in darkness while subjects attempted to fixate an imagined stationary target. Patients with advanced disease (▲). Normal subject (o). Error bars represent 1 SD. After White OB et al., Brain (1983) 106: 555–570.

Table 3. VOR gain in Parkinson patients and controls.

		Patients	
Frequency (Hz)	Controls (n=10)	Mild (n=8)	Advanced (n=6)
VOR–Darkness and mental arithmetic			
0.3	0.68 ± 0.16	0.75 ± 0.29	0.20 ± 0.18 ***
0.5	0.76 ± 0.19	0.78 ± 0.29	0.20 ± 0.21 ***
1.0	0.97 ± 0.13	0.99 ± 0.17	0.50 ± 0.30 ***
VOR–Visible stationary target			
0.3	1.06 ± 0.08	1.13 ± 0.13	0.86 ± 0.15 **
0.5	1.09 ± 0.10	1.17 ± 0.17	0.90 ± 0.20
1.0	1.12 ± 0.09	1.15 ± 0.18	0.95 ± 0.04 ***
VOR–Imagined stationary target			
0.3	0.83 ± 0.12	0.81 ± 0.15	0.30 ± 0.11 **
0.5	0.95 ± 0.08	1.04 ± 0.24	0.50 ± 0.33 *
1.0	1.04 ± 0.10	0.96 ± 0.18	0.65 ± 0.10 **
VOR–Visible moving target			
0.3	0.09 ± 0.08	0.20 ± 0.13 *	0.32 ± 0.16 **
0.5	0.13 ± 0.10	0.32 ± 0.13 **	0.36 ± 0.18 *
1.0	0.35 ± 0.16	0.66 ± 0.21 **	0.62 ± 0.20 **
VOR–Imagined moving target			
		(n=3)	(n=4)
0.3	0.72 ± 0.11	0.63 ± 0.14	0.33 ± 0.14
0.5	0.79 ± 0.06	0.77 ± 0.05	0.18 ± 0.02
1.0	0.89 ± 0.05	1.02 ± 0.23	0.60 ± 0.11

n = No. of subjects. Gain values are the means of the mean VOR gain values for individuals. All P values are derived by the Mann–Whitney U test using the mean VOR gain values of individual subjects
* P < 0.05, ** P < 0.01, *** P < 0.001.

After White OB et al., Brain (1983) 106: 555–570.

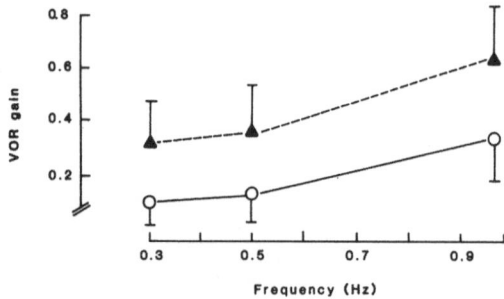

Figure 7. Graph of mean VOR gain obtained while subjects attempted to suppress their VOR by fixating a target moving with their heads. Patients with advanced disease (▲). Normal subjects (o). Error bars indicate 1 SD. After White OB et al., Brain (1983) 106: 555–570.

The paradoxical increase of VOR gain during attempted suppression indicates two things: on the one hand the value of the VOR gain during rotation in darkness appears to be artificially low. Under conditions of visual-vestibular interaction such as suppression, the 'true' VOR gain becomes apparent and indicates structural integrity of the three-neuron reflex arc from the labyrinths to the eye muscles. On the other hand, defective suppression of the VOR is probably related to defective smooth pursuit [11] as has been reported in cerebellar lesions [12] and in multiple sclerosis [13].

2. Progressive supranuclear palsy (PSP)

In 1964 Steele, Richardson and Olszewski were the first to describe this syndrome as an entity. The clinical hallmarks are oculomotor abnormalities, axial rigidity,

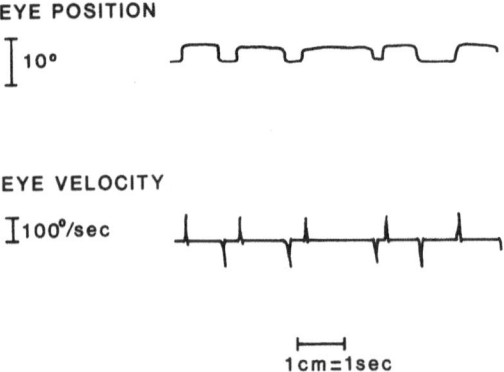

Figure 8. Square-wave jerks during fixation in a patient with progressive supranuclear palsy: riward movements, upward deflection. After Troost BT et al., Ann. Neurol. 2: 397–403, 1977.

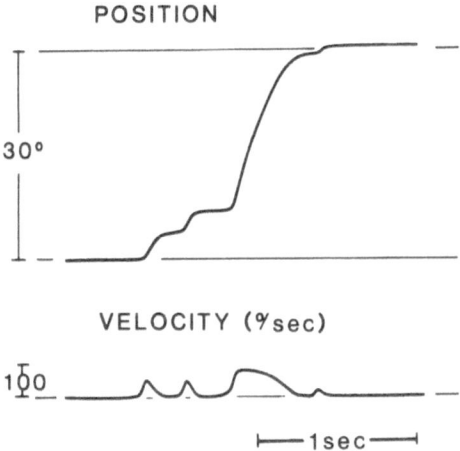

Figure 9. Hypometric refixation saccade toward a target 30 degrees to the right; accomplished in four low-velocity steps. After Troost BT et al., Ann. Neurol. 2: 397–403, 1977.

pseudo-bulbar symptoms and cerebellar and pyramidal signs of the limbs. Vertical eye movement abnormalities are most pronounced. At autopsy, cell loss, neurofibrillary changes and granulovacuolar degeneration and gliosis are found in the basal ganglia and in the brainstem. Symptoms appear between the fifth and the eighth decade. The course is progressive and patients usually die within a few

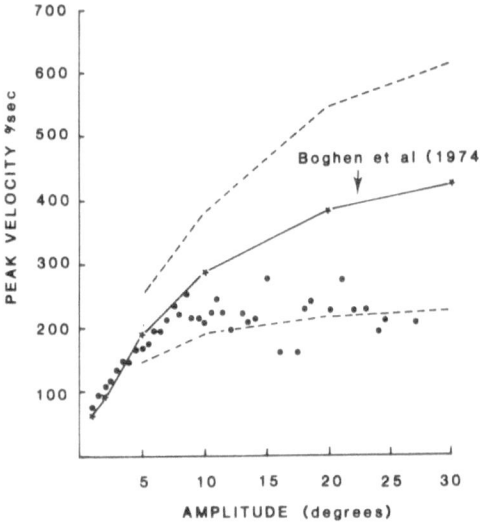

Figure 10. Velocity/amplitude plot of refixation saccades in a patient with PSP. Black circles: mean peak velocities for all saccades at a given amplitude. Black stars and interconnecting lines: mean peak velocity data in normals. Dashed lines indicate 2 standard deviations from the mean established in a previous study. After Troost BT et al., Ann. Neurol. 2: 397–403, 1977.

199

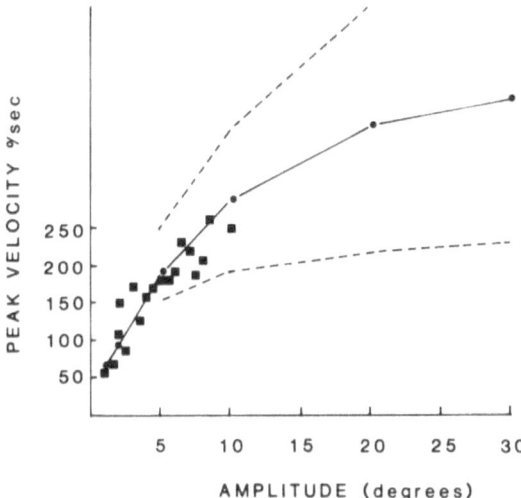

Figure 11. Velocity/amplitude plot of a patient with PSP. Black squares: mean peak velocity values for all saccades at a given amplitude. Patient did not make saccades greater than 10 degrees. Solid and dashed lines same as in Figure 10. After Troost BT et al., Ann. Neurol. 2: 397–403, 1977.

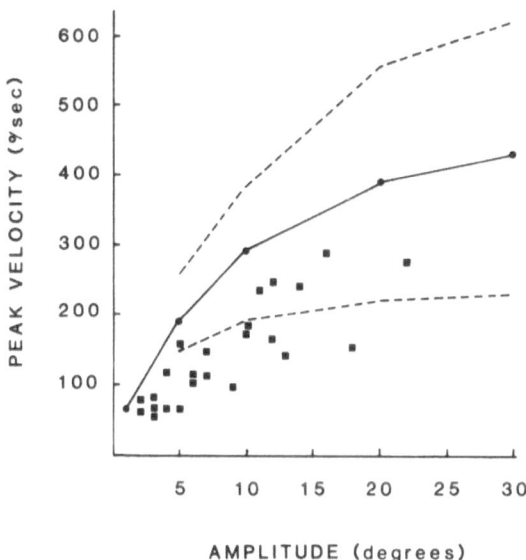

Figure 12. Velocity/amplitude data of a patient with PSP. Black squares: peak velocities for 24 consecutive refixations. Solid and dashed lines as in Figure 10. After Troost BT et al., Ann. Neurol. 2: 397–403, 1977.

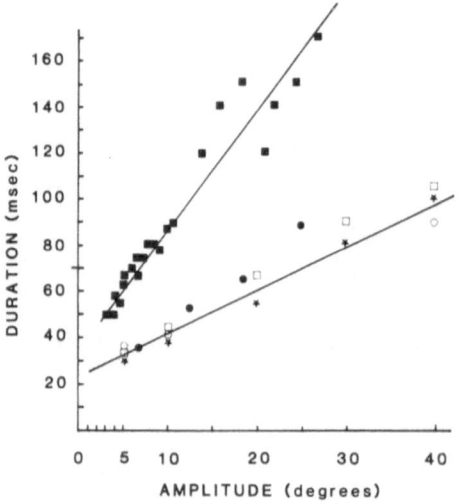

Figure 13. Duration/amplitude plot of data from the same patient with PSP as in Fig. 10, compared with normal subjects. Black squares, represent averaged data from this patient. Normative data from previous studies: black stars, Dodge and Cline, 1901; open squares, Robinson 1964; black circles, Cook et al., 1966, open circles, Bahill et al., 1975. After Troost BT et al., Ann. Neurol. 2: 397–403, 1977.

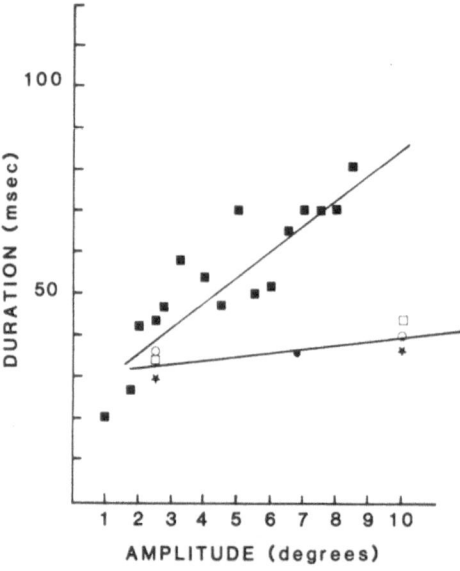

Figure 14. Duration/amplitude data of the same patient with PSP as in Fig. 11. Black squares: averaged data for all saccades at a given amplitude. Normative data same as in Figure 13. After Troost BT et al., Ann. Neurol. 2: 397–403, 1977.

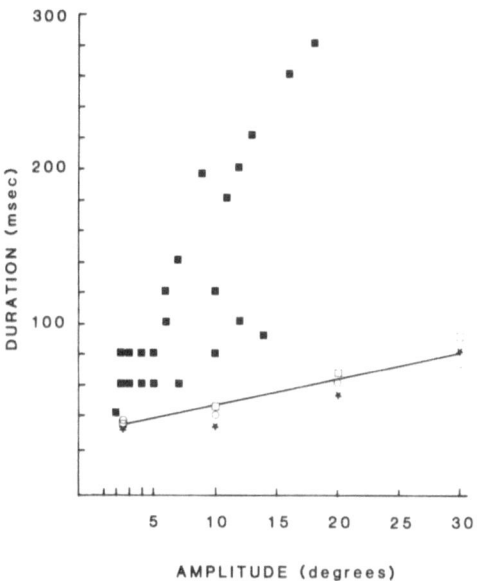

Figure 15. Duration/amplitude data of the same patient with PSP as in Fig. 12. Black squares: individual consecutive eye movements. Normative data same as in Figure 13. After Troost BT et al., Ann. Neurol. 2: 397–403, 1977.

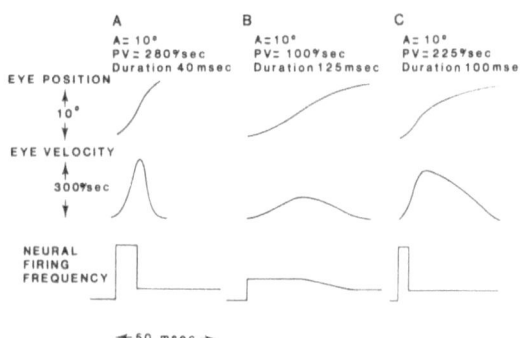

Figure 16. Theoretical analogues of eye position and eye velocity, and histograms of neural firing frequency, which produce normal (A) and possibly produce abnormal (B, C) saccades in patients with progressive supranuclear palsy. (A) Normal 10-degree saccade with peak velocity of 280 degrees per second and duration of 40 msec. Normal 'pulse-step' neural firing frequency is shown. (B) Slow 10-degree saccade: peak velocity 100 degrees per second, duration 125 msec. Defective pulse, virtually 'pulseless' [9]. (C) Long-duration 10-degree saccade: peak velocity near normal at 225 degrees per second. Pulse unsustained. (A = amplitude; PV = peak velocity). After Troost BT et al., Ann. Neurol. 2: 397–403, 1977.

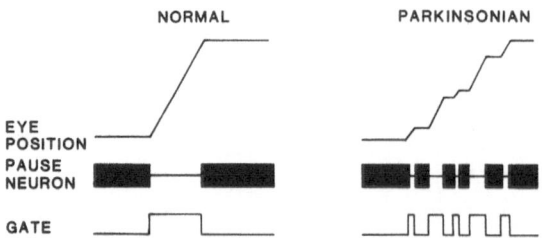

Figure 17. Schematic representation of the saccades of normal subjects and those of parkinsonian patients relative to the hypothetical gate and pause cell function (see text). After Teräväinen et al., Acta Neurol. Scand. 62: 137–148, 1980.

years. The following oculomotor disturbances have been reported.
1. Square wave jerks with a frequency of 1–4 Hz and an amplitude of 0.5–3 degrees (Fig. 8) [14].
2. Hypometric SEM with multiple step saccades (Fig. 9) [16].
3. Decreased SEM velocity (Fig. 10–15) [14, 15, 17].
4. Increased duration of SEM even with normal SEM peak velocity, indicating increased acceleration or deceleration time (Fig. 16) [14].
5. Velocity decrease of the smooth pursuit, with catch up saccades [14].
6. Decreased VOR gain, with defective visual enhancement and defective visual suppression of the VOR [14].
7. Tonic deviation of the eyes with caloric testing [14].

Although dementia has often been cited as a major symptom [17], Fisk et al. [16] found PSP patients to score worse than controls only on mental tests that require visual scanning. They concluded that visual scanning deficits, possibly as a consequence of dysfunction of the superior colliculi, must be considered in assessing the results of mental tasks in PSP patients.

3. Wilson's disease

Wilson's disease is an autosomal recessively inherited disturbance of copper metabolism that results in hepatic and neurologic abnormalities. Clinical hallmarks include rigidity, tremor, pseudo-bulbar symptoms and involuntary movements. A pigmented corneal ring (Keyser-Fleischer) is almost always found in patients with neurologic involvement. Widespread damage of putamen, globus pallidus, caudate nucleus, cortex, thalamus and brainstem has been described. Ocular motor disorders are less frequent in Wilson's disease as compared to Parkinson's disease and progressive supranuclear palsy [20]. A decrease in SEM peak velocity, the absence of the fast component of optokinetic nystagmus, tonic deviation of the eyes on caloric stimulation [18], catch up saccades during smooth pursuit [19], hypermetric saccades [20, 21] and paresis of vertical gaze [23] have been noted. Some investigators report a disturbance of the near reflex (convergence, accommodation and miosis) in Wilson's disease [21, 24]. In normal individuals, the amplitude of accommodation decreases with age from 12 diopters at 8 years of age to 2 diopters at age 50. Klingele et al. [21] reported an accommodation amplitude of 3 diopters in a 22 year old man with Wilson's disease. Curran et al. [24] presented a case of an 11 year old Wilson's disease patient with an accommodation amplitude of only 3 diopters. The patient had normal pupillary responses to light and normal eye movements, except for saccadic intrusions on smooth pursuit.

The disturbances of accommodation and pupillary constriction have been attributed to deposits of copper in the anteromedian part of the oculomotor nucleus [24]. Interruption of cortico-tectal fibers from area 19 and 22 of Brodmann may cause weakness of convergence [21], but the cause of weakness of convergence is not known [21].

4. Huntington's disease

Huntington's disease is an autosomal dominantly inherited disease usually starting in the fourth of fifth decade, although juvenile and senile forms exist. Clinical hallmarks are choreatic movements and dementia. Emotional disturbances are among the first signs. The mean duration of the disease is about 17 years. Cell loss and gliosis are found all over the brain, but are most prominent in the striatum. An increase of SEM latency, decrease of saccadic peak velocity and loss of the fast component of the optokinetic and vestibular nystagmus are obvious in Huntington's disease [32]. Vertical saccades are often more affected than horizontal ones [32]. Patients with advanced disease are capable of making a saccade only after a head movement or after blinking [32]. The latter abnormalities are also seen in oculomotor apraxia [29] and facilitation of eye movements by blinking has also been reported in two patients with brainstem disease [30]. The nature of the blink-saccade synkinesis is not understood. Many saccadic intrusions are seen during smooth pursuit in Huntington's disease. Fixation is interrupted by square wave jerks. A normal person, when instructed to fixate an object, is able to neglect visual stimuli, appearing in the periphery of his visual fields. Patients with Huntington's disease are less able to suppress unwanted visually evoked reflex saccades [32, 34]. The superior colliculi are important in generating saccades to suddenly appearing visual stimuli. The high frequency of distracting eye movements therefore may indicate desinhibition of the superior colliculi in Huntington's disease due to loss of inhibitory influence from the frontal eye fields, the substantia nigra or the nigro-striatal circuit [32, 34].

5. Summary

In summary, in Parkinson's disease, progressive supra nuclear palsy, Wilson's disease and Huntington's chorea, saccadic eye movements show increased latency and decreased peak velocity. Saccadic eye movements are hypometric in all four diseases. In Wilson's disease hypermetric saccades may also be observed. In all four diseases, smooth pursuit is interrupted by saccadic intrusions. Fixation is interrupted by square wave jerks in Parkinson's disease, progressive supranuclear palsy and Huntington's chorea. The gain of the vestibulo-ocular reflex is decreased in Parkinson's disease and progressive supranuclear palsy (Table 4 and 5). The cause of oculomotor abnormalities in extra-pyramidal disorders is not well understood. Descending tracts from the frontal eye fields project to the diencephalon and the striatum [24]. The latter connects through the substantia

Table 4. Eye movement disturbances in Parkinson's disease, progressive supranuclear palsy, Wilson's disease and Huntington's chorea.

SACCADIC EYE MOVEMENTS

Latency increase
Peak velocity decrease
Hypometria, multiple step saccades

SMOOTH PURSUIT

Saccadic intrusion

Table 5. Eye movement disturbances in Parkinson's disease (PD), progressive supranuclear palsy (PSP), Wilson's disease (WD) and Huntington's chorea (HC).

	Square wave jerks	VOR gain decrease	Hypermetria
PD	+	+	−
PSP	+	+	?
WD	?	?	+
HC	?	?	−

+ : present, − : absent, ? : not investigated.

nigra with the superior colliculus [11]. Stimulation of the superior colliculus causes saccades, a combined lesion of frontal eye field and superior colliculus causes slowed and hypometric saccades [28]. Dysfunction of the fronto-nigro-colliculo-reticular pathways is possibly a cause of oculomotor disturbances in patients with extra pyramidal diseases [1]. Dysfunction of the mesencephalic and pontine reticular formation, the common generator of all saccadic eye movements, is another possible explanation. An indication for the latter type of dysfunction may be found in the hypometric SEM with multiple step saccades. Zee and Robinson [28] have suggested that inappropriate activation of pause cells during a saccade may disrupt the saccade. Teräväinen [29] used this model of inappropriate activation of pause cells to explain saccadic hypometria in Parkinson's disease (Fig. 17).

6. Addendum

Bronstein et al. [36], published a study on predictive ocular motor control in patients with Parkinson's disease. They showed a reduced tendency to make anticipatory saccadic eye movements (eye in advance of the target) in these patients. A normal amount of latency decrease on the contrary took place in a predictive smooth pursuit task. The authors explained these results by an increased reliance on visual input in parkinsonian patients. This prevents them from making use of verbal instruction to generate anticipatory saccades. Anticipation in smooth pursuit on the contrary relies on continuous visual information and was found normal. Furthermore, the authors found normal saccadic and smooth pursuit velocity in their patients. They emphasize the normal metrics of saccadic eye movements and of smooth pursuit in mildly and moderately affected patients with Parkinson's disease.

References

1. White O, Saint-Cyr J, Tomlinson R, Sharpe J (1983): Ocular motor deficits in Parkinson's disease. II Control of the saccadic and smooth pursuit systems. Brain 106: 571–587.
2. Bodis-Wolner L, Yahr M (1978): Measurements of visual evoked potentials in Parkinson's disease. Brain 101: 661–671.
3. Pirozzolo F, Hansch E (1981): Ocular motor reaction time in dementia reflects degree of cerebral dysfunction. Science 214: 349–350.
4. Sharpe J, Lo A, Rabinovitch H (1979): Control of the saccadic and the smooth pursuit systems after cerebral hemidecortication. Brain 102: 387–403.
5. Flowers K, Downing A (1978): Predictive control of eye movement in Parkinson's disease. Annals of Neurology 4: 63–66.
6. Buttner-Enever JA, Wadia NH, Sakai H, Schwendemann G: Neuroanatomy of oculomotor structures in olivopontocerebellar atrophy patients with slow saccades. J Neurol, in press.
7. Alvord E, Forno L et al (1984): The pathology of Parkinsonism: a comparison of degenerations in

206

cerebral cortex and brainstem. Advances in Neurology 5: 175–193.

8. Slatt B, Loeffler J, Hoyt W (1966): Ocular motor disturbances in Parkinson's disease. Canadian Journal of Ophthalmology 1: 267–273.

9. Chaco J (1971): Impairment of function of extra ocular muscles in Parkinson's disease. Journal of the Neurological Sciences 15: 251–265.

10. Sharpe J, Herishanu Y, White O (1982): Cerebral square wave jerks. Neurology 32: 57–62.

11. White O, Saint-Cyr J, Sharpe J (1983): Ocular motor deficits in Parkinson's disease. I. The horizontal vestibulo-ocular reflex and its regulation. Brain 106: 555–570.

12. Dichgans J, von Reutern G, Römmelt U (1978): Impaired suppression of vestibular nystagmus by fixation in cerebellar and noncerebellar patients. Archiv für Psychiatrie und Nervenkrankheiten 226: 183–199.

13. Sharpe J, Goldberg H, Lo A, Herishanu Y (1981): Visual-vestibular interaction in multiple sclerosis. Neurology 31: 427–433.

14. Troost B, Daroff R (1977): The ocular motor defects in progressive supranuclear palsy. Annals of Neurology 2: 397–403.

15. Newman N, Gay A, Stroud M, Brooks J (1980): Defective rapid eye movements in progressive supra nuclear palsy. Brain 93: 775–784.

16. Fisk J, Goodale M, Burkhart T, Barnett H (1982): Progressive supranuclear palsy: the relationship between ocular motor dysfunction and psychological test performance. Neurology 32: 698–705.

17. Steele J, Richardson J, Olszewski J (1964): Progressive supranuclear palsy. Archives of Neurology 10: 333–359.

18. Kirkham T, Kamin D (1974): Slow saccadic eye movements in Wilson's disease. Journal of Neurology, Neurosurgery and Psychiatry 37: 191–194.

19. Goldberg M, van Noorden G (1966): Opthalmologic findings in Wilson's hepatolenticular degeneration. Archives of Opthalmology 75: 162–170.

20. Hyman N, Phuapradrit P (1979): Reading difficulty as a presenting symptom in Wilson's disease. Journal of Neurology, Neurosurgery and Psychiatry 42: 478–480.

21. Klingele T, Newman S, Burde R (1980): Accomodation defect in Wilson's disease. American Journal of Ophthalmology 90: 22–24.

22. Leichnetz G (1981): The prefrontal cortico-ocular motor trajectories in the monkey. Journal of the Neurological Sciences 49: 387–396.

23. Gadoth N, Liel Y: Transient external ophthalmoplegia in Wilson's disease. Metabolic and Pediatric Ophthalmology 4: 71–73.

24. Curran R, Hedges T, Boger W (1982): Loss of accomodation and the near response in Wilson's disease. Journal of Pediatric Ophthalmology and Strabismus 19: 157–160.

25. Schiller P, True S, Conway J (1980): Deficits in eye movements following frontal eye field and superior colliculus ablations. Journal of Neurophysiology 44: 1175–1189.

26. Zee D, Robinson D (1979): A hypothetical explanation for saccadic oscillations. Annals of Neurology 5: 405–414.

27. Teräväinen H, Calne D (1980): Studies of parkinsonian movements. 1 Programming and execution of eye movements. Acta Neurologica Scandinavica 62: 137–148.

28. Shibasaki H, Tsuji S, Kuroiwa Y (1979): Oculomotor abnormalities in Parkinson's disease. Archives of Neurology 36: 360–364.

29. Zee D, Yee R, Singel H (1977): Congenital ocular motor ataxia. Brain 100: 581–599.

30. Zee D, Chu F et al (1983): Blink-saccade synkinesis. Neurology 33: 1233–1236.

31. Collin H, Cowey A, Latto R, Marzi C (1982): The role of frontal eye fields and superior colliculi in visual search and non-visual search in rhesus monkeys. Behavioral Brain Research 4: 177–193.

32. Leigh R, Newman S et al (1983): Abnormal ocular motor control in Huntington's disease. Neurology 33: 1268–1275.

33. Albano J, Mishkin M, Westbrook L, Wurtz R (1982): Visuomotor deficits following ablation of

monkey superior colliculus. J Neurophysiol 48: 338–351.

34. Bollen E, Reulen JPH, den Heyer JC, van der Kamp W, Roos RAC, Buruma OJS (1986): Horizontal and vertical eye movement abnormalities in Huntington's chorea. J Neurol Sc 74: 11–22.

35. Melvill Jones G, Gonshor A (1971): Dynamic characteristics of saccadic eye movements in Parkinson's disease. Exp Neurol 31: 17–31.

36. Bornstein AM, Kennard C (1985): Predictive ocular motor control in Parkinson's disease. Brain 108: 925–940.

Eye movement disorders caused by lesions of the cerebral hemispheres

J. VAN GIJN

Lesions of the cerebral hemispheres may affect saccadic eye movements. A *saccade palsy* to the left results from a destructive lesion in the right hemisphere, and vice versa. With unilateral lesions the gaze palsy is transient, at least clinically, with deviation of the eyes to the side of the lesion. Saccade palsy has traditionally been associated with dysfunction of the frontal lobe, but recently the parietal lobe has also been implicated, in particular with right-sided lesions. Some patients with supratentorial haemorrhage, especially in the thalamus, may show contralateral gaze deviation ('wrong-way eyes'), possibly as a result of secondary involvement of mesencephalic structures. Loss of *smooth pursuit movements,* with replacement by saccadic jerks to maintain retinal fixation, is usually associated with ipsilateral occipito-parietal lesions. *Slow reflex eye movements* generated by the vestibular system are rarely affected by hemispheral disease per se. In contrast, optokinetic nystagmus is predominantly a cortical reflex. It is dependent upon both pursuit and saccadic pathways, and may be altered by dysfunction of either system.

The cerebral hemispheres are – by definition – involved in the initiation of all voluntary eye movements, but our knowledge of this process is incomplete. How vertical or vergence movements of the eyes are controlled by the cerebral cortex is largely a mystery, at least in man. Some pieces of evidence exist about disorders of horizontal, conjugate eye movements. The following review is an attempt to fit these pieces into a recognizable shape.

Horizontal eye movements can be distingguished into three categories: 1. saccadic movements; 2. pursuit movements; 3. reflex movements (optokinetic nystagmus, vestibulo-ocular reflexes).

Lesions of the cerebral hemispheres may have different effects on these three systems, depending on the site, size, and age of the lesions. I shall separately consider the disorders of each system, thus following the neurological examination. The emphasis will be on abnormalities that are clinically detectable, rather than on the subtleties of the oculographic examination. Experiments in monkeys that have led to important advances in our understanding of the cortical control of eye movements have been summarized elsewhere [1, 2].

1. Disorders of saccadic eye movements

With *unilateral destructive lesions* of the cerebral hemispheres the disturbances of voluntary gaze are usually transient. More than a century ago Prevost first noted a 'déviation conjuguée' towards the side of the lesion [3]. In the acute phase the patient is unable to execute saccadic movements to the contralateral side, either on command or in search of an object; spontaneous saccades are also absent in that direction. Traditionally, the disorder has been attributed to a dysfunction of the frontal lobe. The concept of a 'frontal eye field' that generates saccades to the contralateral side (Fig. 1) is supported by stimulation experiments during surgery of the brain [4]. A more complex function of the frontal lobe in the control of saccadic eye movements is the suppression of inappropriate saccades [5].

The notion of a frontal eye field has been questioned by some. De Renzi and co-workers performed a prospective study of 436 stroke patients, of whom 120 showed gaze palsy. The presence of this sign was mainly associated with post-rolandic lesions of the right hemisphere, or with left-sided brain damage that involved the entire territory of the middle cerebral artery [6]. Gaze palsy with right-sided lesions also lasted longer (mean 15 days) than with left-sided lesions (mean 8 to 9 days). A weakness in this study is that the site and the size of the lesions was inferred only from the clinical examination. Nevertheless, the conclusions seem to be corroborated by another prospective study of stroke patients – not yet reported in detail – in which it was found that the size of the lesion was more relevant to the occurrence of gaze palsy than the site [7].

Gaze palsies from smaller lesions were particularly associated with dysfunction of the right hemisphere, and with gaze palsies from single-lobe lesions the parietal lobe was involved as often as the frontal lobe [7]. In contrast, frontal lobe lesions appeared more relevant in a smaller study in which computed tomography (CT) was used to verify the lesions in 33 stroke patients with conjugate deviation of the eyes: 26 patients had infarcts or haemorrhages of various sizes involving the frontal lobes, 3 patients showed deeper lesions (internal capsule or thalamus), and in 4 patients the CT scan was normal [8].

The duration of the gaze palsy was rarely longer than 5 days in the two most recent studies [7, 8]. If it exceeded 14 days the explanation was either an exceptionally large lesion [7] or pre-existing damage to the contralateral frontal region [8]. When the gaze palsy begins to resolve the saccades again move the eyes beyond midposition but only transitorily, after which the eyes drift back towards the side of the lesion, which slow movements are interrupted by corrective saccades (gaze-paretic nystagmus to the contralateral side). At a later stage the only difficulty consists in maintaining an extreme eccentric position of gaze to

211

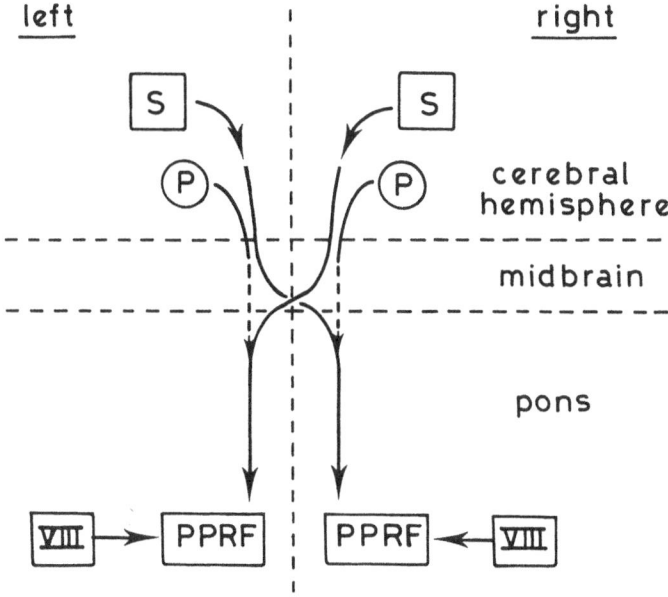

left   right

cerebral
hemisphere

midbrain

pons

Figure 1. Projections upon the pontine paramedian reticular formation (PPRF). S, saccade system; P, pursuit system; VIII, vestibular nuclei (after: Glaser JS, Neuro-ophthalmology. Hagerstown: Harper & Row, 1978).

the contralateral side, and finally no deficit at all is clinically detectable. Electro-oculographic studies, however, may still show slowing or inaccuracy of the saccades directed away from the side of the lesion. After hemispherectomy the abnormalities may be permanent and may also involve saccades to the ipsilateral side, although to a lesser extent [9, 10].

It is clear that the fibre systems from the 'frontal' eye fields to the nuclei in the brainstem (pontine paramedian reticular formation) can be interrupted at levels other than that of the cerebral cortex. Sparing of conjugate eye movements in a patient with complete infarction of the posterior limb of both internal capsules [11] is in keeping with experiments in monkeys suggesting that the pathways for the saccadic eye movements course in the anterior limb of the internal capsule as well as in the thalamus [12]. It is therefore not surprising that deviation of conjugate gaze towards the lesion has been reported in patients with haemorrhages involving either or both of these two structures [8, 12].

It is surprising, however, that haemorrhages may also result in gaze deviation to the contralateral side ('wrong-way eyes' [13]). This phenomenon has been almost invariably associated with thalamic haemorrhage (Fig. 2) [13–15]; the only exceptions are two patients with a frontal lobe haematoma [16, 17]. The Table shows the most relevant clinical features in the 12 patients reported so far. Focal epileptic activity is not an attractive explanation for the paradoxical phenom-

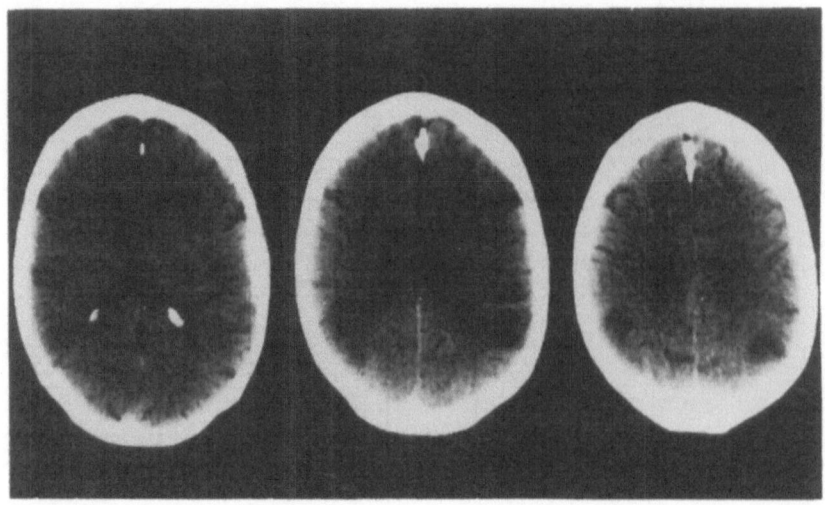

Figure 2. CT scan showing a left thalamic-capsular haemorrhage in a 42 year old hypertensive man, two days after the onset of a right sided hemiparesis with conjugate deviation of the eyes to the right. Some blood has ruptured into the posterior horn of the left ventricle.

enon, as the gaze deviation was never accompanied by other epileptic features, or nystagmus, and the EEG was normal in two patients [14]. A more plausible hypothesis, at least for the patients with thalamic haemorrhage, was suggested by Fisher [13] and assumes a secondary dysfunction of the mesencephalic part of the saccadic system, caudal to its decussation (Fig. 1). In most patients with 'wrong-way eyes' from thalamic haemorrhage the blood had ruptured into the third ventricle and the pupillary reflexes were lost, which is in keeping with such an explanation. Moreover, 'wrong-way eyes' have been reported only with haemorrhages, and never in patients with infarction in the supratentorial compartment.

Table 1. Patients with 'wrong-way eyes'.

	Number of patients	Site of haemorrhage	Rupture into 3rd ventricle	Pupillary reflexes
Fisher 1967 [13]	3	thalamus	3/3	absent
Keane 1975 [14]	3	thalamus	2/3	absent
Walshe et al. 1977 [15]	3	thalamus	?	?
Pessin et al. 1981 [16]	1	frontotemporal	–	present
Sharpe et al. 1985 [17]	1	frontal	–	present
present study (Fig. 2)	1	thalamus	–	present

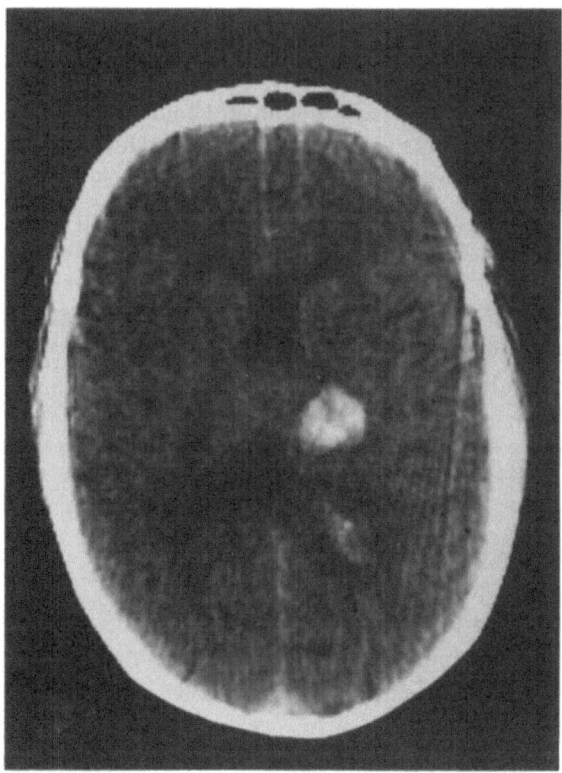

Figure 3. CT scans showing bilateral border zone infarcts in the occipito-parietal area, caused by paroxysmal atrial fibrillation, in a 70 year old man with Balint's syndrome [20]. The scans were made a few days after the onset (by courtesy of Dr. A. Hijdra).

With parieto-occipital lesions resulting in homonymous hemianopia the saccadic eye movements are unaffected, but the patient has difficulty in knowing where to look in the blind hemifield. This results in step-wise searching saccades, later substituted by overshooting or undershooting strategies [18]. The tendency to perform multiple saccades is caused not only by hemianopia per se but also by neglect of contralateral space, associated with a lesion in the parietal lobe [19].

Irritative lesions of one cerebral hemisphere resulting in gaze deviation have been classically associated with the frontal lobe, contralateral to the direction of gaze [4]. However, recent studies attest that epileptic eye and head movements may be directed either ipsilateral or contralateral to the side of the EEG focus [20], and that the seizure activity may originate from posterior cortical areas as well as from the frontal lobe [20, 21].

Bilateral destructive lesions of the frontoparietal cortex or thalamus may result in a general inability to generate saccades on command, with preservation of pursuit and reflex saccadic movements. The patient, in order to succeed in refixation, has to turn the head with a thrust. The concomitant eyelid closure also facilitates saccadic eye movements [22]. Impairment of saccades in both directions may be acquired, usually as part of diffuse diseases of the nervous system, for instance Wilson's disease [23] or spinocerebellar degeneration [24]. A defect of saccadic eye movements may be also a congenital disorder, called 'oculomotor apraxia' [25, 26]. The anatomical defect in this disorder is usually not known.

A particular variety of abnormal voluntary eye movements occurs in patients with bilateral border zone infarcts between the territories of the middle cerebral and posterior cerebral arteries, usually as a result of systemic hypotension. Besides a complex syndrome of perceptual defects (Balint's syndrome) the patient shows inability to attain fixation despite normal saccades [27]. The explanation is that the 'frontal' eye fields generate normal saccades but receive no feedback from the visual cortex, although the patient is not blind (disconnection syndrome; Fig. 3).

2. Disorders of pursuit movements

It is generally believed that pursuit movements are controlled by the ipsilateral hemisphere [28]. This implies that the pathways connecting the cortical 'pursuit centre' with the brainstem nuclei cross the midline either twice or not at all (Fig. 1). Most evidence indicates that the parieto-occipital area of the cerebral cortex is particularly involved in the initiation of pursuit movements.

Following *unilateral lesions* of the parieto-occipital area the pursuit movements to the side of the lesion are no longer performed smoothly, but are broken up by saccades as the point of fixation is falling behind the target [28]. Occasionally acute lesions in the occipito-parietal area are associated with transient loss of pursuit movements to the contralateral side [29]. This may be secondary to spatial neglect, caused by the parietal component of the lesion. In patients who have undergone hemispherectomy years before, electro-oculographic examination demonstrates persistent defects of pursuit movements. These were abnormally slow to the ipsilateral side, and too fast – at least at low speeds – when directed to the contralateral side [9, 10].

The occipitomesencephalic pathways that mediate pursuit movements are probably located in the stratum sagittale internum, which is immediately lateral to the commissural fibres of the tapetum that line the trigone of the lateral cerebral ventricle. Further lateral is the external sagittal stratum, which contains the fibres of the optic radiation (Fig. 4). The close proximity of the efferent, afferent, and commissural fibre systems of the visual cortex near the lateral wall of the trigonal cavity is the reason that hemianopia from parieto-occipital lesions is almost invariably associated with defective pursuit to the same side (whereas pursuit is usually spared in patients with hemianopia from occipital lesions, because the commissural and efferent pathways are intact). Nevertheless, one

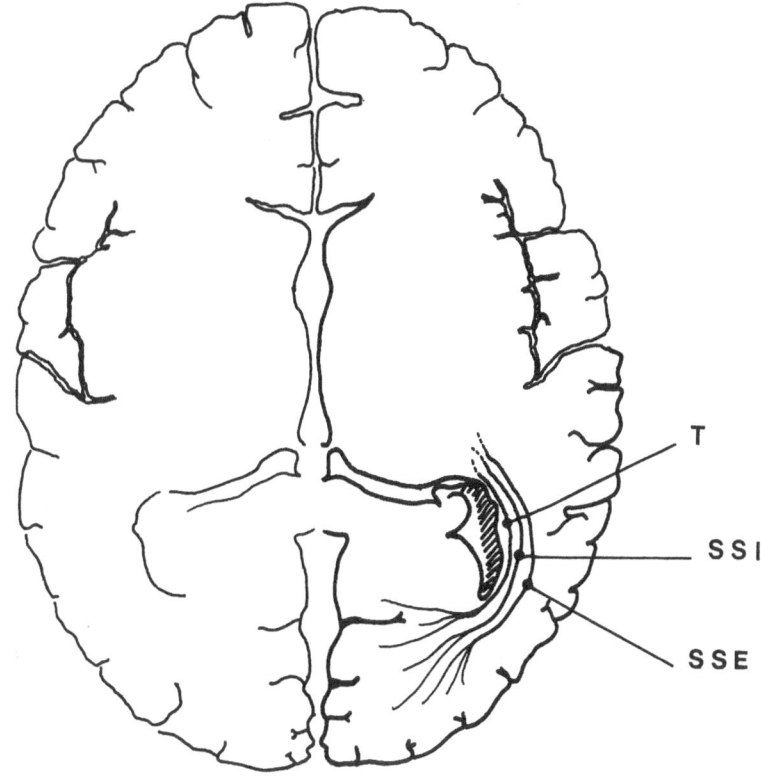

Figure 4. Diagrammatical representation of the fibre structures lateral to the trigone of the lateral ventricle. T, tapetum (to occipital cortex of the opposite hemisphere); SSI, stratum sagittale internum (efferent pathway for pursuit movements, to nuclei in the brainstem); SSE, stratum sagittale externum (optic radiation or afferent system).

patient has been reported who retained normal pursuit despite a haemorrhage that had destroyed most of the three fibre systems lateral to the trigone [30]. The explanation is that either some fibres were spared in the tapetum and internal sagittal stratum, or that other commissural connections transmitted the retinal velocity information from the intact hemisphere to the extrastriate cortex of the 'blind' hemisphere. At the level of the thalamus, the pathway for pursuit movements probably travels closely to the saccadic system, as both ipsilateral pursuit and contralateral saccades may be affected by a single haemorrhage in the posterior thalamus [12, 31].

Bilateral defects of pursuit movements occur when the level of consciousness is impaired, after ingestion of sedative drugs, after diffuse cell loss from various causes, including motor neurone disease [32], or after bilateral infarction of the occipitoparietal cortex [33].

3. Disorders of reflex eye movements

Optokinetic nystagmus is usually tested by means of a striped drum or a tape measure. Under these conditions the reflex is dependent upon visual fixation, and represents a combination of pursuit movements and saccadic movements. In disorders of the saccadic system, testing of the optokinetic nystagmus results in a tonic deviation of the eyes in the direction of the target. If pursuit movements are defective, the optokinetic nystagmus is absent or broken up by saccades [34]. Ter Braak distinguished – in animals – 'active' (cortical) optokinetic nystagmus from 'passive' (subcortical) optokinetic nystagmus[35]. Later he demonstrated that full-field stimulation could generate optokinetic nystagmus in a patient with cortical blindness [36]. The subcortical response shows a gradual build-up, and in normal subjects it is associated with an illusion of self-rotation and after-nystagmus in darkness. In two recently reported patients with parietal lesions, full field pursuit was less affected than foveal pursuit [34].

The *vestibulo-ocular reflexes* are spared in lesions that are confined to the cerebral hemispheres, although electro-oculographic studies may uncover a decrease of voluntary and visual control of the vestibulo-ocular reflex to the side of the lesion [10, 37]. A reported exception were two patients with acute cerebral lesions (without signs of tentorial herniation) who were also treated with anticonvulsant drugs; both had lost their vestibular responses [38].

Acknowledgements

I received valuable comments from Dr. D.S. Zee (Baltimore), Dr. J.D. Meerwaldt (Rotterdam) and Dr. H. Franssen (Utrecht).

References

1. Zee DS (1983): Ocular motor control: the cerebral control of saccadic eye movements. In: Lessell S, van Dalen JWT (eds). Neuro-ophthalmology. Amsterdam: Elsevier, pp·141–56.
2. Zee DS, Tusa RJ, Herdman SJ, Butler PH, Gücer G: The acute and chronic effects of bilateral occipital lobectomy upon eye movements in monkey. In: Keller E, Zee DS (eds). Adaptive processes in visual and oculomotor systems. Pergamon, in press.
3. Prevost JL (1868): De la déviation conjuguée des yeux et de la rotation de la tête dans certains cas d'hemiplegie. Thèse de Paris.
4. Penfield WG, Jasper H (1954): Epilepsy and functional anatomy of the human brain. London: Churchill.
5. Guitton D, Buchtel HA, Douglas RM (1985): Frontal lobe lesions in man cause difficulties in suppressing reflexive glances and in generating goal-directed saccades. Exp Brain Res 58: 455–72.
6. De Renzi E, Colombo A, Faglioni P, Gilbertoni M (1982): Conjugate gaze paresis in stroke patients with unilateral damage – an unexpected instance of hemispheric asymmetry. Arch Neurol 39: 482–6.

7. Mohr JP, Rubinstein LV, Kase CS, Price TR, Wolf PA, Nichols FT, Tatemichi TK (1984): Gaze palsy in hemispheral stroke: the NINCDS stroke data bank. Neurology 34 (suppl. 1): 199.

8. Steiner I, Melamed E (1984): Conjugate eye deviation after acute hemispheric stroke: delayed recovery after previous contralateral frontal lobe damage. Ann Neurol 16: 509–11.

9. Sharpe JA, Lo AW, Rabinovitch HE (1979): Control of the saccadic and smooth pursuit systems after cerebral hemidecortication. Brain 102: 387–403.

10. Estanol B, Saenz de Viteri M, Mateos JH, Corvera J (1980): Oculomotor and oculovestibular functions in a hemispherectomy patient. Arch Neurol 37: 365–8.

11. Chia LG (1984): Locked-in state with bilateral internal capsule infarcts. Neurology 34: 1365–7.

12. Brigell M, Babikian V, Goodwin JA (1984): Hypometric saccades and low-gain pursuit resulting from a thalamic hemorrhage. Ann Neurol 15: 374–8.

13. Fisher CM (1967): Some neuro-ophthalmological observations. J Neurol Neurosurg Psychiat 30: 383–92.

14. Keane JR (1975): Contralateral gaze deviation with supratentorial hemorrhage – three pathologically verified cases. Arch Neurol 32: 119–22.

15. Walshe TM, Davis KR, Fisher CM (1977): Thalamic hemorrhage: a computed tomographic-clinical correlation. Neurology 27: 217–22.

16. Pessin MS, Adelman LS, Prager RJ, Lathi ES, Lange DJ (1981): 'Wrong-way eyes' in supratentorial hemorrhage. Ann Neurol 9: 79–81.

17. Sharpe JA, Bondar RL, Fletcher WA (1985): Contralateral gaze deviation after frontal lobe haemorrhage. J Neurol Neurosurg Psychiat 48: 86–8.

18. Meienberg O, Zangemeister WH, Rosenberg M, Hoyt WF, Stark L (1981): Saccadic eye movement strategies in patients with homonymous hemianopia. Ann Neurol 9: 537–44.

19. Girotti F, Cazazza M, Musicco M, Avanzini G (1983): Oculomotor disorders in cortical lesions in man: the role of unilateral neglect. Neuropsychologia 21: 543–53.

20. Robillard A, Saint-Hilaire JM, Mercier M, Bouvier G (1983): The lateralizing and localizing value of adversion in epileptic seizures. Neurology 33: 1241–2.

21. Thurston SE, Leigh RJ, Osorio I (1985): Epileptic gaze deviation and nystagmus. Neurology 35: 1518–21.

22. Zee DS, Chu FC, Leigh RL, et al. (1983): Blink-saccade synkinesis. Neurology 33: 1233–6.

23. Kirkham TH, Kamin DF (1974): Slow saccadic eye movements in Wilson's disease. J Neurol Neurosurg Psychiat 37: 191–4.

24. Zee DS, Optican LM, Cook JD, Robinson DA, Engel WK (1976): Slow saccades in spinocerebellar degeneration. Arch Neurol 33: 243–51.

25. Cogan DG (1953): A type of congenital ocular motor apraxia presenting jerky head movements. Amer J Ophthal 36: 433–41.

26. Zee DS, Yee RD, Singer HS (1977): Congenital ocular motor apraxia. Brain 100: 581–99.

27. Hijdra A, Meerwaldt JD (1984): Balint's syndrome in a man with border-zone infarcts caused by atrial fibrillation. Clin Neurol Neurosurg 86: 51–4.

28. Daroff RB, Hoyt WF (1971): Supranuclear disorders of ocular control systems in man: clinical, anatomical and physiological correlations. In: Bach y Rita P, Collins CC, Hyde JE (eds): The control of eye movements. New York, Academic Press pp 175–235.

29. Reeves AG, Perret J, Jenkyn LR, Saint-Hilaire JM (1984): Pursuit gaze and the occipitoparietal region – a case report. Arch Neurol 41: 83–4.

30. Sharpe JA, Deck JHN (1978): Destruction of the internal sagittal stratum and normal smooth pursuit. Ann Neurol 4: 473–6.

31. Hirose G, Kosoegawa H, Saeki M, et al (1985): The syndrome of posterior thalamic hemorrhage. Neurology 35: 998–1002.

32. Leveille A, Kiernan J, Goodwin JA, Antel J (1982): Eye movements in amyotrophic lateral sclerosis. Arch Neurol 39: 684–6.

33. Leigh RJ, Tusa RJ (1985): Disturbance of smooth pursuit caused by infarction of occipitoparietal cortex. Ann Neurol 17: 185–7.

34. Baloh RW, Yee RD, Honrubia V (1980): Optokinetic nystagmus and parietal lobe lesions. Ann Neurol 7: 269–76.
35. ter Braak JWG (1936): Untersuchungen über optokinetischen Nystagmus. Arch Néerl Physiol 21: 309–376.
36. ter Braak JWG, Schenk VWD, Van Vliet AMG (1971): Visual reactions in a case of long-lasting cortical blindness. J Neurol Neurosurg Psychiat 34: 140–7.
37. Sharpe JA, Lo AW (1981): Voluntary and visual control of the vestibulo-ocular reflex after cerebral hemidecortication. Ann Neurol 10: 164–72.
38. Rosenberg M, Sharpe J, Hoyt WF (1975): Absent vestibulo-ocular reflexes and acute supratentorial lesions. J Neurol Neurosurg Psychiat 38: 6–10.

Psychogenic eye movements

G. PADBERG

Psychogenic oculomotor disorders are abnormal movements of the external ocular muscles not based upon organic abnormalities. At the same time there must be a psychopathological background, rendering the psychogenic reaction plausible. A conversion reaction in psychoanalytical terms is rare nowadays. Neurasthenic or anxiety reactions occur more frequently, but often the eye movement disorder appears to be the symptom at hand indicating a less well-defined psychological need. This suggests that the line between psychogenesis and malingering is hard to draw at times, and might require specific psychiatric consultations. Psychogenesis implies, that all movements can also be executed at free will. On the other hand, all disorders of eye movement that have been described as psychogenic can also result from organic lesions. Therefore, organic causes have to be excluded before the diagnosis psychogenic eye movements can be considered.

Table 1 shows the various categories that can be discerned; aspects important to the differential diagnosis will be discussed.

Table 1. Psychogenic eye movements

Diplopia
Ptosis
Blepharospasm
Oculogyral crises
Gaze paralysis
Convergence spasm
Divergence spasm
Voluntary nystagmus

1. Diplopia

Diplopia without visible disturbances of eye movement is a frequent complaint. Mono-ocular diplopia is often considered a non organic symptom, but it can occur with optical irregularities between cornea and macula [1]. The diplopia is rarely a full double image, and the distance between the images does not increase in any direction of gaze. Often the images differ in brightness and the diplopia can be relieved by pinhole vision. Mono-ocular diplopia and polyopia have also been described in occipital and parieto-occipital lesions.

Binocular diplopia could be due to a neurotic preoccupation with the physiological diplopia; latent strabism has to be excluded. Malingerers are uncertain about the location of the second image, which can easily be detected [1].

2. Ptosis

An atonic ptosis is mentioned as a skill that can be developed, but is rarely observed, and its existence debated [2]. Electromyographic studies to support the true existence of the atonic psychogenic ptosis have not been reported. A psychogenic ptosis is usually a spastic ptosis. One sees that there is some contraction of the lower eyelid and a lowering of the eyebrow, especially when the ptotic side is compared with the healthy side. Usually the examiner can feel the contraction of the orbicularis oculi if he tries to raise the ptotic eyelid. It is also virtually impossible to maintain a constant ptosis for some time on close observation. If still doubt exists, electromyography might be helpful. Hemispheric lesions [3] and peripheral lesions such as Horner syndrome, oculomotor palsy and myasthenia gravis have to be excluded.

3. Blepharospasm

Since the psychogenic ptosis is in fact a mild degree of blepharospasm, ophthalmological causes of blepharospasm such as orbital and ocular infections or inflammations have to be excluded. Tears do not help to exclude psychogenesis as increased lacrimation has been documented regularly in psychogenic blepharospasm [4]. Blepharospasms, organic or not, may be so severe that they can render the patient functionally blind. Also, stress may increase the frequency of the spasms whatever their causes.

Blepharospasm may be quick and of short duration as in facial tics or dyskinesias. Slower and longer lasting blepharospasms with other dystonic features in the orofacial and cervical region fit the diagnosis of Meige syndrome, in which an organic lesion is rarely found, but which usually respond to drugs such as clonazepam or trihexyphenidyl [5, 6]. Therefore, the diagnosis psychogenic

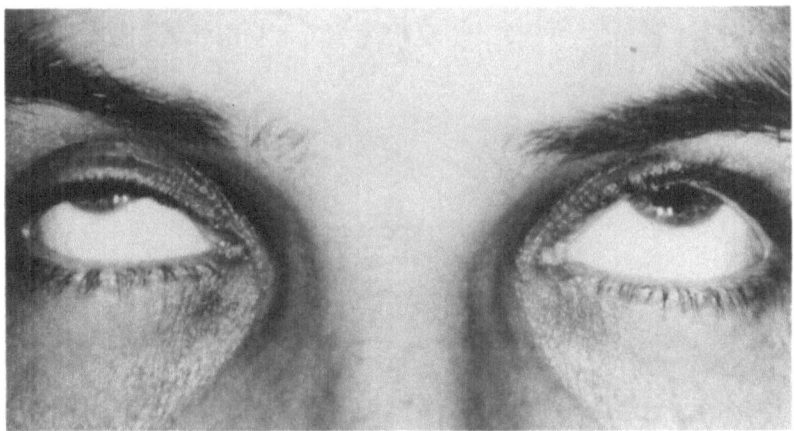

Figure 1. Simulating oculogyral crises.

blepharospasm particularly requires support of the psychiatrist.

4. Oculogyral crisis

In oculogyral crises both eyes conjugately deviate in one direction, usually upward. The crises may last several minutes and occasionally even hours; they have been described in lethargic encephalitis, parkinsonism, neurosyphilis, cranial trauma and with neuroleptics. As with all extra-pyramidal movement disorders, the crises increase in frequency and duration during stress and in emotional circumstances. These movements can be mimicked by looking upward forcefully, or possibly in another way by closing the eyes with the resultant Bell phenomenon and simultaneously contracting the frontales muscles (Fig. 1). Particularly the latter maneuver might easily lead to a partial closure of the eyelids.

5. Gaze paralysis

Psychogenic gaze paralyses are rare and can not be maintained consistently. Usually there is a vertical gaze paralysis on following, while fixation during passive head movements is intact in all directions. An exceptional case of a functional paralysis of horizontal gaze was reported by Troost and Troost [7]. The apparent left-ward gaze palsy in their patient was obtained through spasm of the near reflex. Optokinetic stimulation, passive head rotations and the mirror test revealed full excursion of gaze. In all such cases neurologic causes of supranuclear gaze palsies have to be excluded.

222

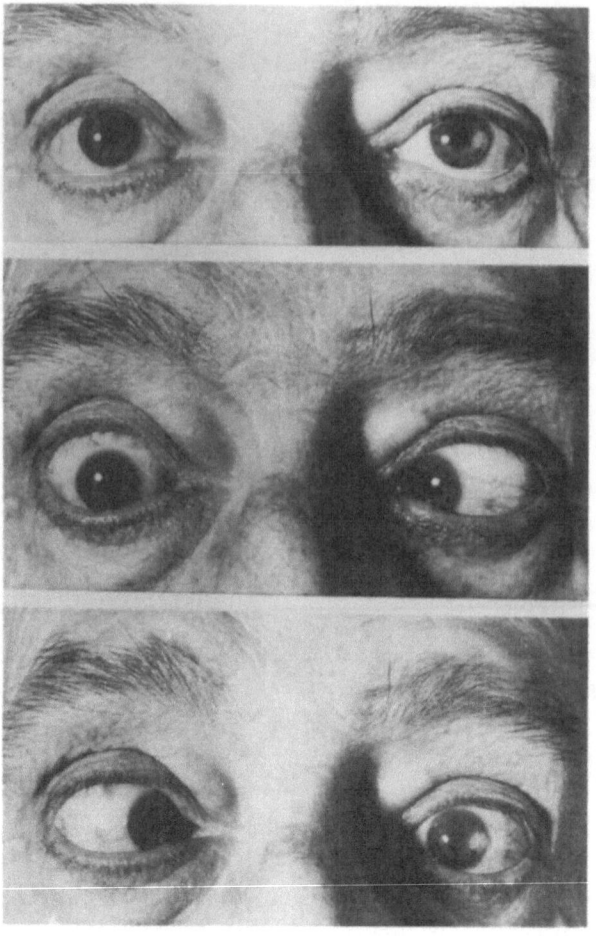

Figure 2. Convergence spasm simulating lateral rectus paralysis.

6. Convergence spasm

Spasm of convergence of psychogenic origin is not a rare phenomenon, and is accompanied by miosis and spasm of accommodation (spasm of the near reflex). Occasionally these patients may demonstrate a dissociated nystagmus which is greatest in the abducting eye. The spasm is usually intermittent, and cannot be maintained unchanged for a long time [8, 9]. Usually there is a full range of motion with only one eye viewing. In combination with movements of gaze it can lead to a bizarre strabism and diplopia. The resulting picture is often confused with a lateral rectus paralysis; the accompanying miosis will help to make the proper diagnosis (Fig. 2). Psychogenic blepharospasm may accompany the spasm of convergence. Organic causes such as trauma, encephalitis and malignancies have to be excluded [10].

7. Divergence spasm

Psychogenic spasm of divergence is extremely rare [2], and has been observed as an intermittent sign only. Spasm of divergence has been described in migraine and in brainstem syndromes of various etiology.

8. Voluntary nystagmus

Voluntary nystagmus is not a true nystagmus, but consists of rapid oscillations that can be evoked voluntary in the horizontal or in vertical direction usually with a mild convergence effort. These oscillations can be maintained for a short while only, and with increasing difficulty on repeated trials. The head is held rigid with the cervical muscles contracted during the nystagmus. Occasionally this 'gift' runs in families [11]. Zahn [12] estimated that approximately 8% of the population will have this talent. Being a voluntary movement, psychopathological conditions can lead to its presentation as an abnormal eye movement.

The diagnosis of psychogenic eye movements is easily suggested, but often difficult to prove, and a lot of energy must go into the exclusion of all possible organic causes of eye movement disorder under question.

References

1. Keane JR (1982): Neuro-ophthalmic signs and symptoms of hysteria. Neurology 32: 757–762.
2. Duke-Elder S, Scott GJ (1971): Neuro-ophthalmology. Vol XII System of Ophthalmology. London, Henry Kimpton.
3. Nutt JG (1977): Lid abnormalities secondary to cerebral hemisphere lesions. Ann Neurol 1: 149–151.
4. Walsh FB, Hoyt WF (1969): Clinical Neuro-Ophthalmology. Ed. 3. Baltimore, The Williams and Wilkins Company.
5. Jankovic J, Ford J (1983): Blepharospasm and orofacial-cervical dystonia: clinical and pharmacological findings in 100 patients. Ann Neurol 13: 402–411.
6. Marsden CD, Lang AE, Sheehy MP(1983): Pharmacology of cranial dystonia. Neurology 33: 1100–1101.
7. Troost BT, Troost EG (1979): Functional paralysis of horizontal gaze. Neurology 29: 82–85.
8. Cogan DG, Freese Jr CG (1955): Spasm of the near reflex. Arch Ophthal 54: 752–759.
9. Cogan DG (1977): Neurology of the ocular muscles. Second edition. Charles C. Thomas, Springfield, Illinois, USA.
10. Guiloff RJ, Whiteley A, Kelly RE (1980): Organic convergence spasm. Acta Neurol Scand 61: 252–259.
11. Aschoff JC, Becker W, Rettelbach R (1976): Voluntary nystagmus in five generations. J Neurol Neurosurg Psychiat 39: 300–304.
12. Zahn JR (1978): Incidence and characteristics of voluntary nystagmus. J Neurol Neurosurg Psychiat 41: 617–623.

Section VI

Treatment

The conservative management of diplopia

C.C. STERK

The aim in the management of diplopia is either to eliminate double vision or to achieve recovery of binocular single vision in the main directions of gaze.

The nonsurgical treatment can be symptomatic i.e. aimed primarily in treating the diplopia for example by giving prism glasses or occlusion; on the other hand the cause of the diplopia can be treated as for example prednison therapy in Graves disease.

1. Occlusion

To eliminate diplopia one eye can be occluded and this may continue until the cause of a paresis is found and if necessary as long as the deviation is variable. The affected eye should be occluded as otherwise pastpointing would be the result.

When the deviation decreases (because of recovery of the affected muscle) and binocular vision is possible in part of the field of gaze occlusion should be given partially or be discontinued giving the fusion reflexes a chance to further decrease the deviation.

If diplopia is only present in a peripheral part of the field of gaze and not in the primary position, sector occlusion can be prescribed and again in front of the affected eye.

As occlusion an eyepad can be used or an occlusion patch. When the patient is wearing glasses one glass can temporarily be taped with various kinds of adhesive tape or nail varnish can be used. If occlusion has to be used for a long period, prescribing an opaque glass may be the solution, though an occluder glass is cosmeticaly even better.

2. Prisms

Prisms change the direction of lightbeams. One prism dioptre changes the course of a lightbeam in such a way that at 1 meter distance it is displaced 1 cm compared with the original course. The direction changes towards the base of the prism causing the image to shift in the direction of the apex.

The relation between the prism strength in prism dioptres and the angle in centigrades is: 7 prism dioptres = 4° centigrade. In average 2 prism dioptres equal 1 centigrade.

The aim of the prism therapy is the recovery of binocular single vision (in contrast with occlusion) in the primary directions of gaze, i.e. straight ahead and looking down.

Indications for prisms

a. Recent paresis awaiting spontaneous recovery or surgery.
b. Long standing paresis in which surgery is not indicated due to poor health, a small concomitant angle or a residual deviation after surgery.
When a muscle palsy exists for some time the deviation will become more and more concomitant.

Restrictions in the use of prisms

An important draw back of prisms as compared with surgery is that the effect of prisms is the same in all directions of gaze. Thus they cannot be used when there are obvious incomitances in the physiological field of gaze and prisms reduce the stimulus for the fusion reflexes to reduce a deviation. Prisms have also no effect in torsional deviations.

Basic principles

1) Restore orthophoria in the most important field of gaze i.e. primary position and depression.

2) Use the lowest prism correction possible which enables binocular single vision.

3) Use only one prism when the deviation is incomitant and place it in front of the affected eye thus avoiding the direction of maximal deviation.

4) Use a different strength if the deviation is markedly variable for near and distance.

5) Reduce the prism strength when the palsy is recovering.

Methods of prescribing prisms

1) When the patient has a refractive error the interpupillary distance can be changed to induce a prism effect. This effect (expressed in prism dioptres) is the strength (in dioptres) multiplied by the eccentration in centimetres. When the glasses have a very low dioptric value the effect of decentration will be minimal. It becomes more complicated when the correction includes a cylinder and especially when the axis of the cylinder is diagonal in regard to the required direction. It will involve some mathematics.

2) Prisms can be incorporated in the glasses. As additional prisms will increase the weight of the glasses a strength of not more than 8 or 10 dioptres is used.

3) Fresnel prisms can be used for the higher strengths, if necessary up to 40 or 50 dioptres. A disadvantage is the effect of a maddox rod they produce when viewing a spot of light.

3. Botulinum toxin

Botulinum toxin has been used by several investigators to weaken eye muscles. The toxin is injected into the muscle that has to be weakened. The method as such has not yet gained a routine place in the treatment of diplopia [1, 2].

4. Different types of diplopia

Exodeviations

Exoforia and convergence insufficiency are deviations in which orthoptic exercises will be given first. The therapy aims at improvement of the convergence mechanism. Physiological diplopia can be used to help the patient recognise when his convergence fails.

In younger patients negative glasses can be described to stimulate accommodation and thus convergence. A disadvantage of prisms is the habituation to them which may increase the deviation. They are however useful in presbyopic patients with a convergence insufficiency.

Esodeviations

A conservative therapy in esodeviation is the use of miotics. The aim is to reduce the accommodative burden on the fusion reflexes. In Leiden we usually use Diflupyl 0.01%. We use it in esotropia of recent onset (no longer than 3 months) before the deviation and suppression have been consolidated. We also use it in intermittent deviations to help recovery. In some cases of a postoperative residal deviations miotics can be given to stabilize the position and enhance orthophoria.

We never use miotics longer than 3 months, because of the possible risk of lensopacification. We usually start with prescribing to use the drops 3 times a week the first month, reducing it to twice a week the second month and only once a week in the third month. We advice to install the drops at night because of the side effects. When after 4 or 6 weeks the effect is small or absent we stop using the miotics.

5. Conditions affecting the eye muscles

5.1 Graves' disease

In Graves' disease the eye muscles loose their elasticity and contractility because of infiltration. Especially the inferior rectus and the medial rectus are often affected. They can contract but cannot relax any more. As these conditions may spontaneously regress, surgical therapy in an early stage is not indicated. The management usually exists in occlusion first of all. In some patients the diplopia can be overcome with prisms. In case there are multiple limitations, or there is a recurrence of the deviation after surgery, prednison can be given (60 mg per day for 2 to 4 weeks gradually decreasing the dosage).

Patients with a malignant exophthalmos (visual loss due to corneal involvement or damage to the optic nerve) also often complain in diplopia because the eye muscles too are affected. When they are treated for their malignant exophthalmos with prednison the eye movements usually improve and their diplopia may disappear. Surgical therapy is possible in case of diplopia when the condition remains unchanged over a period of about 6 months.

5.2 Myositis

Diplopia caused by acute idiopathic myositis can be treated with systemic corticosteroids. This condition belongs in the group of orbital inflammation, as does a pseudo-tumor of the orbit. The resulting diplopia in this last condition can also be treated with systemic steroids.

5.3 Myasthenia Graves

The extra-ocular muscle palsies do not react well to anti-cholinesterase medicines. The ptosis reacts better, but seldom disappears completely. As the symptoms are so fluctuating prisms will seldom help. Biphocal glasses are not very satisfactory either.

Some patients prefer wearing dark glasses, even indoors. Often occlusion of one eye will be necessary. Oosterhuis [3] advices systemic prednison if the above mentioned possibilities are insufficient and if there is no improvement after one year. Regarding the eye muscle paresis the results are fairly good. Some of the patients show a complete remission.

5.4 Muscle palsies

In case of an abducens paralysis occlusion of the affected eye is usually pre-scribed. In case of a paresis only the temporal half of the visual field can be occluded (partial occlusion on glasses). Some patients prefer to adopt a headpos-ture rather than occlude one eye. When the deviation exists for some time and has become more or less concomitant prisms can be used; in mild forms possibly only necessary for distance.

In case of a total third nerve palsy the ptosis prevents the patient from experiencing diplopia. If there is diplopia, occlusion will be the first conservative method of choice. When there is a partial recovery the medial rectus recovers best usually enabling the patient to compensate his exo deviation. The remaining hypotropia can be compensated by holding up the chin. A prism can help reduce the torticollis.

The vertical deviation due to a superior oblique palsy can be treated with prisms.

5.5 Trauma

Diplopia due to orbital fracture and especially due to a blow-out fracture is nowadays not treated surgically immediately. Koornneef [4, 5] is of the opinion that it are not the muscles themselves that become trapped but that it is the system of connective tissue that has been damaged or becomes trapped.

When there is no great dislocation and when there is no enophthalmos to be expected surgery is not carried out. However the eye motility is well documented, a forced duction test is carried out and the patient is instructed to carry out monocular eye movements. After several days the situation is reexamined. If there is no improvement surgery can still be carried out.

References

1. Scott AB (1980): Botulinum Toxin Injection into Extra ocular Muscles as an Alternative to Strabismus Surgery. Ophthalmology 87: 1044–1049.
2. Crone RA, de Jong PTVM, Notermans G (1984): Behandlung des Nystagmus durch Injektion von

Botulinustoxin in die Augenmuskeln. Klin Mbl Augenheilk 184: 216–217.
3. Oosterhuis HJGH (1982): The ocular signs and symptoms of myasthenia gravis. Docum Ophthal 52: 363–378.
4. Koornneef L, Everhard-Halm YS, Oei TH (1980): Fracturen van de oogkas en verschuiving van de indicatie tot behandeling. Ned T Geneesk 124: 2203.
5. Koornneef L (1982): Current concepts on the management of orbital blow-out fractures. Ann Plast Surg 9: 185:200.

Eye muscle surgery in peripheral third, fourth and sixth nerve palsy

M.H. GOBIN

Neurologically determined eye movement abnormalities which can be treated surgically are those due to peripheral oculomotor nerve lesions. It is preferable to classify the ocular motor disturbance with reference to the nerve rather than the muscle paralysis because this is easier to handle. For instance a third oculomotor nerve palsy seldom results in a single eye muscle palsy.

In the past surgery was postponed until the eye deviation was stabilised, this in order to be certain that further improvement was unlikely. Nowadays it has become apparant that excess surgery is easily compensated by fusion reflexes. It is therefore better to treat before irreversible complications occur; for example a paralysis of the lateral rectus muscle leads to a contracture of the homolateral medial rectus giving a pure mechanically limitation of abduction. At present surgery is performed when further spontaneous recovery is unlikely. For example in a paralysis of the lateral rectus muscle, if the esodeviation reduces within a few months from +35° to +5° and abduction obviously improves, complete recovery may be expected and surgery avoided. On the other hand if the esodeviation is only slightly improved after 3 months, surgical treatment is necessary. The Hess-Lancaster test is useful in monitoring eye movements in a graphical way so that evolution of the deviation can easily be followed (Chapter 5).

1. Treatment of a fourth nerve palsy

Of all the eye muscles the superior oblique is most frequently affected being damaged in headinjury or birthtrauma. The latter often improves spontaneously.

A congenital palsy is difficult to diagnose, because it is usually combined with a convergent squint and may give a negative Bielschowsky head tilt test. For this reason a diagnosis can often only be made after correction of the horizontal deviation.

A particular difficult form of congenital paralysis is the one which decompensates in adult life and results in diplopia. Because there is no history of head trauma the ophthalmologist may suspect an underlying neurological cause and refers the patient to the neurologist. There is one clinical sign however which indicates the difference with an acquired palsy: the latter causes such discomfort that the patient may tend to close one eye. This is not seen in decompensated congenital palsy because the patient has learned to eliminate diplopia in early childhood.

Another phenomenon which deserves attention is that a fourth nerve palsy is often bilateral. In asymmetrical palsy the hypofunction of the less affected superior oblique muscle is masked by a vertical deviation. After surgery of the most severe paralysis, paresis of the contralateral superior oblique muscle appears inverting the vertical deviation.

General considerations of the surgery

As a rule, in treatment of a superior oblique palsy we avoid strengthening this muscle but prefer to weaken the antagonist and/or synergist (homolateral inferior oblique muscle or contralateral inferior rectus muscle respectively). Plication or resection of the superior oblique muscle usually does not strengthen the muscle but only shortens the tendon. On the contrary a recession of the contralateral inferior rectus muscle will, in accordance with Hering's law, stimulate the remaining muscle fibres of the paralysed superior oblique leading to reinforcement.

A superior oblique palsy induces a cyclodeviation and/or a vertical deviation. If the cyclodeviation is pronounced weakening of the inferior oblique muscle is advised. Three gradations of weakening are used: posterior myotomy by cutting the posterior part of the muscle, recession implying displacement of the insertion towards the origin thus resulting in weakening of the whole muscle and lastly a desinsertion by detaching the muscle from the scleral insertion (Fig. 1). Normally surgery of both inferior oblique muscles is advised because it is the general experience that surgery on only one muscle may induce contralateral hyperactivation.

If there is no real vertical deviation in the primary position both inferior oblique muscles have to be weakened symmetrically. With a small vertical deviation the inferior obliques are treated asymmetrically, for instance with a posterior myotomy at one side and a recession at the other side. If the vertical deviation is large, especially on downward gaze, the inferior rectus muscle of the lower eye has to be weakened. Here too, a specific grading system is used. With a small vertical deviation a central tenotomy is performed: the central part of the tendon is cut in such a way that the middle part of the tendon is able to retract while the lateral tips of the tendon remain attached to the sclera (Fig. 2). With a marked vertical deviation a recession of the inferior rectus is performed.

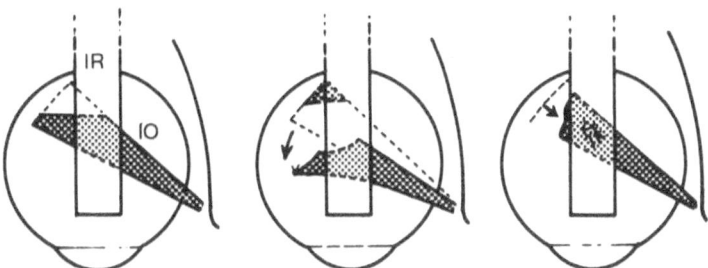

Figure 1. Weakening of the inferior oblique muscle. Left through right: posterior myotomy, ante-ropositioning and desinsertion. The difference between anteropositioning and recession is that in a recession the muscle is not reattached at the equator of the eyeball but backwards in the line of pull of the muscle. For both anteroposition and recession the point of reattachment is midway the lateral and the inferior rectus muscle.

Additional considerations

Recession of the inferior rectus, if combined with contralateral inferior oblique surgery, may result in vertical overcorrection. An other disadvantage is retraction of the lower eyelid, because the inferior rectus is attached to the tarsus, so the lower eyelid is pulled downwards (Fig. 3a + b). Besides this, weakening of a rectus muscle induces some degree of exophthalmos due to widening of the

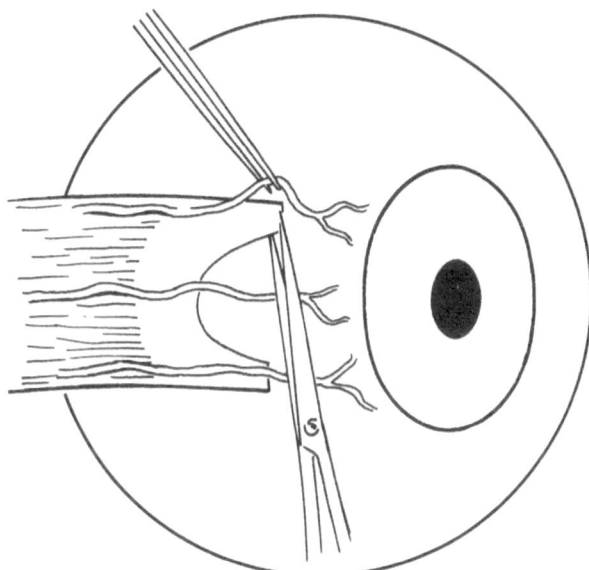

Figure 2. Central tenotomy of the inferior rectus muscle. The middle part of the tendon is cut, the muscle remains attached to the sclera by the lateral tips of the tendon resulting in retraction of the middle part.

236

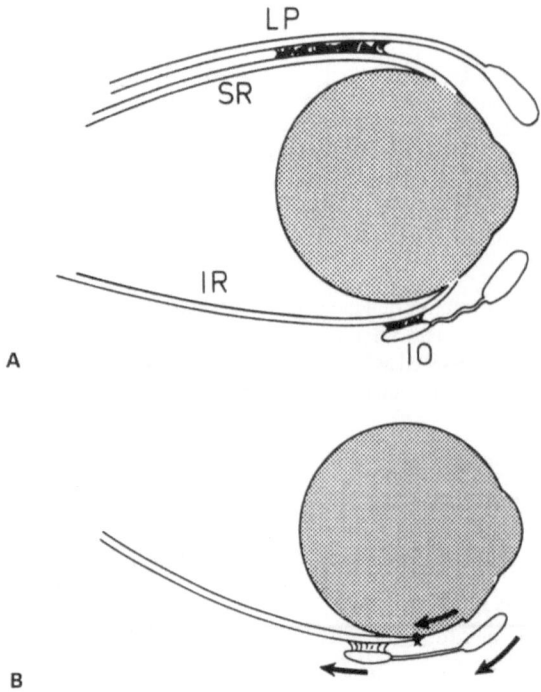

A

B

Figure 3a. The inferior rectus muscle is connected with the tarsus, so that the lower eyelid is pulled down during depression.

Figure 3b. When the inferior rectus is recessed the muscle is moved backwards in a way that the eyelid is pulled downwards. This may result in an apparent hypertropia of the eye, because a white crescent appears underneath the cornea.

palpebral fissure, while weakening of oblique muscles induces enophthalmos and narrowing of the palpebral fissure (Fig. 4a, b + c). Thus weakening of the rectus muscle on one side together with weakening an oblique muscle on the other side may give a disfiguring difference between the width of the palpebral fissures. In order to avoid this, weakening of a homolateral rectus muscle is added to the procedure on the oblique muscle. If an esodeviation is present we will recess the medial rectus muscle; in case of an exodeviation the lateral rectus muscle is recessed. If no horizontal deviation is found in the primary position, a central tenotomy of the medial as well as the lateral rectus muscle will be performed thus avoiding horizontal deviation but resulting in exophthalmos compensating the enophthalmos induced by oblique muscle surgery.

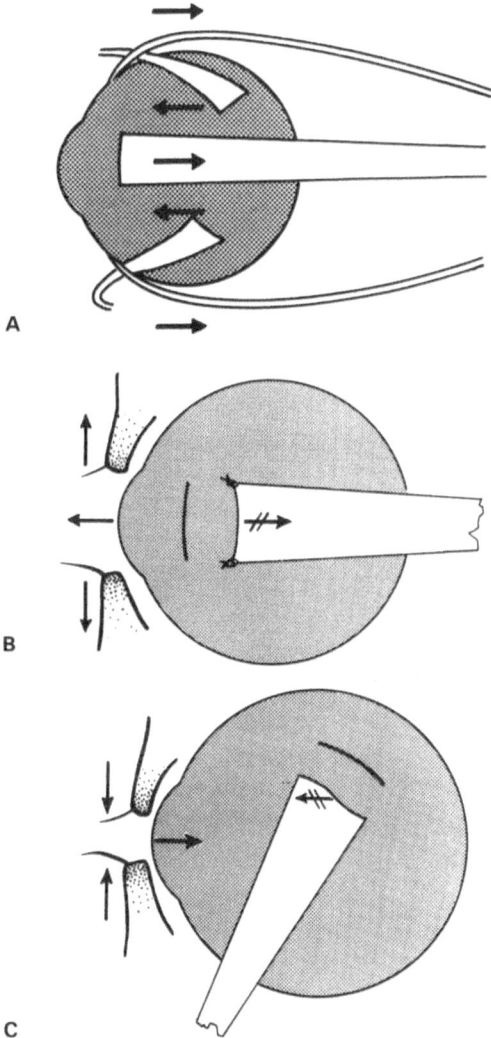

Figure 4a. The rectus muscles pull the eye backwards and the oblique muscles pull the eye forwards.
Figure 4b. Weakening of a rectus muscle results in relative exophthalmos.
Figure 4c. Weakening of an oblique muscle induces enophthalmos.

2. Treatment of a sixth nerve palsy

A sixth nerve palsy has to be distinguished from a Duane syndrome for both disorders show limitation of abduction. The Duane syndrome is of congenital origin usually involving the left eye and generally more common in girls. During adduction there is retraction of the eyeball with narrowing of the palpebral fissure. There is no diplopia and the squint angle in primary position is small.

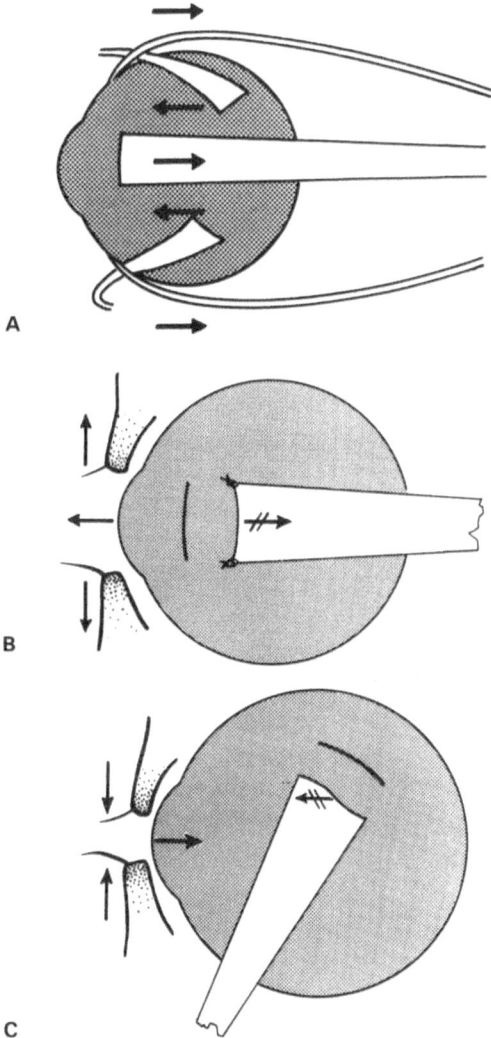

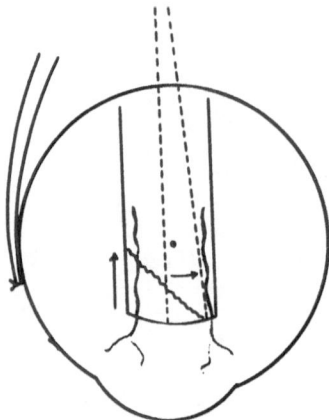

Figure 5. The nasal part of the tendon of the vertical muscle is cut underneath the ciliary vessels, in a way that the tendon remains attached to the sclera by its temporal tip. The line of pull of the muscle is displaced temporal of the rotation centre of the eyeball and obtains an abducting effect.

Frequently an exodeviation is found in the direction of the nonaffected eye. This is pathognomic. In contrast, a sixth nerve palsy gives no narrowing of the palpebral fissure and gives diplopia except in very young children. The deviation in the primary position is large.

General considerations

A sixth nerve palsy is treated by transplantation of the vertical muscles, unless abduction is nearly normalised, in which case we carry out a bilateral 5 mm recession of the medial rectus. This transplantation is done by displacement of the traction line of the muscle to the temporal side changing the direction of pull to that side. In this way the adducting effect of the vertical recti is transformed in an abducting one. if this temporalisation is performed at the superior as well as the inferior rectus muscle they will remain vertically in balance and no vertical deviation occurs.

Here we can also grade our surgery: a nasal tenotomy (Fig. 5) or a turnover of the vertical recti (Fig. 6a + b). In case of a nasal tenotomy the muscle insertion is cut over three-quarters of the width of the tendon, leaving the temporal portion of the muscle attached to the eyeball. The line of pull now runs along the temporal part of the muscle only, instead of its middle. In case of a turning over of the muscle the nasal three quarters of the tendon will also be cut and the nasal tip of the tendon is pulled underneath the muscle and attached to the sclera at the level of insertion of the lateral rectus muscle. This turnover of the muscle results in a more pronounced displacement of the line of pull than a nasal tenotomy.

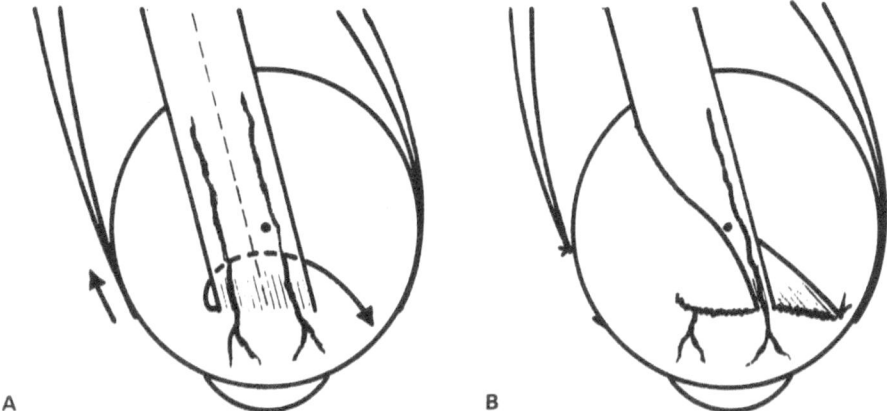

Figure 6a. The nasal part of the tendon of the vertical rectus is cut in a way that the muscle remains attached to the eyeball by means of the temporal tip of its insertion.

Figure 6b. The nasal tip of the muscle is passed between the sclera and the temporal border of the muscle and is reattached at the level of insertion of the lateral rectus muscle. In comparison to a nasal tenotomy the line of pull is displaced more to the temporal side in a way that the abduction effect is more pronounced.

Additional considerations

In addition both the nasal tenotomy and the turnover have the advantage of saving ciliary bloodvessels which run along the border of the vertical rectus muscles. Recession of the medial rectus on the same eye can thus be added with reduced risk of ischemia of the anterior segment of the eye. In order to be efficient temporal displacement of the vertical rectus muscles is always combined with recession of the homolateral medial rectus muscle, which means surgery of three of the four rectus muscles of the same eye. Without the preservation of the temporal ciliary bloodvessels the blood supply of the anterior segment of the eye would become at risk.

Concerning the dosage of surgery, a nasal tenotomy is done if abduction reaches −20 and a turnover if abduction does not reach this extent. As already mentioned above, recession of the homolateral medial rectus and sometimes of the contralateral medial rectus is added (the latter only if the esodeviation in the primary position is large). A bilateral sixth nerve palsy is always treated in two sessions. Operation is first carried out on the most affected eye followed by the other eye 6 months later if necessary.

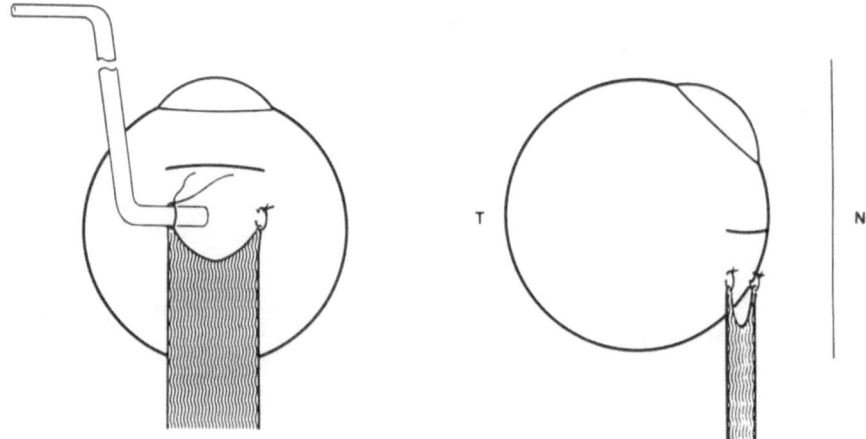

Figure 7. In case of a loop recession the sutures are inserted in the sclera 5 mm behind the original insertion and knotted upon a probe with a diameter of 2 mm. This results in a loop of about 3 mm which allows the middle part of the tendon to retract as far back as 10 mm from the original insertion. The gap between the tendon and sclera is filled up by connective tissue which results in a pseudotendon.

3. Treatment of a third nerve palsy

It may happen that we have to distinguish between a third nerve paralysis and an atypical Duane syndrome. In this syndrome there is a marked limitation of adduction with exodeviation in the primary position. This is however very rare and differentiation from a third nerve palsy can be made as follows: an atypical Duane syndrome is congenital and thus without diplopia; there is also a limitation of abduction; the vertical movements of the eye are normal and in contrast to a third nerve palsy mydriasis, accommodation palsy and ptosis are lacking.

A third nerve palsy may be seen in combination with a fourth nerve palsy, although diagnosis of the latter is hardly possible, because of the absence of a positive headtilt test. The superior rectus muscle is insufficient and has no preponderance over the superior oblique muscle. It does not elevate the eye during Bielschowsky's head-tilt test. A diagnosis can only be made when the patient is asked to look down in abduction where the torsional activity is maximal. The paralysed inferior rectus muscle is not able to counterbalance the torsional effect of the superior oblique muscle; the latter produces a purely intorsional eye movement which is easily seen by means of the perilimbal bloodvessels. In addition the expected hypotropia of the affected eye is absent.

An amazing fact is that the levator palpebrae and the medial rectus muscle may recover whilst vertical eye movements remain restricted.

4. General considerations

The suggested surgical procedure is a bilateral 5 mm recession of the lateral rectus muscle with a large loop on the affected eye (Fig. 7). This loop may be as large as 5 mm, so that the middle part of the muscle can retract about 10 mm. This loop will be placed on the affected eye in order to create an exophthalmos which widens the palpebral fissure and compensates the ptosis.

If there is hypotropia, a recession with a loop of the superior oblique is carried out. If the vertical deviation is large, we add a central tenotomy or a recession of the inferior rectus muscle to the superior oblique muscle weakening on the same side. If the exodeviation is marked we add to our bilateral recession a resection of the medial rectus of the nonaffected eye. A resection of the medial rectus of the paralysed eye has to be avoided, especially if ptosis is present and when a superior oblique weakening is performed. This because it results in further narrowing of the palpebral fissure.

Additional considerations

Because surgery on the oculomotor muscles often influences the palpebral fissure, the ptosis is dealt with in last instance. Once the position of the eye is corrected, ptosis surgery can be performed.

Treatment of disturbances of ocular motility and diplopia

Causal and cosmetic therapeutical possibilities

M. SWART-VAN DEN BERG and R.J.W. DE KEIZER

Methods of treatment in diplopia and disturbances of ocular motility cover the whole area from eyelid to the mid-cranial fossa. Causal therapy and cosmetic possibilities will be discussed. Surgical approach of pathological processes at the root of motility disturbances is taken care of by a team including a plastic (eye) surgeon, an ophthalmologist and a neurosurgeon. Subjects dealt with in this chapter are as listed below: 1) ocular causes of diplopia and motility disturbances; 2) ptosis; 3) orbital disorders.

1. Ocular causes of diplopia and signs of motility dysfunction

Most patients with diplopia demand treatment. It is the task of any (consulted) physician to find a treatment which is suitable for the particular patient. Therapy is twofold: a) resolving the complaints and b) patient's acceptance of cosmetic aspects of a chosen solution.

Treatment abnormalities discussed are: 1.1 astigmatism and corneal opacities; 1.2 anisometropia; 1.3 iridectomy; 1.4 pterygium (symblepharon); 1.5 the contactlens in diplopia caused by disorders of ocular motility.

1.1 Astigmatism

In many cases astigmatism may be corrected by glasses. However, in severe or irregular astigmatism, as in keratoconus or after a corneal perforation, a hard contactlens is usually the choice. A contactlens which then forms the anterior surface of the cornea resolves the astigmatism. In case of an extreme keratoconus it is not longer possible to wear a contactlens and corneal grafting is indicated, as used in corneal opacities. Results are not always predictable and complications may occur [1]. A new method for surgical treatment of astigmatism (and other refractive errors) is the radial keratotomy [1]. Indications for this operation are still disputed.

244

1.2 Anisometropia

As result of a marked difference in refractive error of both eyes (4 dioptres) patients often complain of different image sizes (aniseikonia), even after full correction of the refractive error, however, size differences of about 8% are usually accepted. In other cases full prescription for the eye with the highest refractive error is not possible (for instance: unilateral high myopia; unilateral aphakia). A contactlens usually has a favourable influence on differences in image sizes. For example in aphakia: the postoperative image size after intracapsular cataract extraction in only 10% larger than preoperative whereas 34% larger with a spectacle correction. Furthermore a contactlens extends the whole visual field. In some cases of unilateral aphakia a secondary implant is possible, especially if a contactlens is not well tolerated. The difference in image sizes of the pseudo-phakia and the normal eye is about 3% [2].

1.3 Iridectomy

Monocular diplopia caused by a too large or abnormally located iridectomy may be resolved with a contactlens in which an artificial pupil is painted (Figs 1a and 1b). This also may be helpful in iridodialysis, aniridia, essential iris atrophy and coloboma. The interfering image disappears. However, an expert is required because it is difficult to obtain the right colour contactlens to match the fellow eye.

1.4 Pterygium

Apart from disfiguring the patients, a pterygium can cause diplopia due to astigmatism or disturbances of ocular motility (Figs 2a and 2b), especially if several operations already have been performed and contraction of surrounding tissue has occurred. Shrinking adhesions to caruncle, eye muscles and eyelid (symblepharon) may occur. The standard therapy is local excision, but recurrences may follow many well performed operations (in primary cases even up to 70%). Irradiation (Sr 90) diminishes the rate of recurrences considerably [3]. In severe cases transposition of the pterygium is followed by covering the corneal and scleral defect with a lamellar corneal graft [4] (Figs 3a and 3b). Good motility, visual acuity and cosmetic appearance can thus be obtained.

1.5 The contactlens in diplopia caused by disorders of ocular motility

Contactlenses may be used as treatment in diplopia, resulting from ocular dis-

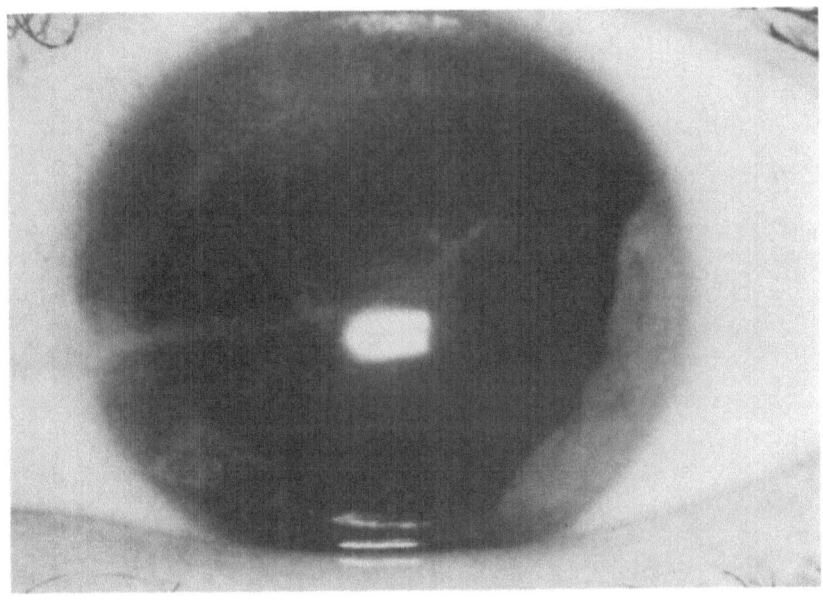

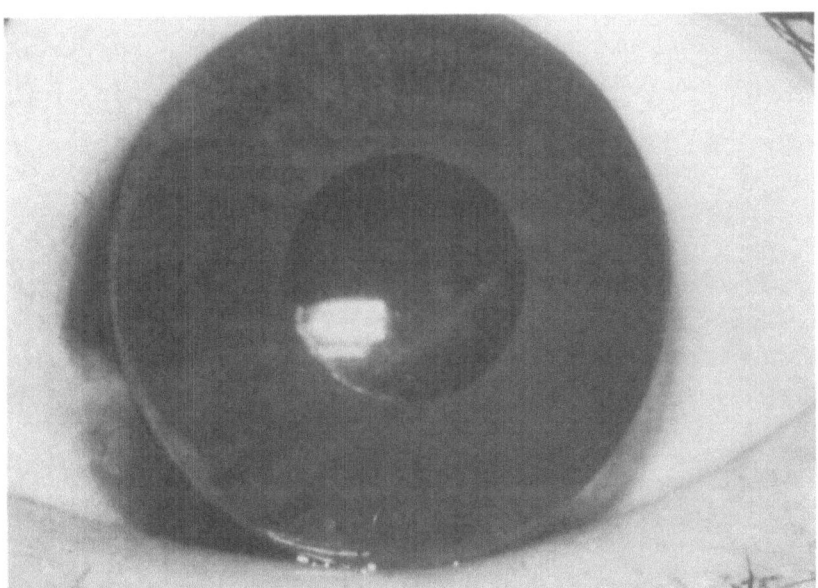

Figure 1A. Traumatic iris coloboma.
Figure 1B. Same eye fitted with a painted contactlens.

246

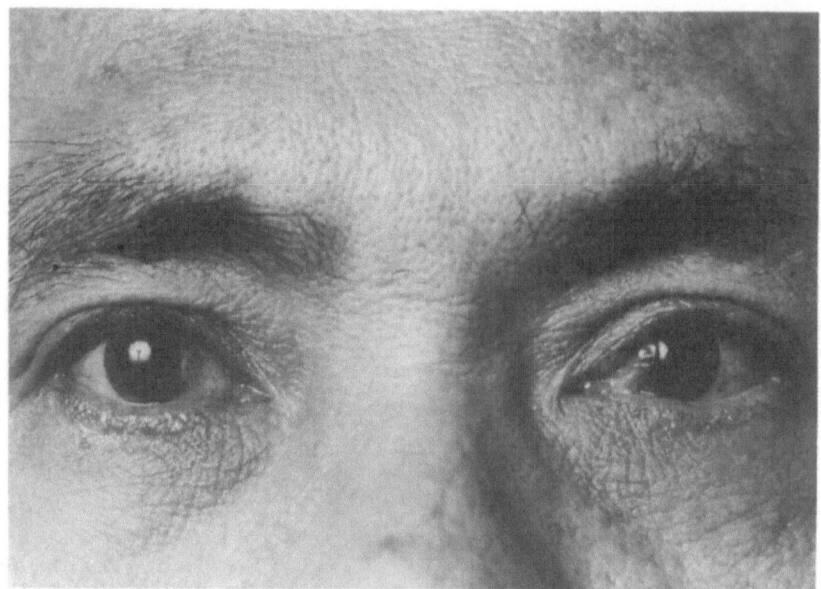

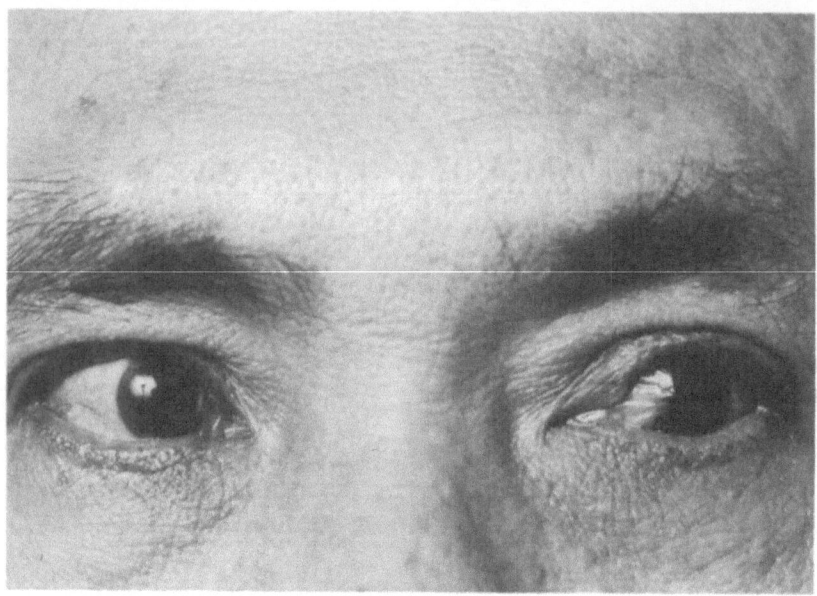

Figure 2A. Severe pterygium of the left eye. The patient looks straight forward.
Figure 2B. Motility disturbances are shown by looking to the left. Abduction of the left eye is difficult.

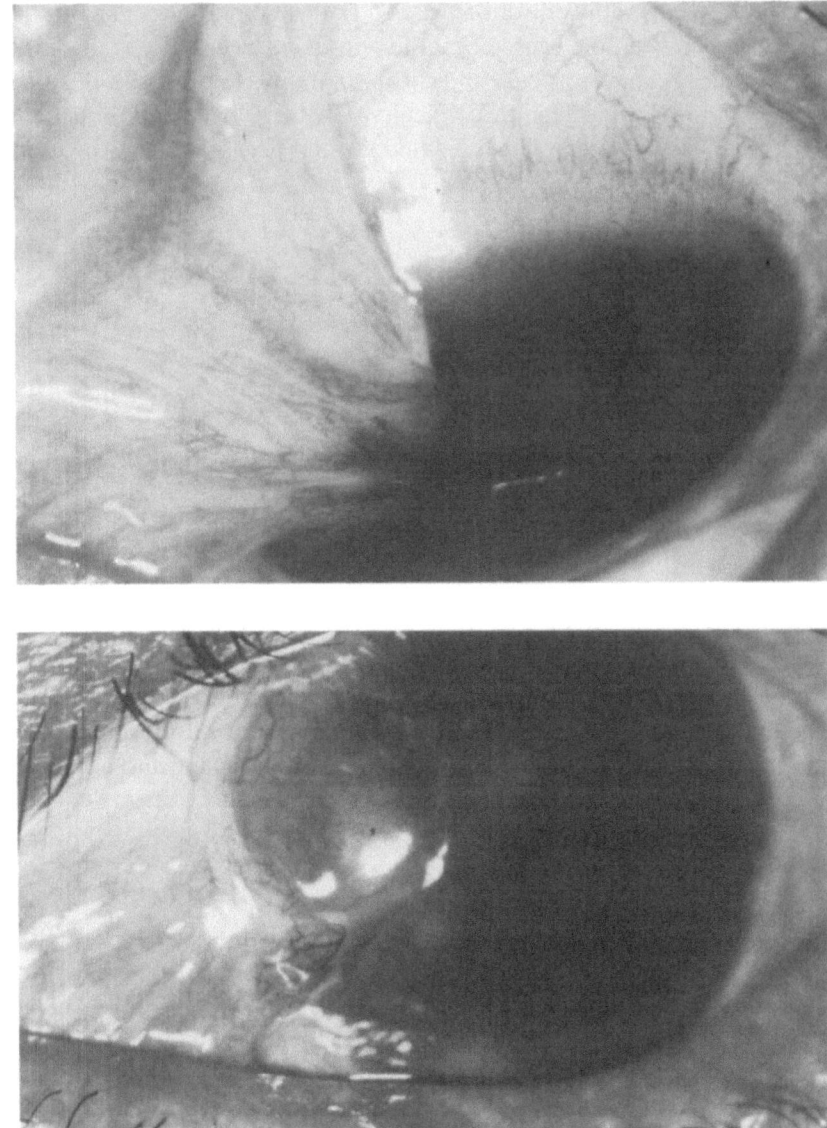

Figure 3A. Severe pterygium before operation.
Figure 3B. Same eye after operation with a lamellar corneal graft.

eases as well as from motility disturbances. The indication to help a patient with a contactlens depends on the cause of motility disturbance and the availability of surgery. If indicated the most easy and cheap solution is to prescribe an aphakia lens (S + 14.00), via which the visual acuity will fade. If this is not sufficient enough a total occlusive lens with a painted iris and black pupil may be used.

2. Ptosis

2.1 Anatomical variations of the palpebral fissure

If small differences in size of the palpebral fissure are observed, one must consider the following:

a) Not to draw the attention of the patient or his family to small differences, which they possibly did not even notify, unless if necessary for diagnostic purposes (e.g.: suspicion of endocrine exophthalmos). Once the difference is noticed, the patient migt be fixed on it.

b) If spectacles are necessary, the lens for the smallest eye should be made as positive as possible (enlargement). In nonspectacle wearing patients glasses can be prescribed in order to obtain an equal palpebral fissure.

c) In evaluation of which muscles have to be attached in strabismus surgery, one should also judge the size of the palpebral fissure. Pre-existing differences in size may be charged in a favourable way, on the other hand care must be taken not to create differences in size. For this reason it might even be necessary to operate more than one muscle.

2.2 Motility disturbances of the upper eyelid (see also chapter 14 'Blepharoptosis')

2.2.1 Conservative treatment of ptosis

If ptosis cannot be surgically treated, cosmetic appearance may be improved by use of a 'ptosis frame'. This is a frame with special hooks supporting upper eyelids. This can only be used for several hours, because the cornea will become dry as blinking of the eyelid is obstructed. Ruben [5, 6] suggests the use of scleral contactlenses. These are more thickened at the edge in order to support the upper eyelid, however, they have no widespread use. These conservative possibilities may also be applied in general muscular disorders, such as myasthenia (mestinon).

2.2.2 Surgical treatment of ptosis

If conservative treatment is not sufficient enough or impossible, surgical treatment must be considered (in a senile ptosis or after III nerve palsy or lesions of m. levator palpebrae or Muller's muscle). The surgical procedure of choice mainly depends on the remaining function of the levator palpebrae muscle, associated abnormalities and the patient's health. Cosmetic aspects and surgical risk for the eye itself should also be taken in consideration. In young children for example it is extremely important to treat a congenital ptosis very early, in case the pupil is covered, to prevent amblyopia. However, in absence of Bell's phenomenon surgical treatment has to be carried out carefully. Lagophthalmos has to be prevented. As for the same reason ptosis must also be evaluated during downward gaze for in several congenital forms the upper eyelid lags behind. Ptosis due to third nerve paralysis should only then be corrected after strabismus surgery has been performed, this from as well as a cosmetic as from an eye motility point of view. Intermittent ptosis as in the Marcus Gunn phenomenon (disappearance of the ptosis while chewing) is usually not surgically treated.

2.2.3 Surgical procedures

Minor ptosis (<2 mm) with 8–10 mm function of the m. levator palpebrae or the presence of a long eyelid: internal tarsoconjunctival muscle resection (Fasanella Servat) or resection of Muller's muscle and conjunctiva (Mustardé's procedure).

Mild ptosis (2–3 mm) with moderate or good levator function. A resection of the levator palpebrae from the conjunctival side or from the skin side (Blascovics' procedure).

Severe ptosis (4–5 mm) with weak or no levator function: m. frontalis slings. This operation is performed with mersilene nonsoluble material (Friedenwald) or fascia lata strips (Crawford).

In bilateral ptosis surgery under general anaesthesia in one session is preferable; this to permit the surgeon accurate and symmetric dosage of shortening. If severe lagophthalmos develops after operation this may be resolved by cleavage of the slings [7].

2.2.4 Disadvantages of different operation techniques

The Fasanella Servat procedure may cause corneal erosions due to the catgut suture. This should be prevented by placing the sutures subconjunctivaly or by inserting a bandage lens.

Resection of the levator palpebrae muscle is a complex surgical procedure, due to dosage of the resection and approach to eyelid structures. General anaesthesia is preferable in these cases. On the other hand local anaesthesia is easier for dosage with regard to the fellow eye. In the USA most ptosis surgery, either monocular or binocular, is done under local anaesthesia using frontal nerve blocks or local infiltration.

In the m. frontalis sling procedures the use of mersilene sutures is not very complex, but may give rise to infections. The use of fascia lata decreases the danger of infection, however, the eyesurgeon has to be familiar with general surgical principles (in the USA lyofascia is obtained in the databank, [8]).

In 12 patients, operated in our clinic by fascia lata technique, the results appeared very satisfactory. Twice a slight lagophthalmos developed which could easily be treated with artificial tears. Once a bacterial infection occurred with full recovery after conservative treatment with antibiotics [9].

2.2.5 Other causes of ptosis

Capillary haemangioma of the forehead and upper eyelid is normally treated conservatively. Treatment of amblyopia induced by astigmatism or partial covery of the pupil by the tumour is essential. If this is not possible, because the eyelid covers the pupil, more aggressive therapy (steroids local or systemic, surgery or radiotherapy) has to be considered, but all of these therapies may result in local or systemic complications.

Facial arteriovenous malformation shows the so called 'growth phenomenon' [10]. This is based on an increasing number of vessels involved in the 'tumorous vascular proces'. If located near the eyelids, ptosis and motility disturbances occur, the latter mainly in orbital involvement. Dislocation of the eyeball causes diplopia which can be treated by embolization of external carotid artery and if necessary oculoplastic surgery has to be done [11].

3. Orbital disorders

In this paragraph disturbed association between eye, eye muscles and orbit is discussed with a focus on the cosmetic aspects. Initially a cause must be determined, whereafter a method of treatment has to be chosen. The items of Graves' ophthalmopathy are described in chapters 9 and 23, orbital trauma in chapter 9 and the vascular disorders in chapter 10. General and posterior located tumours with neurosurgical aspects are described in chapter 25. It has to be said that not each globe displacement results in diplopia for compensation is often achieved and therefore manifest strabismus does not develop. This is mainly noticed in slowgrowing orbital tumours located in the muscle conus (haemangioma, neurofibroma) or arising from the orbital wall (fibrous dysplasia, mucocele). However, if oblique axis or cyclodeviation is induced, diplopia will subsequently develop (e.g. in fast growing malignant tumours).

3.1 Congenital orbital dysplasia

In facial asymmetry as in morbus Crouzon and orbital developmental pathology [12], strabismus surgery and/or orbital surgery depend on age, degree of cosmetic disturbances and motility disturbances. It is important to recognize these facial asymmetries and abnormal ocular motility. Interdisciplinary cooperation is of paramount importance as is to treat this as a team.

3.2 Anterior located secondary orbital tumour

3.2.1 Fibrous dysplasia

Regarding benign (bone) tumours of the orbital wall such as in fibrous dysplasia [13] and reactive hyperostosis, or invasion of the bone in sphenoidal meningioma, cosmetic aspect and motility disturbances are extremely important for the choice of treatment. Fibrous dysplasia is a benign condition, which is progressive in adolescence and loses its activity afterwards. It is a combination of proliferation of fibrous tissue with imperfect osteogenesis. The main signs are dysfiguring, protruding orbital walls or exophthalmos. Due to spongy bone condensations, cystic formations and sclerosis, the orbital capacity has become too small and several foramina are narrowed. The diagnosis is usually made via plain X-ray. In this self-limiting disease an expectative approach is preferred. However, if visual functions are in danger, surgery is required. Dysfiguring cosmetic changes or diplopia are relative indications for surgery. One must realise that exploration without radical extirpation can induce reactivation of the process itself. The team of Moore et al. [14] has a much more aggressive approach and early performs an extensive excision with reconstruction to give a good functional and cosmetic result. This disorders has to be managed by a specialised craniofacial and oph-thalmic team. The more common complication (31%) however in this series is diplopia! Injuries to the trochlea, inferior oblique desinsertion and postoperative oedema or haemorrhage bone grafts may change muscle actions and induce mechanical and motility disturbances [14]. So these procedures change an in principle benign situation, without diplopia, into one with diplopia due to the operation.

3.2.2 Mucocele

A mucocele of the ethmoid and frontal sinus (thick mucous secretion) may expand in the midfrontal part of the orbit (Fig. 4a + b). Most ENT specialists assume that mucoceles are secondary to obstruction of the sinus ostium, inflam-mation, trauma and surgery all may contribute to cyst formation [15]. Tumours are often slow developing so orthophoria with parallel lines of gaze is produced [16]. If otherwise in that region surgery is required expertise and careful explora-tion are requested for trochlea position in prevention of restriction of the superior oblique muscle, the 'Brown's syndrome' and blepharoptosis (Fig. 4c). This kind of surgery needs teamwork of ENT and ophthalmologist. Repositioning of the trochlea is needed to prevent postoperative superior oblique muscle weakness and diplopia.

252

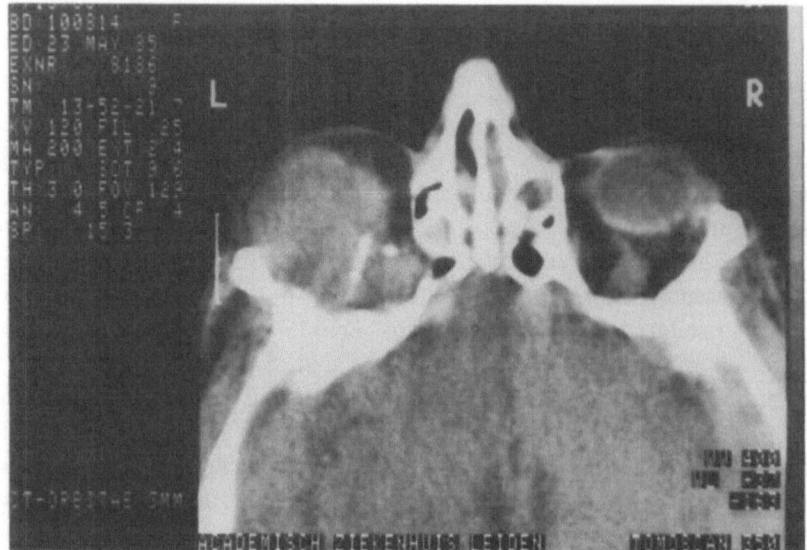

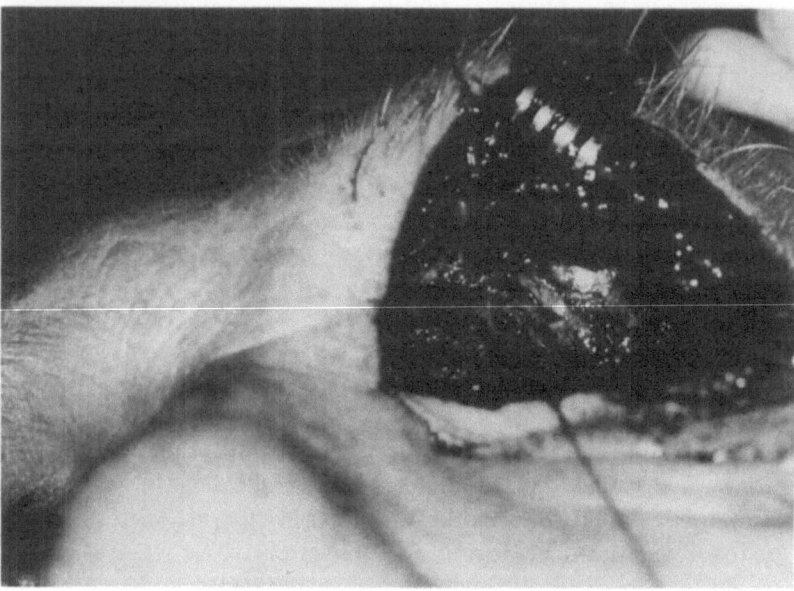

Figure 4A. Axial CT scan of a 70-year-old man with an impressive mucocele of the left orbit and a depression of the eye.
Figure 4B. Surgical view of the giant mucocele.
Figure 4C. Slice of the upper part of the orbit; the trochlear position is located in the mucocele.

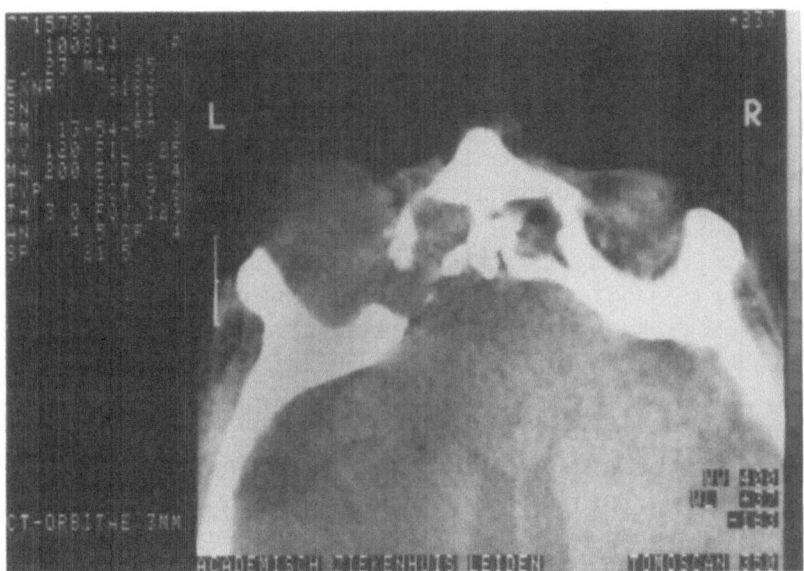

C

3.3 Orbital meningioma

The sphenoid ridge meningioma induces signs and symptoms of the orbit due to space occupation of the ala minor arising from the orbital wall or middle cranial fossa side. A medial localised sphenoid meningioma may cause visual loss (optic atrophy) by direct compression of the optic nerve. The lateral and intermediate located meningiomas can give similar signs but also a superior orbital fissure syndrome and thickening of the temporal bone visible on the outside [17]. Ophthalmoplegia may be caused by nerve palsies or due to mechanical reasons. The diagnosis is based on X ray or CT scan examination; hyperostosis is well visualised on plain X ray, the soft tissue involvement and exact location are demonstrated in contrast-enhanced CT scans. Dependent on neurosurgical exploration and if radical tumour removal is possible sometimes cosmetic procedures such as adnexal and orbital surgery may be necessary [18]. For cosmetic reasons it may be necessary to prescribe special glasses.

The primary optic nerve meningioma predominantly features early visual loss and papil oedema or optic atrophy. The tumour arises between the dural sheath and the pia covering the optic nerve [19]. As the tumour is expanding a big enlargement is restricted by the tough dura so the optic nerve is compressed. Usually the tumour breaks down through the dura into the orbit. This meningioma can cause motility disturbances and this is very surprising since it is an optic nerve tumour! Elevation is mostly restricted probably due to the vigorous contraction of the extra-ocular muscles attempting to overcome the mechanical restriction caused by the thickened and abnormal intraconal optic nerve [19].

If the tumour is not well encapsulated the extra-ocular muscles and also the nerves to the muscles can be invaded. Thus a mechanical or neurogenic cause may elicit the motility imbalance [19, 20]. As therapy of a partially thickened or cuff-like intradural meningioma the tumour can be pulled from the nerve or the nerve can be decompressed. After this surgery with microsurgical techniques, the visual acuity may increase although there is a considerable risk of damage to the optic nerve and its vascular supply.

The highest incidence of this meningioma occurs in the 2nd–4th decade of life but sometimes in the first decade. In children the meningioma seems to be more aggressive so exploration (fine needle aspiration, biopsy) and total extirpation of the tumour and optic nerve are necessary [20, 21, 22]. In the older patients with small tumours a more conservative approach can be used [21]. Careful clinical, CT- and MRI examination [23, 24] and follow-up are necessary. When there is progression causal therapy is carried out, but without enucleation or orbital exenteration [20]. For a cosmetic point of view only the divergent strabismus, in the late, blind situation, is important and strabismus surgery can help.

3.4 Orbital trauma

General considerations and therapeutical consequences (see chapter 9); trochlear trauma and muscle injury caused by sinus surgery; the enlarged orbit.

Trochlear trauma and muscle injury caused by sinus surgery

Trochlear injuries may be caused by an orbital trauma of the superior and medial area or by frontal sinus surgery [25, 26]. Diplopia as a result of a superior oblique muscle imbalance may be induced directly by penetrating wounds or injury of the superior orbital wall. Most ophthalmic centres adopt a conservative attitude in such cases, because they are complicated by multiple trauma, coma and orbital haematoma and in the acute situation it is sometimes difficult to get an optimal surgical view in order to reconstruct multiple pieces of bone around the trochlea. These more conservative centres first remove foreign bodies and at a later stage, if necessary, perform strabismus surgery. Auch Roy-Mainguy et al. [25], however, point out that surgical exploration with primary reconstruction is to be preferred for better results.

Trochlear injuries may also be caused by frontal sinus and neurosurgical exploration. This is more often the case than is generally assumed. Other motility disturbances occurring after frontal sinus, maxillary sinus or ethmoidal sinus surgery may be due to intra-orbital muscle haemorrhages or laceration of the orbital septae. Of course most sinus surgery has no orbital complications, but the ENT surgeon must take care not to enter the orbit. Postoperatively he must pay attention to diplopia. The duty of every ophthalmologist is to take a good medical history from the patient and keep in mind the possibility of a link between sinus surgery and diplopia. Earlier we recorded 8 cases with orbital complaints and motility disturbances, which on stereo X ray revealed defects in the orbital wall caused by sinus surgery. Rosenbaum [26], like other authors, mentions orbital haemorrhage or cellulitis with mechanically induced motility disturbances in some of his cases. In one of our own cases the same orbital complaints we encountered after ethmoid sinus surgery causing orbital emphysema. This gave rise to muscle imbalance which normalised spontaneously after several days.

In every sinus exploration extra-ocular damage has to be prevented because muscular lacerations or fibrous scar tissue around the muscle implicates very difficult orbital- or strabismus surgery. Monocular excercises should be carried out to prevent formation of scar tissue. In a second strabismus operation it is easier to solve these problems, because previous attempts to treat the orbital scar tissue and to dislodge the muscle were unsuccessful [26]. Every surgeon of the facial and orbital walls should know that in some patients the orbital wall is in fact what the name 'papyracea' means: paper thin.

The enlargement of the orbit
One of the main causes of an orbital enlargement is trauma with fractures of the orbital floor or zygoma. The typical signs and symptoms are: enophthalmos, depressed inferior orbital floor, deep upper lid fold and motility disturbances [27]. Motility disturbances and cosmetic disadvantages are usually found to-gether.

In our orbital outpatient department we diagnosed 4 patients with enophthal-mos, who were referred with the chief complaint of vertical diplopia without mention of the enophthalmos. In the medical history there was no trauma but for two cases of chronic sinusitis. The diagnosis of a wide orbital syndrome sensu strictu was made [29]. In patients with the enlarged orbit syndrome, of traumatic or other origin, clinical as well as axial- and coronal CT scan reconstructions have to be made. In close cooperation with an ENT or maxillofacial surgeon reposition of the fractures is to be performed. The traumatic patients should be operated within two weeks after trauma to get good results without difficulties. If this is impossible conservative treatment should be carried out and secondary cosmetic orbital- and strabismus surgery should be performed 6 months after the injury in order to repair the enophthalmos or motility disturbances. Of course a forced duction test has to be performed to detect the cause of the motility problems necessary for the choice of operation technique. Muscle imbalance also can be caused by metastasis, inflammations (Graves' ophthalmopathy!), traumatic haemorrhage, nerve palsy or other shrinking processes. The surgery has to be performed by an ophthalmologist familiar with orbital disorders to prevent orbital complications such as muscle and vascular lacerations. When necessary fibrous strands or special strabismus surgery can be done in a second stage [29]/

In large orbital floor fractures which can induce enophthalmos in the post-traumatic phase teflon plate reconstruction is necessary. If a secondary enlarged

256

orbit is demonstrated as in the wide orbital syndrome multiple teflon balls or dermis fat can be inserted in the deep superior sulcus of the eyelid. The results of this surgery, however, are not exultant [30]. Subperiostal lyodura, teflon or silicone implants gave better results for cosmetic and motility impairment.

References

1. Girard LJ (1981): Corneal surgery. Advanced techniques in ophthalmic microsurgery. Vol. 2. The CV Mosby Co, St. Louis.
2. Leonard P, Rommel J (1982): Lensimplantation. Junk Publ, Den Haag, Chapter IV, pp. 57–95.
3. de Keizer RJW (1982): Pterygiumexcision with or without postoperative irradiation. A double blind study. Doc Ophthalmol 52: 309–315.
4. Dake CL, Crone RA, de Keizer RJW (1979): Treatment of (recurrent) pterygium oculi by lamellar keratoplasty. Doc Ophthalmol 48: 223–230.
5. Ruben M (1975): Contactlens practice. Visual therapeutic and prosthetic. Balliere Tindall, London.
6. Ruben M (1982): A colour atlas of contactlenses. Wolfe Med Publ Ltd, London.
7. Collin JRO (1983): A manual of systemic eyelid surgery. Churchill Livingstone, Edinburgh.
8. Broughton WL, Matthews II JG, Harris DJ (1982): Congenital ptosis. Results of treatment using lyophilized fascia lata for frontalis suspensions. Ophthalmology 89: 1261–1266.
9. van Ganswijk R, de Jong BD, de Keizer RJW (1985): Ptosis correction by means of fascia lata sling. Results in 13 patients. Ophthalmologica 190: 179.
10. French LA (1977): Surgical treatment of arteriovenous malformations. Clin Neur Surg 24: 22–23.
11. de Keizer RJW, van Dalen JTW (1981): Wyburn-Mason Syndrome. Subcutaneous angioma extirpation after preliminary embolisation. Doc Ophthalmol 50: 263–273.
12. Tessier P, et al (1981):Plastic surgery of the orbit and eyelids. Masson Publ Co, New York, chapters 9 and 19.
13. Peeters HJF, Gillissen JPA (1978): Benign tumours of the bony orbital wall. Proc 3rd Int Symp on orbital disorders. Junk Publ, Den Haag, pp. 310–312.
14. Moore AT, Buncic JR, Munro IR (1985): Fibrous Dysplasia of the Orbit in Childhood. Ophthalmology 92: 12–20.
15. Henderson JW (1980): Orbital tumors. 2nd ed BC Decker, New York, pp. 225–231 and pp. 472–486.
16. Crone RA (1973): Diplopia. Excerpta Medica, Amsterdam, pp. 319–320.
17. Bleeker GM (1983): Orbital meningioma. Orbit 3: 3–17.
18. de Keizer RJW (1983): Erkrankungen der Orbita. Augenärztliche Fortbildung. Urban and Schwarzenberg, München, 7/4: 384–385.
19. Wright JE, Call NB, Liaricos S (1980): Primary optic nerve meningioma. Brit J Ophthalmol 64: 553–558.
20. Jakobiec FA, Jones IS (1985): Neurogenic Tumors. In: Clinical Ophthalmology. ThD Duane (ed), Harper and Row, Philadelphia, pp. 31–41.
21. Huber A (1982): Diagnosis and treatment of optic nerve tumours. Orbit 1: 75–85.
22. Wilson WB, Gordon M, Lehman AW (1979): Meningiomas confined to the optic canal and foramina. Surg Neurol 12: 21–29.
23. Koornneef L, Zonneveld FW, Verbeeten B, Blumm R (1984): Direct tri plane scanning of the orbit. Orbit 3: 19–23.
24. de Keizer RJW, Vielvoye GJ, de Wolff-Rouendaal D: MRI in eye and orbital tumors. Orbit (in press).

25. Auch Roy-Mainguy SA, Merlier C, Arnaud B, Fuertes JM (1983): Superior oblique muscle injuries in orbital roof fractures. Orbit 2: 91–98.
26. Rosenbaum AL, Astle WF (1985): Superior oblique and inferior rectus muscle injury following frontal and intranasal sinus surgery. J Ped Ophthalmol Strab 22: 194–202.
27. Gillissen J: Orbital centre personal communication and our own examinations.
28. Cline RA, Rootman J (1984): Enophthalmos, a clinical review. Ophthalmology 91: 229–237.
29. de Keizer RJW, Otto AJ, Brenkman C: The wide orbital syndrome. Orbit (in press).
30. Spivey BE, Allen L, Stewart WB (1976): Surgical correction of superior sulcus deformity occurring after enucleation. Am J Ophthalmol 82: 365–370.

Neurosurgical aspects of tumour induced diplopia

R.T.W.M. THOMEER

Diplopia can result from displacement of structures within the orbit and from ocular nerve palsies of a retro-orbital origin. Every change in the orbital content can lead to diplopia, as well in cases of increase e.g. tumour growth, as of decrease, e.g. loss of orbital fat due to surgery.

Although a mass lesion within the orbit always gives rise to proptosis, this does not hold for diplopia. Especially in cases with slowly growing tumours within the muscle conus (e.g. neurofibratosis) or arising from the orbital bone (e.g. fibrous dysplasia), the patient can remain orthophia as is discussed in the previous chapter. In contrast to the chaos which prevailed in the past, tremendous progress has been made in the treatment of even malignant growths in and around the orbit, due to technical acquisitions and a systemic approach to all of the problems involved. Especially interdisciplinary cooperation is of paramount importance.

1. Orbital tumours

Neoplasms occurring within the orbit can have originated primarily or invade the orbit from surrounding structures. The most frequent examples of invasive tumours are the carcinoma of the paranasal sinus, the sarcoma of the naso-pharynx, and the skull-base meningioma. Primary intra-orbital neoplasms originate from orbital components or by haematogenically spread of malignant tumours. The exact incidence of the individual orbital tumours is not easily to determine, because dates published are obtained in various ways. Those reported by pathologists differ strongly from clinical ones, which is most likely due to selection of material. Clear distinction between primary and secondary (out)-growths may not be useful.

In all cases it is obligatory to determine the exact anatomical position of the tumour as well as its environmental relationship by the use of high-resolution axial and coronal computed tomography (CT) scanning [1]. A subsequent step is taken by biopsy, which by preference should be preceded by carotid angiography.

If a biopsy specimen is needed it is advised to perform a fine needle aspiration for cytological examination [2].

2. Surgical approach of orbital tumours

Modern radiological procedures permit more precise definition of nature, localisation, and anatomical relations of orbital tumours. Interdisciplinary cooperation of ophthalmologists, otolaryngologists, and neurosurgeons promotes choice of the most appropriate route of access in any given case. Surgical aim should be radical extirpation of the tumour, *en bloc,* in malignant cases or piecemeal in meningiomata and other benign processes. Exenteratio of one orbit and resection of part of the skull is sometimes necessary [3, 4]. Today, these combined extirpative procedures can be carried out safely by a joint effort of the disciplines involved. If the lesion is deemed unresectable, a bulk resection is valuable alternative and radiotherapy should then be considered.

Everyone performing this kind of surgery should have a thorough knowledge of the surgical anatomy around and within the orbit. Essentially there are four routes of approach to a primary orbital lesion, i.e. the lateral, superior (transcranial), medial (transethmoidal), and inferior (transmaxillary) routes. Various combinations are also possible [3, 5, 6, 7]. Choice of surgical approach should be determined only by anatomical localisation of the tumour. It has to be said that an initial inappropriate attack on a tumour can eliminate any further chance of definite cure. Because of the size, the great majority of these tumours can be approached via superolateral, lateral, or superior (transcranial) routes.

All approaches demand adequate survey and the possibility of removing the tumour in one session. In addition, it may not lead to a cosmetic or functional defect. Lateral orbitomy was first carried out by Kroenlein [8] a century ago and since then has undergone many modifications. The lateral and superior orbital rims can be removed by an osteotomy remaining pedicled at the temporal muscle (Fig. 1). If the removed bony parts cannot be replaced, as is the case in malignant invasion or after resection of the orbital roof, a plasty with the use of bone cement (Palacos®) easily can be carried out at the end of the procedure and can give good cosmetic and functional results (Figs. 2a and 2b). Others used autologous bone for this purpose [6].

It should be emphasized that all tumours localised in the orbital apex are to be approached by the superior, transcranial route as initially recommended by Dandy [9]. Only this route gives adequate exposure of the optic and ocular nerves. Although less experienced, we agree with Maroon et al. [7] that, if necessary, the optic nerve can be safely dissected free from the chiasm as far as the ocular bulb. Resection of the posterior part of the orbital roof, the medial part of the lesser sphenoid wing including the anterior clinoid process, and transection of

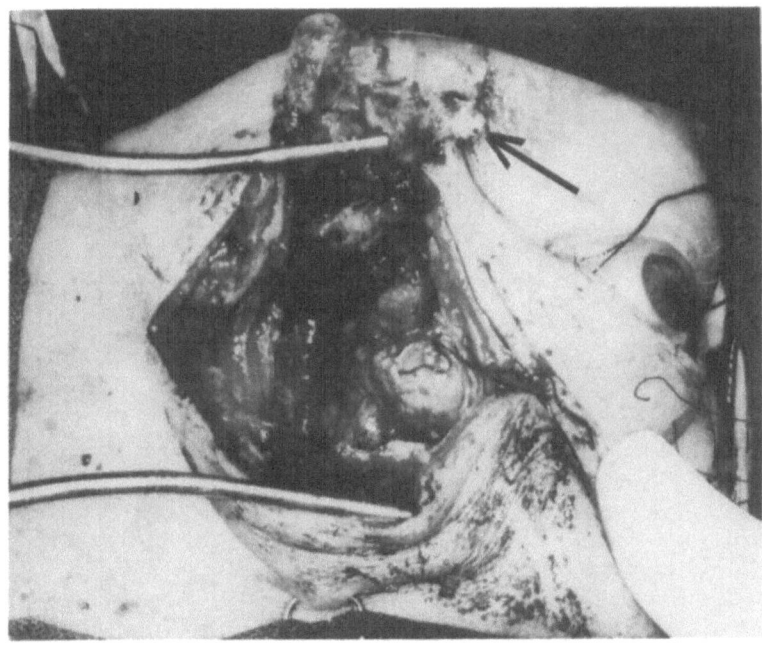

Figure 1. Operative view of lateral orbitotomy for a meningioma. The arrow indicates lateral orbital rim removed, attached to the temporal muscle.

the optic dural sleeve and the annulus of Zinn, can greatly facilitate tumour removal in these areas. Great care must be taken not to sever the trochlear nerve which crosses the surgical field just in front of the annulus underneath the periorbit.

Regardless of the approach some tumours cannot be removed radically e.g. in advanced neurofibromatosis orbitae (von Recklinghausen's disease). If something has to be done in these cases for cosmetical reasons the choice is between intracranial enlargement of the orbital cavity or exenteratio with prothesis (Fig. 3).

3. Middle- and posterior fossa tumours

Eye movement disorders may result from tumours at the skull base behind the orbit due to pressure on one or more ocular nerves. The two exceptions might be the expanding lesser sphenoid wing meningioma which invades the orbit causing mechanical distortion of its contents, and tumours arising from the cranial nerves themselves i.e. the group of neurofibromata. Compared to the other cranial nerves a neurofibroma of an ocular nerve in its retro-orbital span is rare. The skull base behind the orbit can be divided into the middle and posterior fossa separated

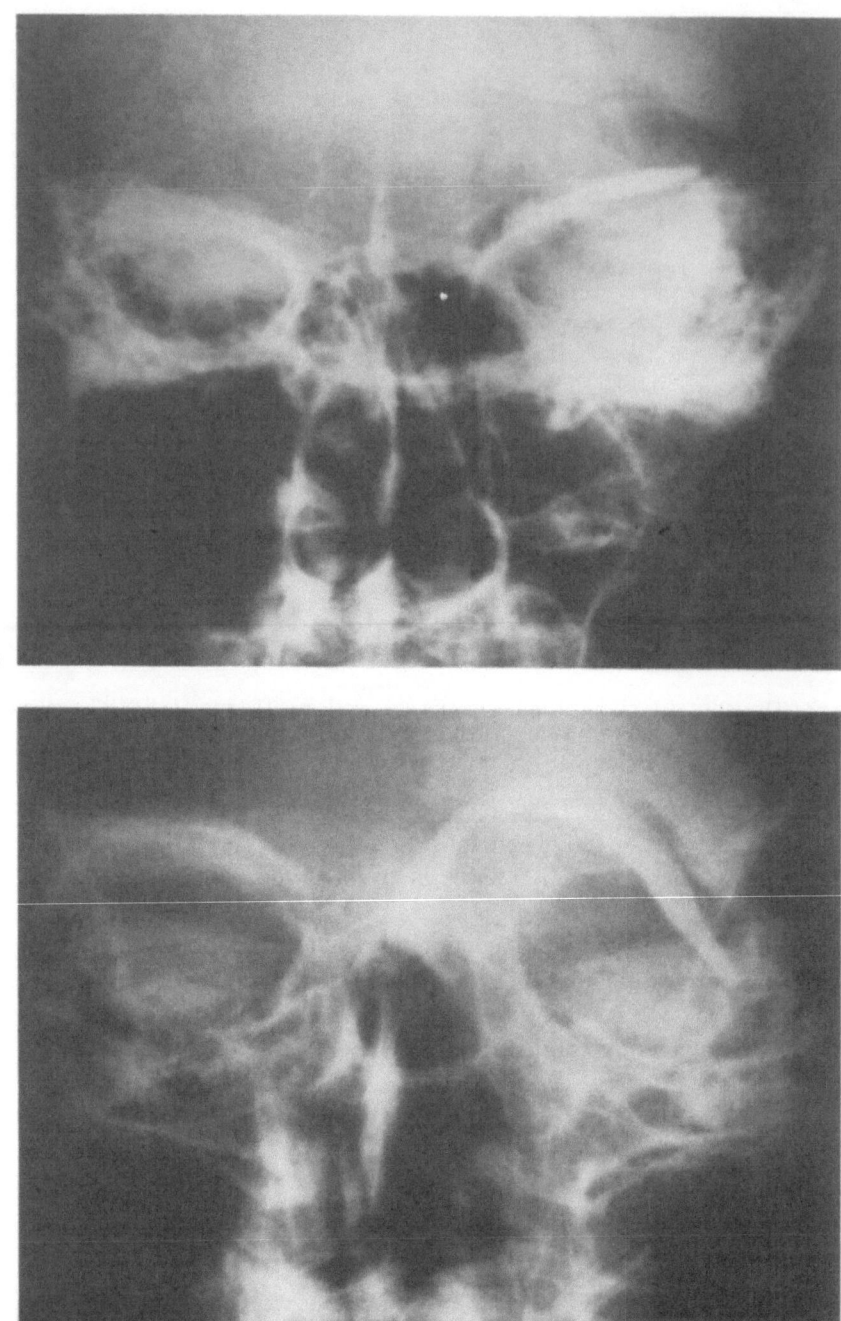

Figure 2A. Plastic reconstruction of orbital roof with bone cement.
Figure 2B. Plastic reconstruction of superior orbital rim and adjacent frontal bone.

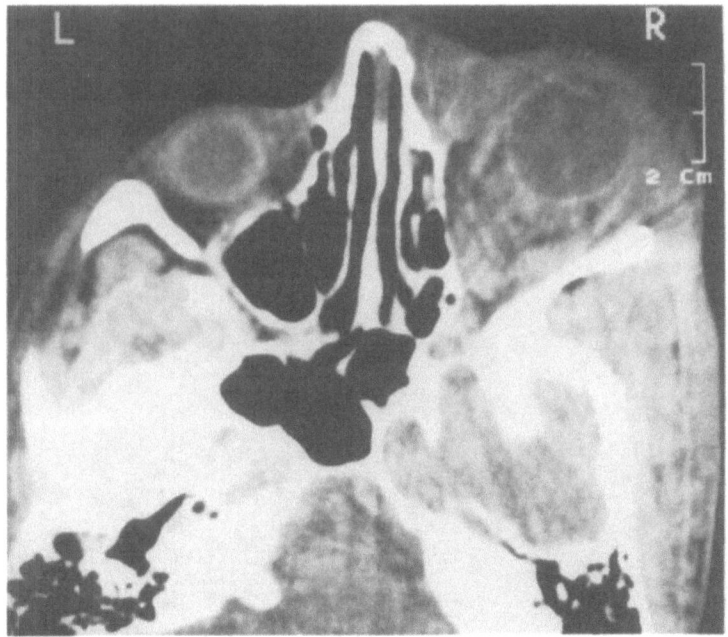

Figure 3. CT scan showing neurofibromatosis orbitae.

by the tentorium (Table 1). By far the most frequently occurring tumour of the medial fossa is the lesser sphenoid wing meningioma (Table 2). Depending on the origin of the tumour a subdivision is made into lateral, intermediate and medial. The conjunction of the periorbita with the intracranial dura at the superior orbital fissure may serve as a route of entry for the already mentioned intra-orbital expansion. In rare cases chordomas, chondromas, and giant aneurysms can compress superior orbital fissure structures [10, 11].

Pituitary adenomas, although histopathologically benign, may invade the parasellar structures and cause palsies of the ocular nerves within the cavernous sinus (Fig. 4). An acute onset of blurred vision or even total blindness whether or not in combination with ocular nerve palsies is very suspect for a bleeding in this tumour, the so called 'apoplexie hypophysaire'. Ocular nerve palsies due to cavernous sinus tumourous invasion can occur without venous congestion of the involved eye and do not exclude this invasion, because venous collateral circulation is able to compensate fully cavernous obstruction. The same is true for cavernous sinus meningiomas [10]. Craniopharyngiomas, such as suprasellar pituitary adenomas, usually compress the chiasm, but can also expand laterally [12, 13]. Any dilated pupil combined with multiple ocular nerve palsies suggests pathology in the cavernous sinus. Epidermoid tumours occur everywhere in the supra- and parasellar regions and more caudally around the brainstem. Although

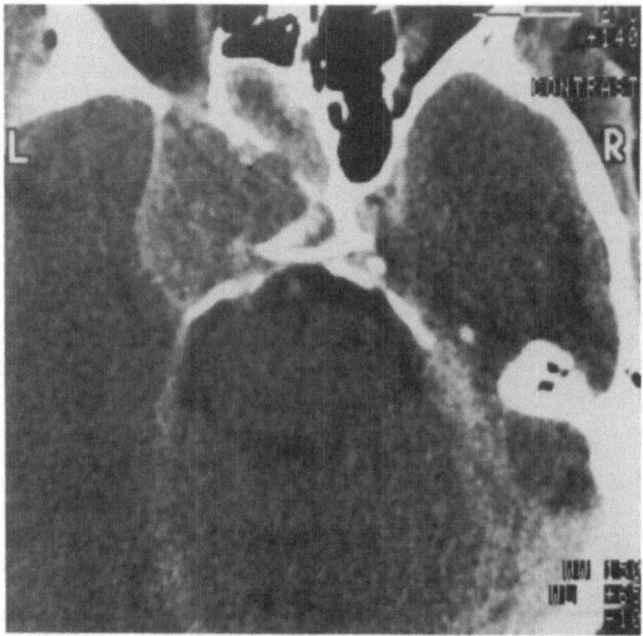

Figure 4. CT scan of pituitary adenoma with parasellar expansion to the left.

benign too in nature, these tumours may even grow around the cranial nerves and vessels instead of simply compressing them, thus complicating a radical excision.

Because of close anatomical relationship between carotid posterior communicating artery and tentorial edge with the oculomotor nerve running in between, it is common in aneurysms at this site, to give oculomotor palsy (Fig. 5). Ocular nerve palsies with an origin in the posterior fossa can be due either to an intraparenchymatous disease process, e.g. pontine glioma, or to an extra-axial

Table 1. Neurosurgical causes of diplopia.

Orbit		
congenital dysplasia		
fracture		
carotid-cavernous fistula		
neoplasm within the orbit		
Retro-orbital lesions		
middle fossa	supra orbital fissure	NN. III.IV,VI
	cavernous sinus	
	tentorial notch	NN. III, IV
posterior fossa		
	(pre) pontine	N. VI

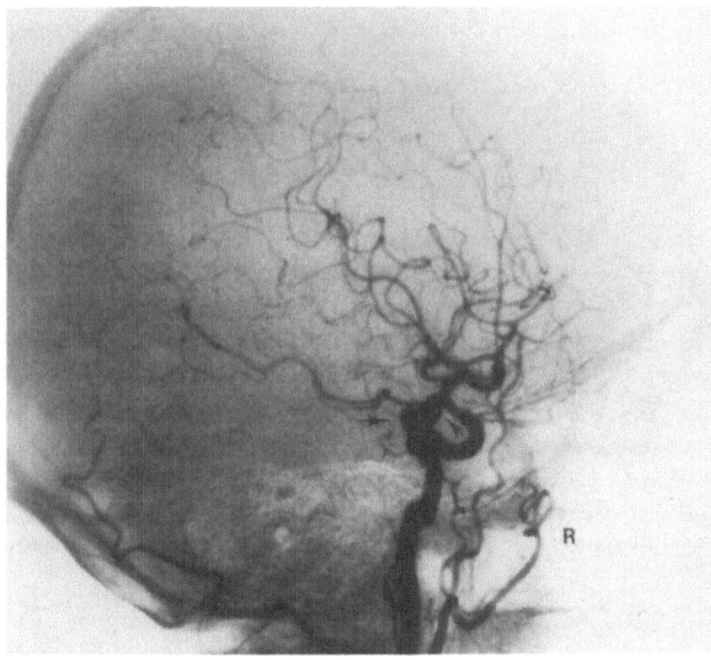

Figure 5. Carotid angiography, lateral view, showing carotid-posterior communicating aneurysm.

tumour compressing the sixth cranial nerve. Most frequently occurring tumours in this region are petrosal-, clival-, and tentorial-notch meningiomas epidermoid tumour, and clival chordoma. Although large cerebellopontine angle tumours (acoustic neuromas) can reach the abducens nerve retroclivally and the oculomotor and trochlear nerves at the tentorial notch, this seldom results in a palsy of these cranial nerves. Chronic intracranial hypertension as in cases of hydrocephalus, may lead to abducens nerve palsies even in the absence of papil oedema.

Table 2. Middle fossa tumours.

Tumours arising from the skull base	Tumours arising at the skull base
Osteoma (-sarcoma)	Meningioma (-sarcoma)
Chondroma (-sarcoma)	Pituitary adenoma
Fibroma (-sarcoma)	Craniopharyngeoma
Chordoma	Epidermoid
Giant cell tumour	Dermoid
Haemangioma	Neurofibroma (N. V)
Fibrous dysplasia (tumour?)	(Aneurysm)
(Plasmacytoma)	
(Metastasis)	

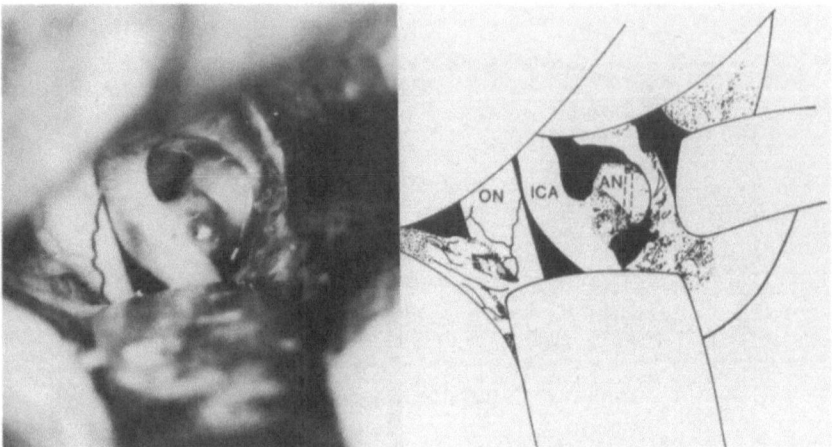

Figure 6. Operative view of right carotid-posterior communicating aneurysm. ON: optic nerve; ICA: internal carotid artery; AN: aneurysm. Dotted lines indicate oculomotor nerve lying directly underneath the aneurysm.

4. Surgical treatment of middle- and posterior fossa tumours

It would go beyond the scope of this chapter to give a detailed description of all of the neurosurgical approaches and techniques in relation to the nature and site of the disease processes associated with retro-orbital pathology. Nevertheless, it seems important to at least comment on the tremendous progress neurosurgery has made since the advent of microsurgical techniques in combination with modern neuro-anaesthesiological modalities.

The vast majority of skull-base tumours that were deemed irresectable, about ten years ago, can be removed radically and safely today. Even in cases of histopathologically benign tumours such as meningioma, it is essential to perform a radical resection at the first session with sparing of the local nerves, because recurrence of a tumour of this kind might also involve contralateral parts of the skull base and eventually make the neo-plasm irresectable, which would mean a real threat [14]. This is also true in other tumours mentioned, with exception of pituitary adenomas. The combination of radiotherapy with rhinoseptal trans-sphenoidal surgery, or in a small percentage of the cases transcranial extirpation of these tumours, gives satisfactory long-term results, notwithstanding non-radical surgery.

Morbidity and mortality of aneurysm surgery have now been reduced to low levels. Aneurysms which cannot be clipped directly, e.g. some infraclinoidal carotid or giant aneurysms of the carotid or middle cerebral artery, can be treated by trapping procedures combined with extra-intracranial bypass surgery (Figs. 7a and 7b) [11, 15, 16]. Tumours extending into both and the posterior fossa may be

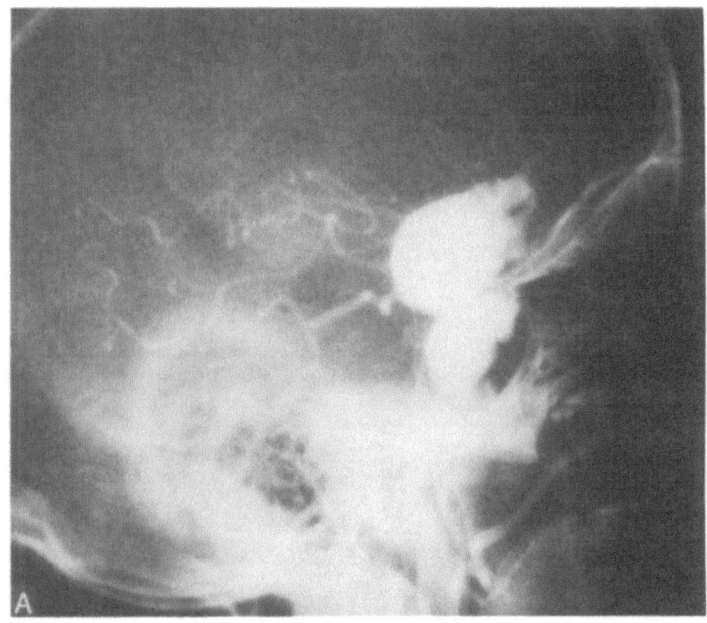

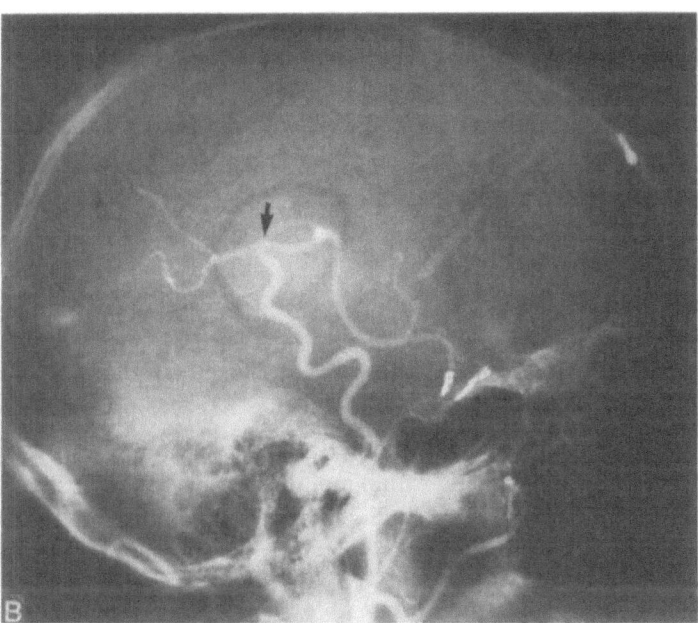

Figure 7A. Giant aneurysm of the internal carotid artery.
Figure 7B. The aneurysm has been trapped (note clips) and an extra-intracranial bypass procedure has been carried out (arrow). A ventricular drain is also visible.

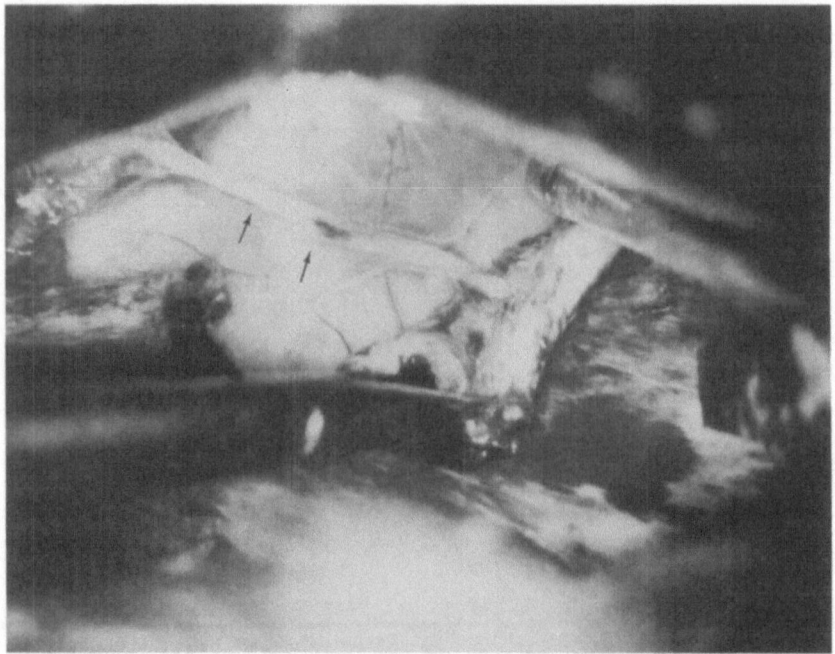

Figure 8. Operative subtemporal view of the tentorial notch. The tentorium has been transected, the frontal part being reflected by the micro-scissors. Arrows show the trochlear nerve stretched over a epidermoid tumour.

resected by transection of the tentorium. Even the very tiny trochlear nerve, which has an intimate relation with the tentorial edge and sometimes enters it early on its way to the cavernous sinus, must be spared (Fig. 8). Today, subtemporo-suboccipital approaches combined with transection of both the tentorium and the transverse sinus make it possible to excise lesions completely, which were formerly considered to be irresectable.

Ocular nerve palsies may be caused by tumour compression but may also result from the surgeon's handling, i.e. the performance of neurolysis. In latter cases, functional recovery is expected within months and general corrective strabismus surgery should not be considered within the first six months after the neurosurgical intervention. The technical standards of strabismus surgery are discussed by Gobin in chapter 23.

References

1. Alper MG (1980): Computed tomography in planning and evaluating orbital surgery. Ophthalmology 87: 418–431.

2. van Heerde P, Peterse JL (1985): Fine needle aspiration of the orbit. Orbit 4: 217–220.
3. Housepian EM (1982): Intra-orbital Tumours. In: HH Schmidek and WH Sweet (eds). Operative Neurosurgical Techniques. Vol 2. Grune and Stratton, New York, pp. 227–244.
4. Jackson IT, Marsh WR, et al (1984): Treatment of tumours involving the anterior cranial fossa. Head Neck Surg 6: 901–913.
5. Alper MG, Aitken PhA (1982): Anterior and lateral microsurgical approaches to orbital pathology. In: HH Schmidek and WH Sweet (eds) Operative Neurosurgical Techniques. Vol 2. Grune and Stratton Publ, New York, pp. 245–277.
6. Cophignon J, Clay C, et al (1974): Abord sous-frontal élargi des tumeurs de l'orbite. Neuro-Chirurgie 20: 161–167.
7. Maroon JC, Kennerdell JS (1984): Surgical approaches to the orbit. Indications and techniques. J Neurosurg 60: 1226–1235.
8. Kroenlein RU (1889): Zur Pathologie und operativen Behandlung der Dermoidcysten der Orbita. Beitr Klin Chir 4: 149–163.
9. Dandy WE (1941): Orbital tumours. Results following the transcranial operative attack. Oskar Piest, New York, pp. 161–164.
10. Trobe JD, Glaser JG, Post JD (1978): Meningiomas and aneurysms of the cavernous sinus. Arch Ophthal 96: 457–467.
11. Peerless SJ, Drake CG (1982): Treatment of giant cerebral aneurysms of the anterior circulation. Neurosurg Rev 149–154.
12. Neetens A, Selosse P 1975 (1977): Oculo-motor Anomalies in Sellar and Parasellar Pathology. Ophthalmologica 80–104.
13. Neetens A, Bultinck R, Martin JJ, Solheid J (1980): Intrasellar adenoma and chordoma. Neuro Ophthalmology 1: 123–135.
14. Derome PJ, Guiot G (1978): Bone problems in meningiomas invading the base of the skull. Clin Neurosurg 25: 435–451.
15. Spetzler FF, Schuster H, Roski RA (1980): Elective extracranial-intracranial arterial by-pass in the treatment of inoperable giant aneurysms of the internal carotid artery. J Neurosurg 53: 22–27.
16. Sundt TM, Piepgras (1979): Surgical approach to giant intracranial aneurysms. J Neurosurg 51: 731–742.

Index

274